Care in a Time of Crisis

Eleonora Rossero

Care in a Time of Crisis

An Ethnography of Coercive Practices in Italian Acute Mental Health Provision

palgrave
macmillan

Eleonora Rossero
University of Turin
Turin, Italy

ISBN 978-3-031-34417-6 ISBN 978-3-031-34418-3 (eBook)
https://doi.org/10.1007/978-3-031-34418-3

This Palgrave Macmillan imprint is published by the registered company Springer Nature Switzerland AG.
The registered company address is: Gewerbestrasse 11, 6330 Cham, Switzerland

Paper in this product is recyclable.

To my father, Oreste

Acknowledgements

Throughout the conduct of the research and the writing of this book, I have received a great deal of support and assistance.

First of all, I am deeply indebted to all of the mental healthcare workers I have met on the field—psychiatrists, nurses, OSS ("Operatori Socio-Sanitari", i.e. health care workers), psychologists, social workers, rehabilitation specialists—who accepted my presence in the first place, patiently answered my countless questions, and shared relevant insights on their everyday practice with me. Also, the emotional support they provided and the life they shared with me on the field, in terms of emotional moments, food, car trips, night shifts, discussions, and personal experience, were of incredible value to me. This book would literally not exist without them.

Also, I owe so much to the mental health service users who accepted my presence in the most delicate situations and allowed me to listen to their stories, which constitute the most precious element of this experience I will never forget in my life.

I am grateful to the sociological research team at the University of Turin that conducted the study "Psychiatric Interventions. About TSO and Mechanical Restraint": the supervisor of my doctoral dissertation, Mario Cardano; Raffaella Ferrero Camoletto; Luigi Gariglio; and Valeria Quaglia. Their scientific support and advice accompanied me as a student and helped me grow as a junior researcher. I must also thank psychiatrists, nurses, and jurists that were part of the interdisciplinary research team, whose insights during our meetings have been incredibly enriching and stimulating for my reflections and development of this work.

I thank Mauro Barisione and Giovanni Semi for their precious advice and critical observations during the early phases of this research, as well as the other Faculty members of the Sociology and Methodology of Social Research (SOMET) programme. Also, I wish to thank Lorenza Magliano and Giovanni Torrente for their careful reading of my doctoral dissertation, as well as Stefan Sjöström and Maria Świątkiewicz-Mośny for their challenging observations during my thesis defence.

I am grateful to my colleagues and friends at the University of Turin and to my SOMET fellows of the XXXIII cohort, with whom I had the opportunity to share this amazing journey. They supported me before, during, and after my fieldwork in every possible way.

I wish to thank my colleagues at Eclectica, who supported me in the writing process and, most importantly, in the transition to another phase of my professional life.

Lastly, my sincere gratitude goes to my family and friends, who provide me with encouragement and love every day.

Contents

About the Author

Eleonora Rossero obtained her PhD in Sociology and Methodology of Social Research at the University of Turin and the University of Milan in 2021. Her research interests concern the sociology of health, and she privileges qualitative research methods. Mental health has been the object of her latest publications, dedicated to the impact of the Covid-19 pandemic on Italian mental health services, the role of interdisciplinarity in the ethnographic study of psychiatric coercive interventions, and Italian de-institutionalization practices and cultures (book review). Besides mental healthcare, she is particularly interested in the narratives of autoimmune diseases: her contribution on this topic includes the article "The Making and Unmaking of Hashimoto's Thyroiditis: On the Mismatch Between Illness and Disease" (2021) and a peer-reviewed monograph on illness trajectories and the process of sense-making about autoimmunity, *Anticorpi anarchici Narrazioni di malattia autoimmune* (2022). She has been a teaching assistant for the Sociology of Health courses at the Department of Clinical and Biological Sciences (University of Turin) and in the interdisciplinary course in Neuroengineering and active ageing (Polytechnic University of Turin). She has been involved as a post-doc researcher in a project on artificial intelligence in the doctor-patient relationship, led by the Fundamental Rights Laboratory (Collegio Carlo Alberto). She is a researcher at Eclectica+ Research and Training in Turin (Italy), where she conducts research and action research on mental healthcare by working closely with health services and professionals.

Abbreviations

ASL	Azienda Sanitaria Locale (local health department)
ASO	Accertamento Sanitario Obbligatorio (mandatory medical assessment)
CSM	Centro di Salute Mentale (mental health centre)
DSM	Dipartimento di Salute Mentale (mental health department)
ED	Emergency Department (Emergency Room + units of observation and semi-intensive care)
ER	Emergency Room
ICU	Intensive Care Unit
MHC	Mental Health Centre
MHD	Mental Health Department
OSS	Operatore Socio-Sanitario (healthcare assistant)
PRN medication	pro-re-nata or "as-needed" medication (as opposed to scheduled medication)
SerD	Servizio per le Dipendenze patologiche (alcohol and drug addiction support services)
SPDC	Servizio Psichiatrico di Diagnosi e Cura (acute psychiatric ward)
TSO	Trattamento Sanitario Obbligatorio (mandatory admission and treatment)

List of Tables

1

Introduction

Abstract In Italy, mental healthcare is currently provided in community and hospital services, namely Mental Health Centres and hospital psychiatric wards called SPDC (*Servizi Psichiatrici di Diagnosi e Cura*). These services have been introduced by Law 180/1978, which symbolically indicates the beginning of a deinstitutionalization process that gradually led to the complete closure of former psychiatric institutions: asylums. While the latter organizations have been sociologically investigated, for example, by the seminal work of Erving Goffman (*Asylums. Essays on the social situation of mental patients and other inmates*, Anchor Books, 1961) and Anselm Strauss et al. (*Psychiatric ideologies and institutions*, Transaction, 1981), little is known about how mental healthcare is provided today in acute wards (Quirk and Lelliott, *Social Science & Medicine, 53*, 1565–1574, 2001). Moreover, most of the available evidence has been produced in the Anglo-Saxon context: UK, USA, and Australia. Literature on the Italian system is limited, except for those contexts representing excellence in terms of restraint reduction and recovery, such as the Trieste model (Mezzina, *The Journal of Nervous and Mental Disease, 202*, 440–445, 2014; Oliveira et al., *Psicologia em Pesquisa, 12*, 24–35, 2018; Okin, *Basaglia's international legacy: From asylum to community*, 2020). In this chapter, I shall introduce the theoretical framework that

E. Rossero, *Care in a Time of Crisis*, https://doi.org/10.1007/978-3-031-34418-3_1

guided my work and define how I wish it to contribute to this under-researched field, providing a brief overview of the structure of the book and of each substantive chapter contribution.

1.1 Exploring Care and Coercive Practices

Psychiatric practice has always entailed a dimension of care and a dimension of custody. Former psychiatric hospitals, or asylums, have been for a long time a symbol of segregation of the mentally insane and otherwise deviant subjectivities from the rest of society. Such places have been the fulcrum of the historical process Michel Foucault called "the great confinement". Their dismantling and the consequent deinstitutionalization process did not abolish coercion, which still represents the oldest and most controversial problem of psychiatric institutions (Steinert et al., 2014). Despite the persistence of coercive practices in this post-asylum era, mental health literature investigating them fails to provide a univocal definition of coercion, and uses the term to refer to a wide range of practices: from undue interpersonal influence to explicit and physical use of force (O'Brien & Golding, 2003). Attempts to clarify the notion of coercion have been advanced by the psychiatrist George Szmukler and colleagues (2015, 2017; Szmukler & Appelbaum, 2001, 2008), who identified a continuum—or spectrum—of what they call "treatment pressures": persuasion, interpersonal leverage, inducement, threat, and compulsion. According to these authors, the term "coercion" is best applied to the last two kinds of pressures: threat and compulsion. This spectrum has then been further developed to include other "coercion-related behaviours" (Lidz et al., 1998), entailing both positive symbolic pressures (such as persuasion) and negative ones (e.g. deception, threat, show of force). Research has also highlighted how formally voluntary interventions are sometimes the result of a combination of persuasion and coercion (Reed & Lewis, 1990). The so-called coercive shadow looming over mental healthcare can lead patients to voluntarily accept medication or hospital admission only to avoid fear, stigma, and humiliation related to compulsory measures (Szmukler, 2017). The distinction between objective and subjective (or perceived) coercion allows to speak about "coerced voluntaries", formally admitted on a voluntary basis but feeling coerced in terms of negative pressures, implicit threats, and poor procedural justice (O'Donoghue et al., 2014), and "uncoerced involuntaries", namely formally involuntary subjects perceiving low levels of coercion (Iversen et al., 2002).

The blurred line between coercion and voluntary acceptance of treatment, together with the difficulty to define and measure coercion, encouraged some scholars to avoid strict definitions and focus on the concrete ways in which coercion is made relevant in everyday clinical practice instead. The work of Stefan Sjöström (2006, 2016) on the micro-level interaction by which coercion is enacted, explored ethnographically as a social practice, provides a theoretically strong example of this situated approach. The sociologist introduces the notion of "coercion context"—inspired by that of "awareness context" coined by Glaser and Strauss in *Awareness of Dying* (1965)—arguing that coercion in psychiatric care represents a sensitive issue concerning human rights and fundamental values, such as patients' autonomy. Psychiatric ward's life is permeated with exceptional activities, such as forcing people to perform body searches and to comply with undesired treatments, sometimes through the use of physical force (Sjöström, 2016). This implies that mental healthcare providers face stress, dilemmas and the need to make these coercive acts acceptable to mitigate their burden (see also the repertoires which practically and discursively make coercion compatible with the provision of care, presented in Chap. 6). The interaction between patients and the staff is always characterized by the intrinsic problem of compliance with medication, rules, ward routines, and the always revisable acceptance to stay in the hospital. In order to handle compliance problems and pursue clinical goals, the staff can strategically invoke a coercion context. The organization of the ward, its locked doors and surveillance activities, plays a crucial function by forcing de facto even voluntary patients to ask for the staff assistance to leave: the setting itself, with its materiality and physical layout, works as a non-discursive element that invokes a coercion context. The tacit possibility that a psychiatrist has to turn voluntary into compulsory treatment, let alone the explicit threat to do it, is part of this coercion context as well, which can deter the patient from leaving without even resorting to formal procedures of involuntary treatment.

In this work, I approached care and coercive practices in their concrete occurrence instead of as decontextualized objects, consistently with Sjöström's situated inquiry. Moving from these assumptions, the following section delves into the aims and questions of the research that forms the basis of this book.

1.2 Aims of the Research

The study's primary purpose is the critical exploration of the deployment of coercive practices—more or less univocally defined as such—and the strategies developed to deal with non-compliant or dangerous behaviour. Moving from the assumption that notions of care and constraint have unstable meanings that vary according to historical and local traditions and ideologies of treatment (Brodwin & Velpry, 2014), I focus on their contextual definitions, as well as underlying meanings, logics, and values about what constitutes a good or at least acceptable practice, and how it is performed in daily work activities. This entails exposing the underlying boundary work (Gieryn, 1983) through which social objects are brought inside a category whereas others are pushed out of that definitional frame (Åkerström, 2002). The definitional processes which label certain interventions as more or less coercive, as good or bad ones, are particularly well suited to be explored in a comparative research design, which I employ to contrast contexts that allegedly provide different answers to the problem of demarcation between acceptable and unacceptable practices: the "restraint" context (where mechanical restraint is used and ward's doors are kept permanently locked) and the "no-restraint" context (which rejects these measures though enacting other coercive interventions).

The ethnographic exploration of such healthcare contexts allows us to ask what is pursued and performed as good, and what, on the contrary, is performed as bad and therefore avoided (Mol et al., 2010). Notions of "good care" and "bad care" pertain to the ethics of care, here intended not as a matter of universal principles, but rather of local solutions to specific problems (ibidem). From this perspective, neither the "restraint" nor the "no-restraint" contexts are explored as intrinsically representing best practices, because this work does not move from a pre-defined normative position. Instead, within each context of care, it aims to explore specific "modes of doing good", namely patterns of ideals, routines, and knowledge oriented towards a specific form of good care (Pols, 2003), shaped (and researched) locally. Since the values at stake and the objects of care are always multiple, care practices are intended as intrinsically problematic, and they deal with tensions and inconsistencies, and they require a constant attempt to hold together what does not necessarily hold together (Law, 2010; Mol et al., 2010). Such tensions in mental healthcare add to the ambivalence experienced by professionals as they negotiate between their preferred self-image as competent healthcare providers, and the necessity to carry out coercive treatments against a person's will (Brodwin, 2014). Psychiatric practice indeed has to do with everyday ethics enacted in the ongoing flow of clinical work, as professionals attempt to define what is right and what is wrong, dealing with the legitimacy of their professional power (Brodwin, 2013).

Given the complexities intrinsic to care and specifically mental healthcare, what is "good" can be ambivalent or difficult to translate into practice. Moreover, various relevant goods or values can be at stake at the same time: therefore, delivered care depends on tinkering with different "goods" (Mol, 2010). The ultimate goal of this work is to explore acute mental healthcare and coercive practices, investigating situated modes of framing and responding to situations of emergency or crisis, and how ideas about "good care" are enacted in daily practice. Moreover, moving from an empirical ethical approach to care (Pols, 2015), the study aims to offer "situated suggestions" to improve acute mental healthcare provision, which consider and compare the different values that the two contexts observed strived and argued for.

1.3 Outline of the Book

After this introduction, a review of the relevant literature is provided in Chap. 2. Research conducted in the fields of sociology, anthropology, and nursing studies, with a specific focus on ethnographic inquiries, is presented. Beginning from the seminal work of Erving Goffman on American asylums as total institutions (1961), the review moves to more recent work and to the contemporary studies of English acute psychiatric wards as permeable institutions, conducted by Alan Quirk et al. (2006). A discussion concerning the notion of coercion and literature on coercive practices is then presented, in order to provide the reader with a description as well as a historical contextualization of (debated) interventions that will be later discussed with respect to the empirical material.

Chapter 3 is dedicated to alternatives to coercive interventions, beginning from a historical overview of the no-restraint movement to contemporary attempts to reduce coercion in psychiatric settings. The chapter also clarifies the perspective from which I have approached care and coercive practices.

In Chap. 4, I provide a reflexive account by describing the methodological path along which the research behind this book has developed. The chapter outlines the research questions which inspired my work, as well as their scientific and societal relevance. A reflexive note considering my experience on the field and my positioning with respect to the object of study is presented.

Chapter 5 deals with the processes of boundary-making which constitute and continuously redraw the map of today's mental healthcare services. Beginning with the definition of the dichotomy between hospital and community care—which has a long tradition in the post-deinstitutionalization, balanced model of mental healthcare—the chapter considers the criteria on which the division of labour among mental health services is performed and maintained in the two contexts studied. These seem to rely on different institutional maps (Strauss et al., 1981), in which the psychiatric ward (SPDC) performs a different function: the only place designated to treat crisis (in the "restraint" context), or one among other places which treats specific cases (such as the so-called onsets) in a context of multi-situated crisis management (this is the case of the "no-restraint" context). Beyond this ideal division of labour between the services, in everyday practice conflicts arise around the allocation of patients, because professionals working in different locations can see the institutional map differently. Therefore, I discuss the shape of the ward (ibidem) and its relation to numerousness and the profile of the admitted population, presenting the notion of *pertinence permeability*. Decisions upon admission and the construction of the "proper patient" are not straightforward and involve a multiplicity of actors: SPDC's professionals, doctors operating in the Emergency Room, and community psychiatrists. Moreover, inter-professional conflicts emerge when doctors' decision does not meet with nursing staff's approval and is contested through a re-categorization of the admitted patient so that s/he can be deemed inappropriate. The heterogeneous strategies employed in negotiations between the different actors involved in performing *circulation work*, as defined by Rhodes (1991), are presented, and each service or unit's bargaining power is discussed. The role of boundary objects connecting the ward and the community is also considered.

Chapter 6 deals with how care and coercion are held together in everyday clinical practice. I discuss how tensions between situated, temporary goals in treating acute patients, and between issues of care and control inherent to psychiatric practice, appear to be practically solved whereby two repertoires: the first one I call *outsourcing coercion*, which excludes coercion from practices and discourses of care and attributes it to different actors (e.g. police forces), and the second one I call *embedding coercion*, entailing the performing of coercion as (good) care whereby four discursive and practical strategies: (i) therapeuticization of coercion; (ii) proceduralization of coercion; (iii) relationalization of coercion; and (iv) multiplication of the objects of care. These repertoires convey different notions of good mental healthcare and result in different attempts to realize it in practice, implying both ideals and their performance or enactments (Pols, 2003; Mol, 2002). The chapter presents pure, ideal, typical versions of these repertoires I separated out for my analysis: in the real world, they are not exclusive of the "restraint" or to the "no restraint" context, but they are adopted transversally, combined, or contaminated with spurious local elements. Moreover, they are employed to perform and talk about different coercive interventions, whether mechanical and other forms of restraint, involuntary treatment, or enforced medication. Besides the description of each pure repertoire and the presentation of empirical data from both contexts in which they are rooted, residual aspects, deviations, and controversial elements are discussed.

The last empirical chapter (Chap. 7) represents a conclusive reflection on ethical stances and values supporting the adoption or rejection of specific restraining measures, notably mechanical restraint and permanently locked doors which differentiate the "restraint" from the "no-restraint" context. Moving from Latour's (Johnson, 1988) notion of nonhuman delegates (in this case, for example, the restraining belts), I discuss how the no-restraint approach tends to oppose delegation and to rhetorically prefer "staying in the relationship" with the acute patient, opting for restraining measures involving human presence such as manual restraint or holding. Findings from fieldwork, though, suggest that delegation and presence are intertwined in both contexts: mechanical restraint does not necessarily rule relationship out (see Chap. 6 on relationalization of coercion), while open-door policy does not necessarily translate into spending more time with patients. Though nonhuman delegates (belts, closed doors, sedative drugs) prescribe withdrawal from relationship, actors can negotiate their behaviour and adjust it to the specific situation, choosing deliberate de-inscription from the vision of the world that is inscribed in those objects (Akrich, 1992; Akrich & Latour, 1992).

To conclude, Chap. 8 presents some situated suggestions (Pols, 2015) for a possible improvement of mental healthcare, which consider local strivings and values and advocate for greater involvement of patients' perspectives on what constitutes good care.

1.4 Terminological Choices

Before concluding this chapter, I wish to clarify the terms I will be using in this book to refer to mental health services and to individuals who access them. Different terms are attached with different meanings and conceptions of the service and the service user, so that the choice between them is not free from relevant implications.

Sociological literature talks—sometimes independently—about psychiatric patients, consumers of psychiatric services, or survivors of psychiatric treatment (Speed, 2006). The "patient" discourse can be indicative of a passive acceptance of a diagnosis and adherence to a medical regimen; it can be employed negatively, indicating an objectified service user as repository of pathology, or positively to absolve patients from blame and sanction for their condition. The "consumer" discourse includes both elements of acceptance and resistance, introducing an element of individual agency in choosing care: the purchasing power. In so doing, it partially moves from the passive patient role, problematizing but still accepting the biomedical model. The "survivor" discourse draws from the anti-psychiatric movement and holds a political connotation, oppositional both to patienthood and to consumerism; it usually entails resistance to medical hegemony and aetiology, proposing alternative ones and highlighting the active role of the individual and the rejection of the sick role (ibidem). Since this study focuses on acute psychiatric settings, where people are sometimes detained and treated against their will, the term "patient" seems in general more appropriate than "consumer/client", which suggests a choice of using the service, or "survivor", which carries a political meaning. Nevertheless, the occasional use of other terms (e.g. "service user" when referring to people in non-acute phases of illness accessing community services) to refer to specific episodes observed on the field will be motivated and contextualized, making explicit the preference of the people involved when relevant.

With respect to the services providing care, the choice between "psychiatric" and "mental health" care reflects two different approaches, the latter term relating to the multidisciplinary delivery of care and to the deinstitutionalization process which prioritizes community over hospital inpatient care. For this reason, preference for one term or the other is sensitive to the context of use: the no-restraint setting in which I conducted fieldwork is very attentive to avoid terminology (and symbols, such as white coats, and of course restraint devices, see also Chap. 5) recalling past practices, preferring "mental healthcare" over "psychiatry", and "service" over "ward". In the empirical chapters I will generally talk about "wards" or "SPDC" for issues of clarity in comparing the two contexts, but I will attune my terminology to participants' practices—which include discursive practices and linguistic choices—making explicit reference to the rationale behind their preferences whenever relevant for my analysis.

References

Åkerström, M. (2002). Slaps, punches, pinches—But not violence: Boundary-work in nursing homes for the elderly. *Symbolic Interaction, 25*(4), 515–536.

Akrich, M. (1992). The de-scription of technical objects. In W. Bijker & J. Law (Eds.), *Shaping technology/building society: Studies in sociotechnical change* (pp. 205–224). MIT Press.

Akrich, M., & Latour, B. (1992). A summary of a convenient vocabulary for the semiotics of human and nonhuman assemblies. In W. Bijker & J. Law (Eds.), *Shaping technology/building society: Studies in sociotechnical change* (pp. 259–264). MIT Press.

Brodwin, P. (2013). *Everyday ethics: Voices from the front line of community psychiatry*. University of California Press.

Brodwin, P. (2014). The ethics of ambivalence and the practice of constraint in us psychiatry. *Culture, Medicine, and Psychiatry, 38*(4), 527–549.

Brodwin, P., & Velpry, L. (2014). The practice of constraint in psychiatry: Emergent forms of care and control. *Culture, Medicine, and Psychiatry, 4*(38), 524–526.

Gieryn, T. F. (1983). Boundary-work and the demarcation of science from non-science: Strains and interests in professional ideologies of scientists. *American Sociological Review, 48*, 781–795.

Glaser, B. G., & Strauss, A. L. (1965). *Awareness of dying*. Aldine.

Goffman, E. (1961). *Asylums. Essays on the social situation of mental patients and other inmates*. Anchor Books.

Iversen, K. I., Høyer, G., Sexton, H., & Grønli, O. K. (2002). Perceived coercion among patients admitted to acute wards in Norway. *Nordic Journal of Psychiatry, 56*(6), 433–439.

Johnson, J. (1988). Mixing humans and nonhumans together: The sociology of a door-closer. *Social Problems, 35*(3), 298–310.

Law, J. (2010). Care and killing: Tensions in veterinary practice. In A. Mol, I. Moser, & J. Pols (Eds.), *Care in practice: On tinkering in clinics, homes and farms* (Vol. 8, pp. 57–72). transcript Verlag.

Lidz, C. W., Mulvey, E. P., Hoge, S. K., Kirsch, B. L., Monahan, J., Eisenberg, M., et al. (1998). Factual sources of psychiatric patients' perceptions of coercion in the hospital admission process. *American Journal of Psychiatry, 155*(9), 1254–1260.

Mezzina, R. (2014). Community mental health care in Trieste and beyond: An "open door–no restraint" system of care for recovery and citizenship. *The Journal of Nervous and Mental Disease, 202*(6), 440–445.

Mol, A. (2002). *The body multiple: Ontology in medical practice*. Duke University Press.

Mol, A. (2010). Care and its values. Good food in the nursing home. In A. Mol, I. Moser, & J. Pols (Eds.), *Care in practice: On tinkering in clinics, homes and farms* (Vol. 8, pp. 215–234). transcript Verlag.

Mol, A., Moser, I., & Pols, J. (Eds.). (2010). *Care in practice: On tinkering in clinics, homes and farms* (Vol. 8). transcript Verlag.

O'Brien, A. J., & Golding, C. G. (2003). Coercion in mental healthcare: The principle of least coercive care. *Journal of Psychiatric and Mental Health Nursing, 10*(2), 167–173.

O'Donoghue, B., Roche, E., Shannon, S., Lyne, J., Madigan, K., & Feeney, L. (2014). Perceived coercion in voluntary hospital admission. *Psychiatry Research, 215*(1), 120–126.

Okin, R. (2020). The Trieste model. In T. Burns & J. Foot (Eds.), *Basaglia's international legacy: From asylum to community* (pp. 317–331).

Oliveira, T. T. S. D. S., Fabrici, E. P., & Santos, M. A. D. (2018). Structure and functioning of a mental health team of Trieste in its members' perspective: A qualitative study. *Psicologia em Pesquisa, 12*(2), 24–35.

Pols, J. (2003). Enforcing patient rights or improving care? The interference of two modes of doing good in mental health care. *Sociology of Health & Illness, 25*(4), 320–347.

Pols, J. (2015). Towards an empirical ethics in care: Relations with technologies in health care. *Medicine, Health Care and Philosophy, 18*(1), 81–90.

Quirk, A., & Lelliott, P. (2001). What do we know about life on acute psychiatric wards in the UK? A review of the research evidence. *Social Science & Medicine, 53*(12), 1565–1574.

Quirk, A., Lelliott, P., & Seale, C. (2006). The permeable institution: An ethnographic study of three acute psychiatric wards in London. *Social Science & Medicine, 63*(8), 2105–2117.

Reed, S. C., & Lewis, D. A. (1990). The negotiation of voluntary admission in Chicago's state mental hospitals. *The Journal of Psychiatry & Law, 18*(1–2), 137–163.

Rhodes, L. A. (1991). *Emptying beds: The work of an emergency psychiatric unit.* University of California Press.

Sjöström, S. (2006). Invocation of coercion context in compliance communication—Power dynamics in psychiatric care. *International Journal of Law and Psychiatry, 29*(1), 36–47.

Sjöström, S. (2016). Coercion contexts: How compliance is achieved in interaction. In A. Molodynski, J. Rugkåsa, & T. Burns (Eds.), *Coercion in community mental health care: International perspectives* (pp. 131–142). Oxford University Press.

Speed, E. (2006). Patients, consumers and survivors: A case study of mental health service user discourses. *Social Science & Medicine, 62*(1), 28–38.

Steinert, T., Noorthoorn, E. O., & Mulder, C. L. (2014). The use of coercive interventions in mental health care in Germany and The Netherlands. A comparison of the developments in two neighboring countries. *Frontiers in Public Health, 2,* 141.

Strauss, A., Schatzman, L., Bucher, R., Ehrlich, D., & Sabshin, M. (1981). *Psychiatric ideologies and institutions.* Transaction.

Szmukler, G. (2015). Compulsion and "coercion" in mental health care. *World Psychiatry, 14*(3), 259–261.

Szmukler, G. (2017). *Men in white coats: Treatment under coercion.* Oxford University Press.

Szmukler, G., & Appelbaum, P. (2001). Treatment pressures, coercion and compulsion. *Textbook of community psychiatry,* 529–544.

Szmukler, G., & Appelbaum, P. (2008). Treatment pressures, leverage, coercion, and compulsion in mental health care. *Journal of Mental Health, 17*(3), 233–244.

2

On Coercion in Inpatient Psychiatric Settings

Abstract The chapter introduces the notion of coercion, the way in which it has been defined in relevant literature, and the historical debates concerning its use in psychiatric practice. Available data from national and international contexts on involuntary treatment and several restraining measures—such as mechanical, manual, chemical, and environmental restraint—are presented.

2.1 Coercion in Psychiatric Settings: An Introduction

Psychiatric practice always revolved around the dual imperatives of care and custody. The historical process called by Michel Foucault (2006a) "the great confinement" gradually led to the rise of the asylum, the architectural symbol of the old psychiatric power where coercion and segregation from society were accomplished (Brodwin & Velpry, 2014). The closure of the asylums and the deinstitutionalization process did not abolish coercion, which remains common practice even in today's post-asylum era. In the following paragraphs, I will try to circumscribe the concept of coercion, identify practices employed within contemporary

E. Rossero, *Care in a Time of Crisis*, https://doi.org/10.1007/978-3-031-34418-3_2

psychiatric care which can be labelled as coercive, and navigate the debate around their legitimacy, justification for their application, and suggested alternatives according to previous research in the field. The scientific literature review here provided includes quantitative and qualitative studies, both national and international, selected after careful consideration of their methodological quality (Hanji, 2017).

2.1.1 What Counts as Coercive? Defining and Justifying Coercion

Coercion is the oldest and most controversial problem of psychiatric institutions (Steinert et al., 2014). It is both a complex and a delicate issue, for it raises relevant clinical, ethical, and legal questions (Menegatto & Zamperini, 2018). The application of coercive interventions is usually justified within medical discourse as a mean to help the patient overcome the crisis s/he is experiencing and regain his/her rationality (Kaltiala-Heino et al., 2000). The fact that some patients' disturbed behaviour may be dangerous to themselves or others can result in a paternalistic approach to mental healthcare, according to which patients have to be protected from themselves (Richter & Whittington, 2006). The opinion suggesting that patients usually lack insight into their illness further justifies the adoption of compulsory measures. Albeit undesirable, coercive interventions are sometimes considered inevitable to manage violent, suicidal, or otherwise potentially harmful behaviour: a necessary evil to ensure safety (Perkins et al., 2012). Erving Goffman's *Asylums* (1961, p. 77) provides us with an example of how psychiatric staff working in asylums viewed such interventions as necessary sacrifices to preserve a higher good, such as patient's life and integrity. The sociologist describes how, to manage suicidal or self-harming behaviour, the asylum staff could feel it is necessary to keep inpatients under continuous surveillance, to force-feed them, to curtail the freedom of their hands, or even to tie them to a chair.

Despite its longstanding relation to psychiatric care and its extensive use in mental health literature, a specific definition of coercion is not always provided, and the term is often used to refer to a wide range of practices, from undue interpersonal influence to an explicit and physical use of force (O'Brien & Golding, 2003).

An important attempt to clarify the notion of coercion and get to a more precise understanding to orient research in the field has been made by the psychiatrist George Szmukler and colleagues (2015, 2017; Szmukler & Appelbaum, 2001, 2008). In order to reduce moral connotation and draw relevant distinctions between a broad set of practices, Szmukler chooses to talk about "treatment pressures"—aimed at inducing by different means a reluctant patient to accept treatment—which are not necessarily coercive (Szmukler & Appelbaum, 2008). The authors identify a continuum of treatment pressures, which I detail in Table 2.1, made of five elements: persuasion, interpersonal leverage, inducement,

Table 2.1 Spectrum of treatment pressures according to Szmukler and Appelbaum (2008)

Persuasion	An appeal to reason. Benefits and risks of the treatment are openly discussed with the patient, whose arguments are respected.
Interpersonal leverage	Adherence to treatment may be reached using some kind of interpersonal pressure that the psychiatrist is able to exercise on the patient, such as exploiting his/her emotional dependency.
Inducement Threat	Both inducements and threats involve conditional propositions: *if* the patient accepts (does not accept) treatment A, *then* the psychiatrist will (will not) do X. The distinction between the two forms of treatment pressures requires establishing a baseline, namely the position in which the patient would have been if the offer has never been made. In the case of inducements, declining does not make the patient worse off: if, for example, s/he was offered a payment in exchange for accepting treatment, his/her rejection does not imply deprivation of any kind. In the case of threat, declining does make the patient worse off if, for example, refusing treatment leads to involuntary admission and so to a temporary deprivation of freedom.
Compulsion	Compulsory measures such as involuntary hospitalization, outpatient commitment, and compulsory treatment imply the use of force sustained by legal statute.

The authors further specify their model by distinguishing threats and unwelcome predictions. Predictions are statements of facts over which the psychiatrist has no control. If s/he accurately presents the risks that the patient will take in refusing or interrupting medication, making a reasonable prediction of an unwelcome event in which the psychiatrist will not be an agent, that is not a threat and therefore cannot be considered "coercive" threat, and compulsion. According to them, the term "coercion" is best applied to the last two kinds of pressures: threat and compulsion.

Szmukler and Appelbaum's spectrum of treatment pressures has been employed to conduct research on non- (or less-) coercive interventions, otherwise labelled as informal coercion (Hotzy & Jaeger, 2016; Jaeger et al., 2014). The study highlights how in acute inpatients settings, such as psychiatric emergency wards where formal coercion is prevalent, knowledge and ability to identify informal coercion is low among nurses; it further suggests specific training for mental healthcare professionals about factual and ethical dimensions of informal coercive interventions.

Different scholars (Lidz et al., 1998) adopted a similar spectrum approach but widened the number of "coercion-related behaviours": (1) persuasion, (2) inducement, (3) threats, (4) show of force, (5) physical force, (6) legal force, (7) request for a dispositional preference, (8) giving orders, and (9) deception. Persuasion, inducement, and request for a preference are further categorized as positive symbolic pressures, as opposed to negative symbolic pressures such as threat, deception, giving orders and show of force (which lies in a grey area between threat and actual imposition of force). At the maximum level of coercion, we find legal and physical force, which completely deprive the patient of the possibility to refuse treatment.

Other studies prefer a more extensive definition of coercion with the explicit intent to identify as ethically problematic a number of practices that form part of the taken-for-granted everyday work of mental healthcare workers, who should apply the principle of least coercive care necessary to fulfil their therapeutic goals (O'Brien & Golding, 2003). The authors suggest that not only forcing somebody to do something against their wishes counts as coercion, but also manipulating their wishes does. This means that besides those practices which are commonly considered coercive—compulsory hospitalization, use of physical force, restraint, forced medication, seclusion—they also include those behaviours aimed at manipulating someone's decision-making, such as deception, restricting access to information, and providing false ones. This is consistent with Reed and Lewis' (1990) study on negotiation of voluntary admission in Chicago mental hospital, usually obtained through a combination of persuasion and coercion. The strategy consists in presenting the advantages of voluntary admission to the patient in order to convince him to accept it and sign (persuasion), suggesting that he will stay in hospital longer if involuntarily admitted even though it is not necessarily the case, keeping information from him (e.g. the possibility to interrupt involuntary treatment before it expires), and threatening to commit him if he does not sign (coercion).

A further, relevant distinction in the scientific literature about coercion in psychiatric settings is that between objective and subjective (or perceived) coercion. Perceived coercion refers to the subjective experience of feeling coerced, namely the perception of a strong pressure on one's will or of a threat when no threat was actually intended. Such occurrence is strongly tied to the coercive shadow that looms over mental healthcare: patients worry about compulsion that might occur if they do not comply, leading them to "voluntarily" accept medication or hospital admission only to avoid fear, stigma, and humiliation related to compulsory measures (Szmukler, 2017). Attempts to operationalize and measure levels of coercion perceived by the patient at the time of hospitalization have been made by developing the Admission Experience Interview, whose application in a US study indicates that approximately 10% of legally voluntarily admitted patients felt coerced, while 35% of those involuntarily admitted did not feel coerced (Hoge et al., 1997). Further research conducted in Europe (Ireland) using the same assessment tool shows that the amount of "coerced voluntaries"—who are formally admitted on a voluntary basis but feel coerced in terms of negative pressures, implicit threats, and poor procedural justice—can be quite relevant: 22% of voluntarily admitted patients experienced equal levels of coercion to those who are admitted involuntarily (O'Donoghue et al., 2014). Conversely, it has been documented that formally involuntary subjects can perceive low levels of coercion, being defined as "uncoerced involuntaries" (Iversen et al., 2002).

The blurred line between coercive measures and patients' voluntary acceptance of treatment, and the consequent difficulty to define and measure coercion, encouraged some scholars to get past clear-cut classifications and focus their research on the concrete ways in which coercion is made relevant in everyday clinical practice. Stefan Sjöström (2006, 2016) proposes a theoretical understanding of the micro-level interaction by which coercion is enacted, after having ethnographically studied those social practices that are constructed as coercive (or non-coercive) within the specific settings in which they take place. The sociologist introduces the notion of "coercion context", inspired by that of "awareness context" coined by Glaser and Strauss' *Awareness of Dying* (1965). The latter refers to the varying degrees of information that terminally ill patients possess about their health status and chances of survival: four awareness contexts are identified, from closed awareness, where the patient does not know about his/her terminal diagnosis, to open awareness, which allows for honest discussion between the patient and the clinician. The social function of the co-creation of different awareness contexts is related to the sensitivity of the topic—terminal illness—which poses an interactional problem to the therapeutic relationship. Similarly, Sjöström argues, coercion in psychiatric care represents a sensitive issue as it concerns human rights and fundamental values such as patients' autonomy. Psychiatric ward's life, he maintains, is permeated with exceptional activities such as forcing people to comply with rules and treatments, performing body searches, restraining patients, and administering injections using physical force (2016). Mental healthcare workers who are confronted with the arduous task of exercising coercion face stress, dilemmas, and the need to make coercive acts acceptable and mitigate their burden. On the patients' side, different awareness contexts may occur according to the possessed level of knowledge about their legal status, rights, laws, and procedures. A context of closed awareness seems to be present in the hospital setting: patients can be unaware of legislation about compulsory admission and uncertain about their status and rights, primarily because of the physical layout of the ward (e.g., closed doors, ready-made beds for restraining patients) and the strict norms which regulate life in the ward regardless of the formal regime (voluntary or involuntary) of those admitted to it.

The interaction between patients and the staff is characterized by the intrinsic problem of compliance, not only with medication but also with rules, ward routines, and the always revisable acceptance to stay in the hospital. In order to handle compliance problems and pursue their clinical goals, the staff can take advantage of the uneven distribution of information and strategically use the law to invoke a coercion context. A convincing example of this strategic acting is the communication method that Sjöström calls "stalling": whenever a voluntary patient asks to be discharged despite the professional opinion that s/he should stay—which is a relatively frequent occurrence—the staff can make use of the patient's lack of knowledge about his/her rights and behave *as if* s/he cannot leave the ward without their permission, by asking him/her to wait and think it through, or telling him/her that first s/he has to talk to a doctor. The organization of the ward with its permanently locked doors plays here a crucial function, by forcing de facto even voluntary patients to ask for the staff assistance to leave: *it is the setting itself with is materiality and physical layout which works as a non-discursive element that invokes a coercion context.* The tacit possibility that a psychiatrist has to turn voluntary into compulsory treatment, let alone the explicit reference to it in the form of threat, is part of this coercion context as well, which can deter the patient from leaving without even resorting to formal procedures of involuntary treatment. Strategic information management and limitation of patients' coercion awareness context is, according to this perspective, the main resource mental healthcare workers have to achieve compliance about medication and staying at the hospital, and to maintain social order within the ward. An example observed on my own field, about how information pertaining to coercion can be kept from patients limiting their awareness about their status, is the strategy of not communicating the expiration of their involuntary treatment (which lasts seven—renewable—days, information they might not be aware of), so that the person does not know she is formally free to leave the hospital as a voluntarily admitted patient.

The present work agrees with Sjöström's approach to a situated inquiry which investigates coercion in its concrete occurrence instead of as a decontextualized object. This means that attention is paid to the contextual deployment of coercive practices—more or less univocally defined as such—and to locally developed strategies to shape and deal with problems (e.g. non-compliant or dangerous behaviour). I have focused on contextual definitions of coercion and care, on underlying meanings, logics, and ideas about what constitutes a good or at least acceptable practice, and how good care is performed in daily working activities. We know that notions of care and constraint have unstable meanings that vary according to historical and local traditions and ideologies of treatment (Brodwin & Velpry, 2014). The definitional processes which label certain interventions as more or less coercive, as good or bad ones, are particularly well suited to be explored in a comparative multi-situated ethnography, which contrasts contexts that provide different answers to the problem of demarcation between acceptable and unacceptable practices. The purpose is to expose the underlying boundary work (Gieryn, 1983) which brings some social objects inside while excluding others from that definitional frame. The last paragraph of Chap. 3 will delve deeper into the notion of situated coercive practice as the point of departure of this work.

Before moving to it, though, I provide an international overview on coercive practices such as compulsory treatment and the most common forms of restraint currently in use, in a synchronic as well as a diachronic perspective. The review highlights how such practices are legitimized by portraying them as forms of treatment or care, sometimes downplaying the dimension pertaining to behaviour control.

2.2 Involuntary Admission and Treatment

Involuntary admission and treatment are one of the few forms of coercive intervention in the healthcare system (Lincoln, 2006). This is the consequence of a profound change of modern psychiatric care, whose focus moved from custodial to curative goals. Judicial authority, which once had power over the custody of the mentally ill, today represents a guarantor of their rights. These are protected by current western legislation, which considers compulsory treatment an exceptional measure. At the international level, a number of human rights documents provide context and guidance, such as the Principles for the Protection of Persons with Mental Illness (1991), the European Convention for the Protection of Human Rights and Fundamental Freedoms (1950), the Declaration of Hawaii (1983), and the Ten Basic Principles for Mental Health Law published by the World Health Organization (1996). The latter justify involuntary admission if the patient is suffering from a severe mental disorder and compulsory treatment is necessary in the interest of the patient's health or safety, or the protection of other persons.

Despite the international framework, national laws which regulate compulsory hospitalization vary markedly from country to country according to different traditions, cultures, and resources. Drawing from WHO recommendations, the procedure is usually founded on one or two of these elements: (i) the presence of a mental illness which can be properly treated within a hospital setting and (ii) the potential danger to oneself or others. The basic requirement is that the patient suffers from a mental disorder, which is defined differently across jurisdictions despite the availability of international classification systems, the DSM-5 and the ICD-10 (Zhang et al., 2015). The inclusion of substance abuse, mental retardation, and personality disorders is contentious (ibidem). The second most common requirement for involuntary hospitalization is threatened or actual danger to oneself or others. This dangerousness criterion is sufficient on its own to justify compulsory treatment in some jurisdictions (Finland, Greece, Ireland, and Portugal), while in the UK, Denmark, and Ireland it is not the only essential requirement (ibidem). The need for treatment is an additional criterion stipulated in the UK, Italy, Spain, and Sweden. Table 2.2, a re-elaborated version of Hatling et al. (2006), summarizes the criteria for involuntary admission in European countries.

As highlighted by other recent reviews on involuntary treatment around the world (Saya et al., 2019), Italy, along with Spain and Sweden, are the only countries which do not formally consider danger to oneself or others a criterion for forced hospitalization. Outside of Europe, the criterion of dangerousness is present in the legislation of most countries—such as New Zealand, Australia, some Canadian jurisdictions,

Table 2.2 Criteria for involuntary admissions according to National Laws or Acts (Hatling et al., 2006)

Criteria	EU countries
Mental illness and danger	Austria, Belgium, France, Germany, Luxemburg, Netherlands
Mental illness, danger or need for treatment	Denmark, Finland, Greece, Ireland, UK, Portugal, Norway
Mental illness and need for treatment	Italy, Spain, Sweden

most states in the USA, China, and Japan— in either broader or more detailed acceptations which specify the nature of potential harm (physical, bodily, suicidal behaviour, deterioration, or reduced capacity of the person to take care of him/herself).

Besides criteria for involuntary treatment, countries vary in their established procedures as well. Differences concern the person entitled to make the application (family member, guardian, psychiatrist), the number and qualification of assessors for the applicability of the involuntary admission criteria, the maximum duration of the measure (unspecified or, when specified, ranging from seven days to two years), and the possibility to provide involuntary treatment outside the hospital (community compulsory care, possible in the UK, Norway, the USA, Canada, Australia, and New Zealand).

Epidemiological data on the international practice of compulsory admission are scarce, also because of varying definitions and heterogeneous methods used to collect them (Salize & Dressing, 2004). Despite the efforts to limit forced hospitalization through reforms, rates of compulsory admissions appear to have increased, and this could be a consequence of the tendency to reduce the average duration of stays in psychiatric inpatient facilities at the expense of more frequent readmissions (de Stefano & Ducci, 2008).

A small study on patients' experience of involuntary psychiatric care suggested contrasting perceptions of restricted autonomy (in terms of both liberty and agency), violation of physical integrity and human value, disrespect, but also feelings of being protected and cared for (Johansson & Lundman, 2002). Olofsson and Jacobsson (2001) describe involuntarily hospitalized patients' feelings of not being involved in their own care, not receiving information on treatment, and being treated as criminal or as inferior kind of human beings. Negative accounts of involuntary admission also express a sense of meaninglessness due to the sole focus of treatment on medication and lack of activities, so that the stay in hospital is perceived as a pointless form of storage (Wyder et al., 2013). Generally speaking, factors negatively influencing the experience are power imbalance with the staff, feeling unsafe, episodes of restraint, lack of information and involvement in treatment decisions, and scarce meaningful activities; on the contrary, positive factors are participation in own care, flexibility of ward rules, sense of safety, good relationships with staff and other patients, having the opportunity to talk and feel listened to (ibidem).

2.2.1 Involuntary Admission and Treatment in Italy: "Trattamento Sanitario Obbligatorio"

Involuntary medical treatment ("*Trattamento Sanitario Obbligatorio*", TSO) in Italy is regulated by Law 833/1978, which established the entire National Health Service. The three conditions under which involuntary admission can be adopted are dictated in article number 34 of Law 833/78. The measure should take place in a hospital regime only in those cases where: (1) psychic conditions are such as to require urgent therapeutic intervention, (2) treatment is not consented to by the patient, and (3) circumstances do not allow the adoption of timely and adequate measures in an outpatient regime. Contrary to legislation in many other countries (see Table 2.2), Italian law does not consider danger represented by the mentally ill subject among the motives for compulsory admission. This is in direct contrast with the first national legislation on asylums enacted in 1904, which was not concerned with illness but with dangerous social behaviours that psychiatric institution had to incapacitate (Donnelly, 1992). For this reason, the law represents the purging of psychiatry's traditional and legal responsibility for social control (Betti, 1989), which nevertheless does not seem to have completely disappeared from today's psychiatric practice and conceptions associated with psychiatry's role in our societies.

From a historical point of view, individuals described as mentally ill have been considered a possible danger to themselves or others up until 1978. Accordingly, their compulsory admission to psychiatric hospitals was authorized by Judicial or Public Safety Authorities. On the contrary, Law 180/1978 and then Law 833/1978 frame involuntary admission as an exception to the voluntariness of medical treatment, an extreme solution to be applied only when other means of obtaining consent have failed. Moreover, the coercive intervention must always be respectful of individual dignity and Constitutional rights. The regulation of forced treatment has been one of the central topics in the debates of the health commission discussing the content of the law, initially criticized by Franco Basaglia himself and compared by one deputy to a form of medical arrest (Foot, 2015). Due to the little time available (Law 180 was discussed and accepted in only twenty days, through a special procedure), a spirit of collaboration and negotiation prevailed, and Basaglia changed his position though acknowledging the limitations of the law. In fact, the historic reform resulting from that debate is centred around the *voluntary* nature of treatment. Moreover, mandatory measures, allowed in very special circumstances only (see the following paragraphs), are framed as therapeutic acts aimed at taking care of the person's mental health rather than protecting society. Danger, once prejudicially associated with mental illness, disappeared from the text of the law, and the only legal figure entailed in the procedure—the tutelary judge—has the duty to prevent abuses and ensure that the involuntarily treated person's constitutional rights are not violated. Indeed, besides regulating involuntary admissions and treatments, the law sets down some principles which represented a paradigmatic change: it acknowledged those suffering from mental illness as people, guaranteeing their human and civil rights, and providing them health care in a general hospital rather than in special, isolated psychiatric facilities. As the Italian historian Valeria Babini observes (2011), the law shows a secular and modernizing nature in that it removes every reference to the patient's dangerousness and to "public scandal", framing the psychiatric patient as an "ill" citizen like any other. The content and the origin of the Italian psychiatric reform, born within the same institutions it meant (and then managed) to close down—asylums—qualify it as unique on the international scene. The city of Trieste, in particular, has become a symbol of the reform, a centre of pilgrimage for critical psychiatrists, and a model for community-oriented services recognized as such by the World Health Organization (Tone, 2015).[1]

[1] It is important to acknowledge that changes introduced by the reform in 1978 have been the result of a polycentric process, which has its origin in Gorizia—where the first group of radical psychiatrists formed around Franco Basaglia—but later spread across Italy. Turin, Naples, Venice, Genoa, Perugia, Arezzo, Parma, Ferrara, Trieste: in these and many other cities anti-institutional psychiatric movement developed, carrying forward a different version of change with its own specificities (Foot, 2015).

Consistently with the medical framework set by the psychiatric reform in 1978, the procedure to initiate an involuntary treatment in Italy entails a motivated proposal from a physician, sustained by a second physician working in a public structure. The proposal is then transmitted to the mayor, who will authorize the placement of the patient and notify the Tutelary Judge within forty-eight hours. During fieldwork, I have observed how involuntary admission does not necessarily take place at the end of this procedure, but the patient can be accompanied to the hospital right after the proposal or, in cases of emergency, while it is being formulated (e.g. the ER doctor proposes the TSO and the ward's psychiatrist sustains it, while the patient is already at the hospital and about to be transferred to the psychiatric unit; then, the mayor and the Tutelary Judge ratify the intervention).

Involuntary medical treatment cannot exceed seven days, at the end of which an extension of seven additional days can be requested if the conditions of the patient do not allow his/her voluntary treatment or discharge from hospital. The renewal is once again proposed by two physicians, transmitted to the mayor, and approved by the Tutelary Judge. Interruption of the involuntary treatment before its natural expiration (seven days) is always possible and requires the notification of the abovementioned institutional figures as well.

Law 833/1978 regulates a second measure, that of "*Accertamento Sanitario Obbligatorio*" (ASO), a compulsory psychiatric evaluation aimed at assessing the health condition of a person and the possible need for admission and treatment. The measure has to be motivated and authorized through the same procedure required for involuntary medical treatment. The adoption of the measure should always pursue the collaboration and consensus of the person, who can accept the treatment offered by mental healthcare staff: for this reason, involuntary medical treatment does not automatically follow.

Most recent data show that involuntary admissions in Italy in 2020 have been 5.398, corresponding with 7.1% of total admissions of that year in public psychiatric wards (Ministry of Health, 2021b). Rates of involuntary admissions, which can be seen as an indirect measure of therapeutic efficacy of programmes implemented by Mental Health Departments, vary significantly between the different Italian regions, with a national figure of 1.1 for every 10,000 inhabitants (ibidem). These rates are significantly lower than previous years, due to the disruptive effect of the Covid-19 pandemic on hospitals and health services, and the reduced admissions in psychiatric units registered in 2020 (Piccinelli et al., 2022; Rossero, 2022). For this reason, Table 2.3 provides a comprehensive overview of available data and the regional distributions of involuntary admissions from 2017 to 2020, but rates related to 2019 are shown to avoid biased information (Ministry of Health, 2021a).

We can observe from these data that involuntary admission rates for the two regions considered in this study—Piedmont and Friuli Venezia Giulia—are respectively 1.1 (in line with the national rate) and 0.4 (the

Table 2.3 Regional distributions and rates of involuntary admissions in Italy (Ministry of Health, 2021a, 2021b)

	Involuntary admissions per year				Rate/10,000
Region	2017	2018	2019	2020	inhabitants (2019)
Piemonte	474	401	406	336	1.1
Valle d'Aosta	27	21	17	25	1.6
Lombardia	938	926	818	716	1.0
P.A. Bolzano	20	15	18	19	0.4
P.A. Trento	62	80	66	48	1.5
Veneto	395	322	331	255	0.8
Friuli Venezia Giulia	36	43	42	69	0.4
Liguria	201	205	215	182	1.6
Emilia Romagna	929	910	921	810	2.5
Toscana	220	230	204	129	0.6
Umbria	194	213	222	190	3.0
Marche	178	245	261	166	2.0
Lazio	541	545	387	318	0.8
Abruzzo	223	246	233	204	2.1
Molise	24	26	16	27	0.6
Campania	489	402	307	179	0.6
Puglia	751	657	613	437	1.8
Basilicata	31	20	20	15	0.4
Calabria	359	314	239	162	1.5
Sicilia	1.203	1.245	1.098	857	2.6
Sardegna	313	341	303	254	2.1
Italy	**7.608**	**7.407**	**6.737**	**5.398**	**1.3**

lowest rate in Italy together with P.A. Bolzano and Basilicata region).[2] Further data on other elements of mental healthcare provision in the two contexts—such as number of acute beds, resources allotted to mental healthcare, and average duration of hospitalization—are provided in Chap. 3, which describes the methodological choices and the rationale behind the selection of these regions.

2.3 Restraint and Its Multiple Forms

Broadly speaking, the term "restraint" consists in reducing a person's free movement. It is used in both medical (emergency medicine, geriatrics, orthopaedics, psychiatry) and non-medical (law enforcement) areas, but it is particularly controversial in psychiatry because it is usually employed against the person's will, and its very same need is doubtful (Negroni, 2017). The variegated set of restraining measures has a long history in psychiatry, as they have always been used in different settings to manage violent or agitated people (Holmes et al., 2004). Before the advent of the asylum and of psychiatry as a medical discipline, mental illness was dealt with within the family. Treatment at home usually included restraint, as accounts of that time from both Europe and the USA reveal. Edward Shorter (1997) recounts how an insane but peaceful person living in the countryside was generally let to run loose, whereas a troublesome one could be chained down in the stable or in an isolated room, becoming a victim of a crime of sequestration that authorities may find out years later. Severely ill people were confined not only at home, but also in workhouses or alms-houses, under restraint or in cages (ibidem). In the first half of the nineteenth century, even after Pinel's unchaining of the insane at Bicêtre (1806), a wide set of restraining instruments were in use: the fixed chair (fixed to the wall and to which the patient was

[2] These data are based on hospital discharge records ("*Schede di Dimissione Ospedaliera*") and therefore may not include involuntary admissions performed in Community Mental Health Centres of Friuli Venezia Giulia. Since patients can be involuntarily admitted to the SPDC and then transferred to the MHC, it is very likely that some of them have been considered in the official report based on hospital discharge records. In Piedmont, all of the involuntary admissions are performed in psychiatric hospital wards and are therefore registered in the ministerial report.

attached), the moving chair (moving about due to the patient's restlessness), finger-glove garments (fitting the person tightly to keep their hands pressed against their thighs), straitjackets, muffs, handcuffs, wicker caskets (in which patients were enclosed), and even dog collars (Foucault, 2006b). Forced isolation in darkened rooms was also practised, maintaining its therapeutic effect due to desensitization (see Paragraph 2.3.4).

Today, restraint is still employed to manage disturbed behaviour in acute mental health settings, and it is accomplished by a variety of means: physical (or manual), mechanical, pharmacological, and environmental. All of these measures attract moral valuations, but their use differs greatly between countries, and not every method is adopted in every country. Table 2.4, derived from Whittington et al. (2006, p. 147), represents the frequency of use of different kinds of restraining measures in acute psychiatric settings of twenty-five countries around the world, based on the responses of at least one resident expert in each country. The authors consider mechanical restraint (movements are restricted or prevented by belts, handcuffs or other equipment), manual restraint (or "hands-on" restraint, which usually precedes other kinds of interventions), seclusion (enforced isolation in a bare, unstimulating environment), net bed (lockable metal frame bolted to the patient's bed), enforced medication (or rapid tranquillization through injected drugs), and pain compliance (pressing or holding of limb which deliberately makes every movement painful for the patient).

Data show how interventions can be extremely common (such as enforced medication, mechanical and manual restraint) or rather rare (net bed and pain compliance), while even neighbouring countries can differ significantly in their preferred practices to deal with the disruptive behaviour of acute psychiatric inpatients. The authors acknowledge that these data only represent the visible tip of the iceberg, since a wide range of unrecorded manoeuvres used by the staff to coerce patients remains invisible. Nevertheless, they can provide a general idea of the distribution of better defined and widely known coercive measures in a situation of scarce reliable, comparable, and systematic epidemiological data (Sashidharan et al., 2019).

A quantitative study (Steinert et al., 2010) on the international incidence of restraint and seclusion confirms a huge variety in the type,

Table 2.4 Use of coercive measures in acute psychiatric settings (Whittington et al., 2006, p. 147)

Country	Mechanical restraint	Manual restraint	Seclusion	Net bed	Enforced medication	Pain compliance
Australia	Occasional	Regular	Regular	Never	Regular	Never
Austria	Regular	Occasional	Occasional	Regular	Regular	Never
Canada	Regular	Regular	Regular	Never	Regular	Never
Czech Republic	Regular	Regular	Regular	Never	Regular	Never
Finland	Regular	Occasional	Regular	Never	Regular	Never
France	Occasional	Regular	Regular	Never	Regular	Never
Germany	Regular	Regular	Regular	Never	Regular	Never
Greece	Regular	Regular	Regular	Never	Regular	Never
Iceland	Never	Regular	Never	Never	Regular	Never
Ireland	Never	Regular	Regular	Never	Regular	Occasional
Italy	Regular	Regular	Never	Never	Regular	Never
Japan	Regular	Regular	Regular	Never	Regular	Never
Netherlands	Occasional	Regular	Regular	Never	Regular	Never
New Zealand	Occasional	Regular	Regular	Never	Regular	Not specified
Norway	Regular	Regular	Occasional	Never	Regular	Never
Portugal	Occasional	Regular	Regular	Never	Regular	Never
Slovenia	Occasional	Regular	Never	Never	Regular	Never
Spain	Regular	Regular	Never	Never	Regular	Never
Sweden	Regular	Regular	Occasional	Never	Regular	Never
Switzerland	Regular	Regular	Regular	Never	Regular	Regular
Taiwan	Regular	Regular	Regular	Never	Regular	Never
Thailand	Never	Regular	Regular	Never	Regular	Never
Turkey	Occasional	Occasional	Occasional	Never	Regular	Never
UK-England and Wales	Occasional	Regular	Regular	Never	Regular	Never
UK-Scotland	Occasional	Regular	Regular	Never	Regular	Occasional
USA	Regular	Regular	Regular	Never	Regular	Never

duration, and frequency of these measures, with the two most diverse countries being the Netherlands (average duration of seclusion: 300 hours; average duration of rarely used mechanical restraint: 1182 hours),[3] and the UK (seclusion rarely used; mechanical restraint not allowed; average duration of a physical restraint episode: 20 minutes). The other countries considered (Austria, Finland, Germany, Japan, New Zealand, Norway, Spain, and Switzerland) fall between these two extremes, and most of them use mechanical restraint. Iceland represents an exception as it is a small country where seclusion and restraint have been abolished decades ago. The authors conclude that since Western mental health services are similar in terms of resources and populations at risk, the different use of coercive measures is probably based on culture, traditions, and local policies. Moreover, definitions of coercive interventions differ from country to country: in the UK, "restraint" means physical restraint, whereas mechanical restraint is considered unethical and is not used. In all other countries mechanical restraint is in use, and in an unknown proportion of cases, it requires (unrecorded) physical restraint to be initiated.[4] Definitions of involuntary medication differ as well, and other freedom-restricting measures whose coercive nature is controversial are in use. This is consistent with an understanding of coercion as a continuum which encompasses several practices with different degrees of influence, locally construed as more or less acceptable according to the clinician's and the patient's experience of the situation (Olsen, 2003).

The reasons behind this heterogeneity have been addressed by Bowers et al. (2004). The authors underline how containment methods give rise to strong emotions and are frequently associated with the "abhorred past of psychiatry": methods that are not used in a given country tend to be

[3] These data are related to seclusion and restraint orders gathered by the Dutch Health Inspectorate and do not provide information on the number and duration of discrete seclusion or restraint episodes. Nevertheless, the discrepancy between practice in the Netherlands and the UK remains significant, also because Dutch psychiatric professionals consider mechanical restraint and seclusion less invasive and less threatening of personal integrity than involuntary medication (whose use is restricted by the Dutch mental health legislation), while in the UK mechanical restraint is not allowed (Steinert et al., 2010).

[4] This has been observed on the field too: while mechanical restraint was reported in the patient's clinical record and, in some Piedmontese wards, in a dedicated register, physical restraint preceding the initiation of mechanical restraint was not registered. More generally, no national registers of mechanical restraint episodes and duration exist in Italy (see Paragraph 2.3.1).

regarded as typifying that barbaric kind of psychiatric practice and therefore rejected. Their study on the training paths of psychiatric nurses in the UK concluded that relative evaluations of containment methods are a product of national cultures and values, which are then reflected in psychiatric practice. These findings raise questions with respect to infra-national differences of orientation towards the acceptability of containment methods. This concerns the Italian context, characterized by a general approval of mechanical restraint, except for the relevant case of no-restraint services, which firmly reject this measure associating it with the psychiatric power exercised in the asylum (Rossi & Toresini, 2015; see also Paragraph 2.3.1). Issues of what is preferable between different coercive practices and the values behind such preferences will be discussed in Chap. 6.

The last international study on coercive interventions that is worth mentioning is the EUNOMIA (European Evaluation of Coercion in Psychiatry and Harmonization of Best Clinical Practice) research project, funded by the European Commission (Kallert et al., 2005). The study has been conducted in twelve countries—Bulgaria, Czech Republic, Germany, Greece, Israel, Italy, Lithuania, Poland, Slovak Republic, Spain, Sweden, and the UK—which are considered to be at different stages of the psychiatric reform processes: from areas with a strong community orientation and a low rate of inpatient psychiatric beds (such as Italy) to contexts relying on hospital-based mental health services (e.g. Germany and Poland). The research focused on involuntarily admitted patients, but also underlined how voluntary admissions sometimes entail a degree of coercion (Kallert et al., 2011). Results reveal that almost 40% of involuntarily treated patients experience at least one coercive measure among seclusion, restraint, and forced medication (Kalisova et al., 2014). These measures are applied in all countries participating in the EUNOMIA project, although with wide variations with respect to frequency, type, and legal background (Raboch et al., 2007). Markedly different practices concerning the use of coercive measures are deemed to reflect differences in societal attitudes, clinical traditions, and treatment customs in individual psychiatric facilities (Raboch et al., 2010). The EUNOMIA study group acknowledged coercive psychiatric treatment as a rarely studied issue and called for further research to identify factors in clinical practice, including staff-patient interactions, which may influence the adoption of coercive interventions (ibidem).

2.3.1 *Contenzione*: Mechanical restraint

Mechanical restraint restricts patients' movement or completely prevents them from moving by means of belts, handcuffs or other devices. In acute care facilities, it has been a common practice for decades. The reasons for the application of this measure are usually patient-oriented, relating to patients' safety (prevention of falls and self-harm), agitation or violence (protection of other patients and the staff), behavioural control (in case of restlessness, confusion and altered mental status), wandering (usually for older patients), and support (e.g. helping the patient to fall asleep) (Evans & FitzGerald, 2002). These reasons are consistent with the ones expressed in the restraint context by participants to the study presented in this book. Other reasons pertaining to the use of mechanical restraint are also staff/organization-related, such as the need to compensate for insufficient staff members, the will to punish, or in case of non-compliant behaviour (ibidem).

Nurses play a key role when it comes to mechanical restraint, since they usually initiate the procedure in emergency situations, and they are involved in the care of restrained patients (Goethals et al., 2012). Moreover, even if the decision to restrain should be taken by the psychiatrist after clinical assessment, nurses usually appear to be the key informants describing the patients' conditions and events that could lead to their restraining, or even the key decision-makers (Kontio et al., 2010). The decision-making regarding mechanical restraint is characterized by an inbuilt ethical conflict concerning the will to preserve a therapeutic relationship, and the need to weight a patient's best interest against other people's best interests (ibidem). Strategies to hold together the performance of care and coercive practices will be extensively discussed in Chap. 5. Despite the moral distress associated with mechanical restraint and other restrictive practices, nurses also expressed fear that these measures could be reduced or eliminated without providing alternative means whereby maintaining a safe ward was possible and that they could be blamed in case adverse events happened (Muir-Cochrane et al., 2018).

Besides raising ethical dilemmas, mechanical restraint has been described as an unpleasant, challenging, and risky procedure for those who employ it: the team performing it, which is usually made of less than five people and generally nurses, is exposed to physical and psychological harms (Vedana et al., 2018). Several injuries to the patient have been found related to mechanical restraint, from infections, contractures and pressure sores to cardiac arrest, thrombo-embolism, and even death (Kersting et al., 2019). In order to minimize risks and orient these procedures, recommendations, guidelines, and codes of practice have been produced in many countries (Whittington et al., 2006). One of the most authoritative guides is that developed by the National Institute for Clinical and Health Excellence for the UK (2015), available online. It recommends using restraining techniques only when de-escalation techniques have failed, for no longer than necessary, never to punish, inflict pain or humiliation, and regularly assessing the patient's condition using the least intrusive level of observation necessary. Moreover, the guidelines suggest staff training about restrictive interventions, adequate number of staff, resuscitation equipment always available, and immediate post-intervention debrief to address potential physical harm and emotional impact of the event on the staff, other patients, and possible witnesses. Guidelines and attempts to regulate the performance of mechanical restraint from a technical and procedural point of view are related to the strategy of proceduralization of coercion, discussed in Chap. 6, Sect. 6.3.2.

Available literature tells us that mechanical restraint is hardly ever used alone, without the administration of sedative drugs, and if so, it is usually considered unacceptable (Negroni, 2017). Moreover, it is usually preceded by manual restraint which allows for the application of restraints (Whittington et al., 2006). The use of combinations of restrictive measures adds to the already difficult quantification of restraint rates, which vary greatly between countries also because of inconsistent definitions and data collection techniques (Oster et al., 2016). A recent systematic review conducted by Beghi et al. (2013) on restraint use in psychiatry worldwide found a prevalence between 3.8% and 20% of hospitalized patients, which is consistent with previous reviews. The reviewers conclude that, despite the attempts to reduce the use of restraint and introduce alternatives, it is still widely used in psychiatric wards of many countries.

In Italy, mechanical restraint is widely used to manage aggressive, violent, or disruptive behaviour. Since data on registered restraints are not systematically gathered and analysed at a central level, its incidence can only be estimated: for every 100 admissions 20 mechanical restraints are practised, and 11% of inpatients are mechanically restrained (Ferioli, 2013).

From a legal point of view, mechanical restraint raises questions because it is not mentioned in Law 833/78 regulating involuntary admission and treatment, nor in other specific regulations. This legal vacuum opens for debate and doubts about the lawfulness of mechanical restraint. The justifying hypotheses for its application are those foreseen in the penal code, articles 52 ("legitimate defence") and 54 ("state of need"). Alternative orientations argue for the ethical and constitutional illegitimacy of mechanical restraint, which could be prosecuted as abduction and private violence (articles 605 and 610 of the penal code). With respect to soft law acts, the National Bioethics Committee in 1999 observed "the frequent use of even prolonged restraint" in most of the Italian psychiatric wards and recommended a drastic reduction of this practice, to be used only for exceptional cases and emergency (CNB, 1999). The same Committee denounced a "remnant of asylum culture" and called for it to be overcome (CNB, 2000). Nurses' deontological code (Codice Deontologico delle Professioni Infermieristiche, 2019, art. 35) states that mechanical restraint is not a therapeutic act, but a precautionary one to be used in a state of need to protect the patient and the staff. In 2010, the interregional conference "*Conferenza delle Regioni e delle Province autonome*" defined mechanical restraint as an anti-therapeutic act and set as its goal to eliminate it by concrete measures aimed at gradually reducing its use. In 2017, a national investigation conducted by the Committee for Human Rights (*Senato della Repubblica*) to verify the application of these recommendations revealed a highly heterogeneous situation: only five regions had produced guidelines and were actively monitoring the phenomenon of mechanical restraint; some regions registered local initiatives but no regional strategies; four others had not developed any programme; one region never transmitted any update about its progress (Algostino, 2020).

Among the local initiatives advanced to reduce or eliminate mechanical restraint in Italy, a group of mental health services formally founded in 2013, the association called "Club SPDC no-restraint" (Rossi & Toresini, 2015).[5] The association embraces the abolition of mechanically restraining measures and the open-door policy, explicitly identifying as its cultural references the work of John Conolly (1856) and that of Franco Basaglia, whose refusal to sign the register of mechanical restraints in the asylum of Gorizia in 1961 is defined as the founding act of the no-restraint movement in Italy (ibidem). The "Club" aims at providing visibility to the no-restraint practice, sharing knowledge and supporting the transition of those services which intend to embrace the no-restraint method, as well as legally assisting victims subjected to "existential and biological harms deriving from mechanical restraint" in Italian psychiatric wards (ibidem). In 2015, the association had 21 SPDC members, while in its online spaces it maintains to represent 5% of Italian psychiatric wards.[6]

The strategies implemented by these services to deal with acutely disturbed people are usually developed according to contextual specificities, such as the availability of mental health centres open twenty-four hours a day and with a "good emergency filter capacity", as noted by the National Bioethics Committee (CNB, 2015, p. 16). The strength of community services and the orientation of the whole Mental Health Departments represent a fundamental element for the reduction of restraining measures, as we can read from the speech given by Giovanna Del Giudice at the Eighth Conference of the "Club SPDC no-restraint" (2015): "It seems to us that it is more appropriate to talk about no-restraint [Mental Health] Departments rather than wards: mechanical restraint affects the whole Department, its organizational features, cultures, operational styles, the relationship between the different roles, and with the broader

[5] SPDC is the acronym for *Servizi Psichiatrici di Diagnosi e Cura*, indicating the acute psychiatric wards located in Italian general hospitals, and introduced in 1978 after the gradual closure of former psychiatric hospitals.

[6] https://180gradi.org/salute-mentale/180gradi/spdc-no-restraint, accessed on 26th November 2022.

community".[7] These considerations contributed to the choice I made to include in this study community services as well as hospital psychiatric wards (see Chap. 3) and to investigate the relations and mutual representations between them (see Chap. 4).

In such polarized context, mechanical restraint in Italy is a controversial issue, debated from both legal and ethical perspective. Tragic events such as the death of Francesco Mastrogiovanni in 2009 and Giuseppe Casu in 2006 (see Del Giudice, 2015), both mechanically restrained, contributed to the discussion, and a national campaign called "*…e tu slegalo subito*" (which can be rendered into "untie him/her now") has been launched to raise awareness on this practice and promote change towards its abolition.[8] Nevertheless, scientific research in this field is scarce, and practices implemented in the no-restraint contexts are mainly discussed among specialists and not always supported by empirical evidence (Mauceri, 2017). To the best of my knowledge, only one national survey on Italian psychiatric inpatient facilities—*Progress Acuti*—has been conducted so far by the Italian National Institute of Health in 2004 (see Dell'Acqua et al., 2007). A report focused on the practice of mechanical restraint in Italian psychiatric wards—*Contenere la contenzione meccanica in Italia*—has then been published in 2017, providing the basis for future research aimed at developing guidelines to contain (and ultimately eliminate) mechanical restraint (Mauceri, 2017).

---

[7] The quotation is the author's translation from page 17 of the proceedings of the Eighth Conference of the "Club SPDC no-restraint" (2015), available on the website of the national campaign "…e tu slegalo subito" for the abolition of mechanical restraint: http://www.slegalosubito.com/wp-content/uploads/2017/11/Atti-VIII-Convegno-SPDC-No-Restraint.pdf, accessed on 26th November 2022.

[8] Such episodes can be interpreted and employed to criticize mechanical restraint *tout court*, or they can be read as examples of inefficient health service and abuse: lack of monitoring of vital parameters, violation of human rights, and abandonment of the restrained patient point more to the conditions in which restraint has been practised than on the practice itself. Episodes of mechanical restraints observed on the field did not resemble such tragic conditions, even though the practice is associated with both physical and psychological suffering patients used to express.

2.3.2 *Contenimento*: Holding or Manual Restraint

Manual restraint is a physical intervention intended to hold a person immobile or limit her/his voluntary movement by using body contact as the only source of restraint. This practice is sometimes referred to as physical restraint, even though the expression is sometimes intended to include mechanical restraint (i.e. using devices such as belts) as well. To avoid confusing terminology, I will try to avoid the use of "physical restraint" as much as possible, preferring "manual restraint" instead.

The use of manual restraint on people with mental disorders is usually a response to violent behaviour, but it can also be adopted in case of attempts to abscond, agitation, self-harm, and refusal of medication (Bowers et al., 2012). The measure often underpins or precedes others: mechanical restraint, seclusion, and forced medication often rely on manual restraint as a first step (Whittington et al., 2006). The practice entails some risks, in terms of injuries (both to the patient and the staff), as well as more serious harms due to continuous struggle and increased risk of patient mortality when s/he is pressed in a prone position on the floor (ibidem). Bowers et al. (2012) found that the use of manual restraint is increasing. In their study on a sample of 136 acute psychiatric wards in England, manual restraint was "a regular feature of life on all the study wards", along with show of force (i.e. a number of staff assembled in front of the patient, implicitly or explicitly threatening to manually restrain them or force them to undergo treatment, unless they comply voluntarily). Despite its prevalence, a lack of data has been noticed, because research is usually scarce, small scale, based on reports of violent incidents, and not specifically focused on manual restraint (Stewart et al., 2009). A review of the available data found that episodes of manual restraint last around ten minutes, with about half involving the restraint of the patient on the floor in the prone position. With respect to manually restrained patients' characteristics, they tend to be younger, male, and involuntarily admitted (ibidem). Research on the subjective experiences of this practice for patients and staff defined manual restraint a "trauma for all", preceded by disturbed ward atmosphere and poor communication, and followed by feelings of anger, distress, frustration, and embarrassment (Bonner et al., 2002).

Manual restraint is sometimes referred to as holding, a term which carries a therapeutic connotation. Yannis Gansel and Samuel Lézé (2015) investigated the concept through a genealogical approach, whose findings are of particular interest to this work. They explain how, in the 1960s, the British psychoanalyst Wilfred Bion elaborated the concepts of "container" and "contained" to describe a key element of a child's mental development, that of maternal care, which can be seen as an *enveloping act* that gives body limits to the child. These concepts have then been applied by child psychiatrists to justify a bodily practice called "packing therapy", used to treat agitated autistic children, bringing together their body as it lacks containment, giving them a secure feeling of unity while contrasting the distressing feeling of being in pieces (Saget, 2009). A theory inspired by psychoanalysis has been used to justify a practice of bodily constraint, which has as its ultimate target the mind: constraint goes from being a "pure action of concrete control" to "an immaterial act of care" (Gansel & Lézé, 2015). Similarly, restraint (*contention* in French) restores body limits of the subject in mental distress (who suffers from a lack of *contenance*) and at the same time pacifies the violent person. The use of physical force is converted into legitimate and therapeutic restraint as the actors verbalize and explain its necessity, distinguishing it from punishment (ibidem).

A similar terminological difference can be found in Italian between "*contenzione*" and "*contenimento*". While the first term is generally used to refer to the physical act of restraining a person's movement (through mechanical—*contenzione meccanica*—chemical or environmental means), the notion of "*contenimento*" is associated with both de-escalation techniques and manual restraint (or holding), and it takes on a different connotation associated with care. The following excerpt I translated from an Italian report on mechanical restraint clarifies this difference (Mauceri, 2017, pp. 162–163).

> The containment [*contenimento*] of distress, as opposed to the immobilisation implied by restraint [*contenzione*], it's precisely the goal pursued, in their variety, by the relational practices adopted by no-restraint SPDC

> [psychiatric wards] to deal with acute psychiatric crisis (Rossi & Toresini, 2015). The purpose of containment (holding), according to the meaning attributed in 1958 by the English psychoanalyst Winnicott—to hold in one's arms, to protect, to care for—implies sensorial-affective-cognitive practices such as touching, speaking, encourage, show 'presence'. […] The use of force, which has sometimes to be employed in no-restraint SPDC, is temporary and combined with communication strategies that explain to the patient the meaning of the staff's action.

The quotation highlights the same shift in meaning explained by Gansel and Lézé (2015): the transformation of a physical act (holding) into a form of care by referring to psychoanalytical concepts, and the therapeuticization of that act by means of relation and communication that illustrates staff's motives for its application. The "pure action of concrete control" is here represented by mechanical restraint, a mere act of immobilization which, according to its opponents, holds no therapeutic value. "*Contenimento*", on the contrary, is "an immaterial act of care" and protection performed through "sensorial-affective-cognitive practices"; the use of force it implies is always temporary and explained to the patient. This distinction is crucial to everyday practices of no-restraint settings, such as those included in the present study (see Chap. 6, and specifically Excerpt 6.15 and its discussion).

2.3.3 The Sedative/Curative Divide: Pharmacological Restraint

A form of intervention entailing the forced (non-consenting) administration of medication in emergency situations is commonly called in modern psychiatric practice "rapid tranquillisation", defined as all medication given in the short-term management of disturbed/violent behaviour (NICE, 2005, p. 100). Because of the coercive nature of such a measure and its purpose of limiting a person's freedom of movement as well as controlling his/her behaviour, this intervention is sometimes referred to as pharmacological, or chemical, restraint.

From a historical perspective, mental hospitals have always been in need for sedation. The first chemical agents used for this purpose were opiates, hyoscine, and digitalis, substituted by chloral after its synthesis and the discovery of its sedative properties in 1869 (Healy, 2000). Chloral, along with barbiturates, bromides, and anticholinergic agents, remained in use until the half of the twentieth century (ibidem). Such drugs were employed principally as chemical containment besides physical treatments such as electroconvulsive therapy (ECT), or in a combination of the two, for example, to allow the transportation of agitated patients from their homes to the hospital for tranquillization through ECT: it is reported how "many acutely excited schizophrenics" were successfully calmed down by means of electrically induced convulsions administered as they were admitted to the hospital (Meyer-Gross et al., 1954, p. 287).

The half of the twentieth century saw the introduction of antipsychotic drugs, some of which specifically advertised for the control of aggressive behaviour and agitation (Allison & Moncrieff, 2014). Illustrations published in medical journals in the 1950s and the 1960s showed advertisements for antipsychotic drugs (e.g. trifluoperazine). Some commercial ads portrayed old instruments (e.g. a "squirrel cage" used for calming patients in the eighteenth century, appeared in the *Journal of Mental Science*, 105, January 1959) to suggest that the advertised drug could replace physical confinement of the patient. Others, sometimes explicitly targeted for people with a diagnosis of schizophrenia or psychosis, promoted trifluoperazine to treat violent and hostile behaviour, adopting a more therapeutic wording by referring to the restoration of insight and the establishment of the relationship with the mental healthcare staff (Stelazine advertisement appeared on the *British Journal of Psychiatry*, 111, June 1965).

During the 1960s and 1970s, more antipsychotics came onto the market and continued to be advertised for the control of behavioural disturbance, increasingly associated with the reduction of the symptoms and opportunity to render the patient more amenable to other treatments (Allison & Moncrieff, 2014). It is the case of the already mentioned Stelazine advertisement (1965), but also of chlorpromazine, associated with the promise to make the patient "more sociable and more receptive to psychotherapy" (advertisement published on *Mental Hospitals*, 11 (5), 1960). Interestingly, the aims of this work is the fact that such drugs were usually presented as alternatives preferable to other forms of restraint. A particularly eloquent advertisement (*Hospital & Community Psychiatry*, 18(9), 1967) depicted a half-closed door of a "restraint closet", where one could see hanging several straps and belts used to practise mechanical restraint. The caption below explicitly suggested that the introduction of antipsychotics, specifically chlorpromazine, helped making those tools "obsolete", replacing them in the management of disruptive behaviour. Preference to treat aggressive behaviour with antipsychotics instead of physical measures is reported in publications of that period as well, which make explicit reference to drugs as chemical restraint (Fann & Linton, 1972). The authors underline how negative side-effects, such as rigidity and the Parkinsonoid state, are not deleterious in situations of emergency, and that antipsychotic drugs represent an "excellent alternative" to physical measures (ibidem, p. 479).

By the 1980s, haloperidol had gradually taken over from chlorpromazine as the most frequently used drug to treat agitated patients. The growing spread of the term "antipsychotics" instead of "tranquillizers" reflects the acknowledgement of their effects on the disease *underlying* the disturbed behaviour (King & Voruganti, 2002). The focus on disease-specificity and the portraying of emergency sedation as part of a wider therapeutic process obscure the actual purpose of such medications—to rapidly calm the violent and aggressive patient—and the properties which make them effective chemical restraints (Allison & Moncrieff, 2014). On a conceptual level, chemical restraint is not synonymous with forced therapy or involuntary treatment: the latter terms are related to a specific diagnosis and wish to treat the underlying disease even without the patient's consent, while the former merely aims to manage a patient's behaviour, without having a broader therapeutic function (Negroni, 2017). Nevertheless, *the terminological distinction fails to solve the disagreement on whether medications administered in emergency situations to ameliorate agitation constitute treatment or a form of restraint.* Since antipsychotics require days to weeks to exhibit their positive effects on symptoms of psychosis, clinicians can make use of their side-effect profiles to achieve rapid sedation without immediately intervening on the underlying pathology (Currier, 2003). Such sedation—which can range from a reduction of agitation of a patient that remains at least partially responsive to complete unconsciousness—seems to be at the same time a wanted short-term outcome and a side-effect of the therapeutic treatment: we might call it a *deliberate collateral-effect* of the administration (see also Chap. 5, specifically the discussion concerning Excerpt 5.1).

At the extreme ends of the controversy around the "restraint *versus* treatment" nature of forced medication, we see two polarized positions. On the "treatment" side, psychotropic agents are said to be designed to promote sedation by decreasing anxiety, restoring moods, and improving cognitive abilities by restoring reality testing, so that they ultimately have to be considered a form of treatment (Crumley, 1990). On the side of "restraint", we find critical views such as that of the psychiatrist Thomas Szasz, who defined antipsychotics as chemical straitjackets, denying their function of therapeutic agents (Szasz, 1957). The controversy ultimately reflects the debate around the double mandate of psychiatry—cure and control—which characterizes other restraining measures as well: the therapeutic effects of manual restraint in restoring limits and pacifying the violent person (see the previous paragraph) and the beneficial effects of desensitization achieved through seclusion (see next paragraph).

Besides the lack of agreement on what (if anything) constitutes chemical restraint, the extent to which forced medication is used is difficult to determine, also because national data providing incidence rates do not exist (Currier, 2003). Available literature suggests that it is frequently used, also in combination with other measures such as mechanical or physical restraint which facilitate the non-consensual administration of drugs (Negroni, 2017). We know that in contemporary psychiatric practice, haloperidol is the psychotropic drug most often employed to manage aggression (Goedhard & Heerdink, 2017). Benzodiazepines, such as short-acting lorazepam and midazolam, are used as well because of their anxiolytic and sedative properties, alone or in combination with haloperidol (ibidem). Atypical antipsychotics such as olanzapine appear to be as effective as haloperidol, with the advantage of having a decreased risk of extrapyramidal side effects.[9] As to the mode of administration, current recommendations suggest considering oral or inhaled medication first, resorting to intramuscular injection if the patient refuses oral therapy or a faster onset is needed (ibidem).

In the following chapters, I will use the expression "chemical restraint" to refer to those administrations guided by a behavioural control purpose, while by "forced medication", I will refer to the intramuscular injection of drugs (either sedative or curative) which would have otherwise (i.e. with the collaboration of the patient) been administered on a voluntary basis as part of a long-term treatment programme. At times, during fieldwork, the distinction between the dual purpose of medication has been difficult for me to tell, either because both objectives—immediate tranquillization and long-term treatment—were pursued at the same time, blurring their boundaries, or because I was unfamiliar with the effects of each psychotropic drug. I asked mental healthcare professionals for clarification every time I have not been able to understand the underlying logic of their pharmacological choices, and the topic has been directly addressed in individual interviews to engage them in a specific reflection (see again, for example, Excerpt 6.1 in Chap. 6).

2.3.4 Locked Versus Open-Door Wards: Environmental Restraint

Seclusion entails the temporary removal of an individual, without his/her consent, to a locked environment which s/he is not permitted to leave. This measure differs from mechanical restraint (which does not remove all social contact from the patient), time out (temporary isolation which the patient agrees with), and so-called open seclusion (the door is left open, but the patient is not free to leave) (Alty & Mason, 1994).

[9] These include acute dyskinesia (uncontrolled, involuntary movements), tardive dyskinesia (with a delayed onset after prolonged use of antipsychotics, sometimes permanent), Parkinsonism (tremor, bradykinesia, rigidity, and postural instability), akinesia (loss of ability to move muscles voluntarily), akathisia (feeling of physical restlessness), and neuroleptic malignant syndrome (a life-threatening reaction to antipsychotic drugs characterized by fever, altered mental status, muscle rigidity, and autonomic dysfunction, resulting in labile blood pressure, tachypnea, tachycardia, sialorrhea, diaphoresis, skin pallor, and incontinence).

Historically, the primary example of a similar procedure comes from the second century A.D., when in a paper entitled *Madness or Insanity* the Greek physician Soranus of Ephesus described how to calm down a mentally ill patient by placing him in a quiet room and restrain him by massaging his limbs in order to not upset him (Hodgkinson, 1985). The description seems to refer to a form of smooth manual restraint, implying that the patient is not left alone, as opposed to today's practice of seclusion.

In the nineteenth century, in England, seclusion and restraint were attempted to be separated—the former being considered a humane alternative to the latter—by John Conolly, who introduced padded-rooms, with floor and walls covered in soft material and without any furniture but pillows (see Paragraph 2.4.1). The psychiatrist argued for its therapeutic effect due to the desensitized environment, attempting to frame seclusion as a form of treatment as well as of control.

Seclusion was regulated for the first time in 1890 by the Lunacy Act, imposed under public pressure to establish legal control over psychiatric admissions of private patients (Takabayashi, 2017). The new legislation introduced a registry called "Medical Journal" to be kept by the superintendent of the asylum, in which at least once a week there should be recorded the number of patients of each sex, those under seclusion or restraint, deaths, injuries and episodes of violence to patients since the last entry; for both seclusion and restraint, reasons and period had to be stated, as well as means by which restraint was applied (Lunacy Act, Section 31, 1890).

English legislation in the post-war years increasingly registered a recognition of the rights of the insane, first in the Mental Health Act of 1959, then in the one of 1983. During the 1980s, the number of journal articles about seclusion denotes increased public awareness internationally, also due to the lawsuits brought by patients who had been secluded or restrained. A relevant example from the USA is the Boston State case (1979), whose legal debate centred around whether a patient has the right to refuse medication (including seclusion) in non-emergency situations: the Federal Judge recognized this right and deemed forced medication on a secluded patient inacceptable since the refusal to take medication would not have precipitated an emergency of an already restrained patient (Alty & Mason, 1994). In the UK, several inquiry reports of those years were concerned with seclusion, investigating the death of secluded patients (Prins et al., 1993), or allegations of physical and sexual abuse on patients while in seclusion (Blom-Cooper et al., 1992). In the former case, the Committee of Inquiry did not call for the abolition of seclusion but recommended a specific procedure for its practice and the suitability of the seclusion room. In the latter case, the Committee defined the seclusion unnecessary and recommended its "phasing-out and ultimate ending"; the use of seclusion was then reviewed by the Special Hospitals Service Authority, which considered alternative practices, but concluded that seclusion could not be completely eradicated at that time (Exworthy et al., 2001).

Today's mental healthcare in the UK is regulated by the Mental Health Act of 1983. The Code of Practice last reviewed in 2015 established the criteria seclusion rooms have to meet—such as reinforced windows to provide natural light, furniture limited to bed, pillow, mattress and blanket, and a clock visible to the secluded patient to avoid disorientation—and set the least restrictive option as one of its guiding principles. Nevertheless, monitoring conducted by a Care Quality Commission reported patients spending hundreds of days in seclusion (the longest one being twenty-three months) and found that some hospital seclusion facilities were unfit for seclusion (CQC, 2015, 2016).[10]

Literature on the contemporary use of seclusion in the UK shows that the measure is usually initiated in the case of aggression (physical or verbal, self-directed and hetero-directed), exacerbation of psychiatric symptoms (delusions, confusion, disturbed behaviour), absconding and medication refusal (Bowers et al., 2017). The same study also revealed a process of substitution: hospitals without a seclusion room (one-quarter of UK acute psychiatric hospitals) managed disturbed behaviour through heightened adoption of other techniques, such as coerced intramuscular

[10] "Examples of poor practice include: a lack of respect for the privacy and dignity of patients in seclusion; inadequate furnishing (so that patients are kept in a bare room with only a mattress or blankets for comfort); little or no access to toilets; inadequate clothing for patients; and patients being disturbed by staff playing a radio or talking loudly in the observation area. Other problems include rooms either always being too hot (which may be a particular problem if the room has padding on walls) or too cold; or that are dirty (in some cases made dirty by a previous patient and not cleaned properly between uses)" (CQC, 2016, p. 1).

medication, constant observation in a separate room, PRN medication,[11] and calls to the police, as well as seclusion in rooms not dedicated for that purpose and therefore at risk of harming.

Moving from the Anglo-Saxon (where seclusion was more regulated and debated) to the international scene, literature about seclusion has addressed a number of related issues. First of all, the impact of seclusion on those who have personally experienced it is associated with feelings of sadness, fear, abandonment (Holmes et al., 2004), trauma (Frueh et al., 2005), and punishment (Meehan et al., 2000). The nurse-patient relationship has been found exposed to negative effects of seclusion, due to a perceived loss of autonomy and trust, as well as feelings of isolation, reported by people subjected to such a measure (Hoekstra et al., 2004). Nurses' attitudes towards seclusion entail a belief in its beneficial outcomes (Meehan et al., 2000); nonetheless, it is considered ethically problematic, thus constituting an element of distress (Lind et al., 2004). The latter issue is explored in a recent Norwegian study (Haugom et al., 2019) addressing the relationship between treatment and control during seclusion, which produces ethical challenges for the mental healthcare staff. These were related to the negative feelings expressed by secluded patients, to the use of seclusion in conjunction with mechanical restraints, and to the seclusion of voluntarily admitted patients treated as involuntary ones. The study also highlights the burdensome work performed by the staff to balance patients' best interests and those of other people in the ward and to control violent behaviour in their daily working life.

A framework which draws together the major theoretical constructs of seclusion has been advanced by Thomas Mason (1994), who identifies three basic rationales for the adoption of this measure: therapeutic intervention, containment, and punishment. Mason's framework specifies each rationale's component dimensions, ordered along a benevolent-malevolent continuum (e.g. from paternalism to revenge/sadism). The three rationales identified by Mason seem to represent the red thread

[11] PRN medication is an abbreviation for the Latin *Pro re nata*, indicating prescribed medication which is not administered according to a schedule, but according to the patient or mental health worker only if needed.

connecting all of the coercive measures, whose "therapeutic *versus* controlling" purpose is debated: this was the case for manual restraint (see Paragraph 2.3.2) and antipsychotic medications (see Paragraph 2.3.3).

Besides seclusion, environmental restraint is also performed through the locking of acute wards' doors. Locked wards, from which the inpatients cannot leave without the permission of the staff, can be considered a form of environmental restraint in that they impede individuals' free movement outside of the unit. Acute psychiatric treatment is usually performed in locked wards, regardless of the legal status of those admitted to them (Hochstrasser et al., 2018). Frequency and reasons for locking ward doors have been investigated to a limited extent only (Haglund & von Essen, 2005). A literature review conducted in 2009 (Van Der Merwe et al., 2009) found only eleven empirical studies on this topic. Door locking of psychiatric wards has returned to be increasingly common in the UK after decades—specifically the 1960s and 1970s—of door opening (Bowers et al., 2010). A Swedish study (Haglund et al., 2007) revealed that 73% of Swedish psychiatric inpatient wards were locked, 81% of which were not caring for involuntarily admitted patients, even though the Swedish mental health laws do not state that wards hosting committed patients have to be locked. Similarly, a small correlation between involuntary admission and treatment in a locked ward was found in a census investigation of five European countries (Rittmannsberger et al., 2004). In Italy, a study conducted in 2004 by the Italian National Institute of Health on a sample of Italian psychiatric wards showed that almost 80% of them keep their doors locked permanently (Dell'Acqua et al., 2007).

The prevalence of locked wards, let alone their spread registered in the UK and possibly elsewhere, may reflect the increased focus on risk assessment and management, which encourage defensive instead of defensible psychiatric practices (Ashmore, 2008; Simpson et al., 2003) as a form of protection against organizational blame (Crowe & Carlyle, 2003). This has been noticed on the field, in the restraint context, where doors are now permanently locked and permissions for inpatients to temporarily exit the ward with a nurse—once frequent—have been increasingly reduced to avoid risk and legal responsibilities in case of adverse events. Moreover, door locking reflects the putative correlation between mental disease and risk of violence, even though diagnosis is not a sufficiently good predictor for aggressive behaviour, which in turn might be aggravated by restrictions (Schneeberger et al., 2017). In fact, the main rationale for locking psychiatric wards is safety: closed doors allow to regulate patients and other persons' possibility to leave and enter the ward, so that the practice can be seen as protecting both the patients from the community outside and the community from the patients (Haglund et al., 2007). Arguments for locked doors include prevention of absconding, reducing access of unwanted individuals and illegal substances, increasing the time that staff can spend in therapeutic activity instead of door-guarding, avoiding the stigma of being returned to the ward by the police, and reassuring relatives of vulnerable patients (Rae, 2006). On the other hand, arguments against locked doors include the creation of a custodial rather than therapeutic ambience, feelings of powerlessness and dependency, increased frustration and aggression, risk of staff not engaging with patients, workload resulting from controlling entry and egress, and indiscriminate adoption of a restricted measure for all of the patients, even those who are less seriously ill (ibidem). During my research, many of these arguments have been encountered. In the no-restraint context, the open-door policy was sustained by referring to decreased tension in the ward, and to the fact that healthcare workers should not be in charge of a custodial function (see Chap. 5.2 about the strategic segregation of care and coercion and their attribution to different actors). Moreover, the activity of surveilling the entrance was generally portrayed as an occasion to actively engage with patients in the common spaces of the ward (e.g. the hall). Nevertheless, in cases of elevated workload or risks, doors have been temporarily closed, and the introduction of the open-door policy raised some perplexities (see Chap. 5.1.2), denoting it as a topic which is not free from controversies and open discussion in specific situations.

Research suggests a possible reduction in involuntary measures associated with the introduction of an open-door policy. Data collected in 21 German hospitals from 1998 to 2012 reveal that aggression, restraint, and seclusion are less frequent in open wards, possibly because of a therapeutic approach focused on relationships rather than patient coercion and control (Schneeberger et al., 2017). A six-year, hospital-wide study in Basel registered a continuous reduction, even though in small numbers, of seclusion (from 8.2 to 3.5%) and forced medication (from 2.4 to 1.2%) after the implementation of an open-door policy (Hochstrasser et al., 2018). Absconding, defined as leaving the ward against medical advice, was found to be reduced in an evaluation study concerning the introduction of an open-door policy in an acute psychiatric ward in Berlin (Lang et al., 2010).

Locking policies seems to vary between countries, hospital and wards, being mainly based on local traditions (Huber et al., 2016). Pollmächer and Steinert (2016) drew attention to the variety of practices which are likely to lie on the continuum between always locked and always open wards, implying that strategies of temporary opening (or closing) are in place and should be investigated. In the no-restraint context included in this study, the hospital ward where fieldwork was conducted lay between the two extremes: after a period of introduction of the policy for a few hours a day, doors are currently open twelve hours a day (from eight to twenty) and locked at night. The same is true for the Community Mental Health Centres considered. In the restraint context, doors of the ward were permanently locked.

References

Algostino, A. (2020). Per una interpretazione costituzionalmente orientata della contenzione meccanica. In M. Cardano, A. Algostino, M. Caredda, L. Gariglio, & C. Pardini (Eds.), *La contenzione del paziente psichiatrico. Un'indagine sociologica e giuridica*. Laboratorio dei Diritti Fondamentali. il Mulino.

Allison, L., & Moncrieff, J. (2014). 'Rapid tranquillisation': An historical perspective on its emergence in the context of the development of antipsychotic medications. *History of Psychiatry, 25*(1), 57–69.

Alty, A., & Mason, T. (1994). *Seclusion and mental health: A break with the past*. Springer.

Ashmore, R. (2008). Nurses' accounts of locked ward doors: Ghosts of the asylum or acute care in the 21st century? *Journal of psychiatric and mental health nursing, 15*(3), 175–185.

Babini, V. (2011). Curare la mente. Dall'universo manicomiale al "paese di Basaglia". In C. Pogliano & F. Cassata (Eds.), *Scienze e cultura dell'Italia unita*. Einaudi.

Beghi, M., Peroni, F., Gabola, P., Rossetti, A., & Cornaggia, C. M. (2013). Prevalence and risk factors for the use of restraint in psychiatry: A systematic review. *Rivista di Psichiatria, 48*(1), 10–22.

Betti, M. (1989). Italia e U.S.A. Legislazione psichiatrica a confronto. In G. C. Davison & J. M. Neale (Eds.), *Psicologia Clinica*. Zanichelli.

Blom-Cooper, L., Brown, M., Dolan, R., & Murphy, E. (1992). *Report of the committee of inquiry into complaints about Ashworth Hospital, 1, Cm 2028-1*. HMSO.

Bonner, G., Lowe, T., Rawcliffe, D., & Wellman, N. (2002). Trauma for all: A pilot study of the subjective experience of physical restraint for mental health inpatients and staff in the UK. *Journal of Psychiatric and Mental Health Nursing, 9*(4), 465–473.

Bowers, L., Alexander, J., Simpson, A., Ryan, C., & Carr-Walker, P. (2004). Cultures of psychiatry and the professional socialization process: The case of containment methods for disturbed patients. *Nurse Education Today, 24*(6), 435–442.

Bowers, L., Cullen, A. E., Achilla, E., Baker, J., Khondoker, M., Koeser, L., et al. (2017). *Seclusion and Psychiatric Intensive Care Evaluation Study (SPICES): Combined qualitative and quantitative approaches to the uses and outcomes of coercive practices in mental health services*. NIHR Journals Library.

Bowers, L., Haglund, K., Muir-Cochrane, E., Nijman, H., Simpson, A., & Van Der Merwe, M. (2010). Locked doors: A survey of patients, staff and visitors. *Journal of Psychiatric and Mental Health Nursing, 17*(10), 873–880.

Bowers, L., Van Der Merwe, M., Paterson, B., & Stewart, D. (2012). Manual restraint and shows of force: The City-128 study. *International Journal of Mental Health Nursing, 21*(1), 30–40.

Brodwin, P., & Velpry, L. (2014). The practice of constraint in psychiatry: Emergent forms of care and control. *Culture, Medicine, and Psychiatry, 4*(38), 524–526.

CNB – Comitato Nazionale di Bioetica. (1999). *Treatment of Psychiatric Patients: Bioethical Problems. The National Bioethics Committee's Statement concern-*

ing the Council of Europe White Paper on the treatment of psychiatric patients. English document. Retrieved November 26, 2022, from http://bioetica.governo.it/en/opinions/opinions-responses/icb-opinion-on-the-council-of-europe-white-paper-on-the-treatment-of-mentally-ill-patients/

CNB – Comitato Nazionale di Bioetica. (2000). *Psychiatry and mental health: Bioethical guidelines outline and recommendations.* English document. Retrieved November 26, 2022, from http://bioetica.governo.it/media/3361/p46_2000_psychiatry-and-mental-health_en.pdf

CNB – Comitato Nazionale di Bioetica. (2015). *La contenzione: problemi bioetici.* English document. Retrieved November 26, 2022, from http://bioetica.governo.it/media/3534/p120_2015_medical-restraint_en.pdf

Codice Deontologico delle Professioni Infermieristiche. (2019). Italian document. Retrieved November 26, 2022, from https://www.fnopi.it/archivio_news/attualita/2688/codice%20deontologico_2019.pdf

Conolly, J. (1856). *The treatment of the insane without mechanical restraints.* Dawsons of Pall Mall.

CQC. (2015). Mental Health Act 1983 monitoring visit. Nominated Individual: North Region. Visit date: 1 December 2015. Visit reference: 35303.

CQC. (2016). Brief guide: Seclusion rooms. Direct link. Retrieved November 26, 2022, from https://www.cqc.org.uk/sites/default/files/Brief_guide_Seclusion_Rooms.pdf

Crowe, M., & Carlyle, D. (2003). Deconstructing risk assessment and management in mental health nursing. *Journal of Advanced Nursing, 43*(1), 19–27.

Crumley, F. E. (1990). Chemical restraint? (Letter). *American Academy of Child and Adolescent Psychiatry, 29*, 982–983.

Currier, G. W. (2003). The controversy over "chemical restraint" in acute care psychiatry. *Journal of Psychiatric Practice, 9*(1), 59–70.

de Stefano, A., & Ducci, G. (2008). Involuntary admission and compulsory treatment in Europe: An overview. *International Journal of Mental Health, 37*(3), 10–21.

Del Giudice, G. (2015). *…E tu slegalo subito: sulla contenzione in psichiatria.* Collana 180, Alpha beta.

Dell'Acqua, G., Norcio, B., de Girolamo, G., Barbato, A., Bracco, R., Gaddini, A., Miglio, R., Morosini, P., Picardi, A., Rossi, E., Rucci, P., & Santone, G. (2007). Caratteristiche e attività delle strutture di ricovero per pazienti psichiatrici acuti: i risultati dell'indagine nazionale "Progress Acuti". *Giornale Italiano di Psicopatologia, 13*, 26–39.

Donnelly, M. (1992). *The politics of mental health in Italy*. Routledge.
Evans, D., & FitzGerald, M. (2002). Reasons for physically restraining patients and residents: A systematic review and content analysis. *International Journal of Nursing Studies, 39*(7), 735–743.
Exworthy, T., Mohan, D., Hindley, N., & Basson, J. (2001). Seclusion: Punitive or protective? *Journal of Forensic Psychiatry, 12*(2), 423–433.
Fann, W. E., & Linton, P. H. (1972). Use of perphenazine in psychiatric emergencies: The concept of chemical restraint. *Current Therapeutic Research, Clinical and Experimental, 14*(8), 478–482.
Ferioli, V. (2013). Contenzione: aspetti clinici, giuridici e psico-dinamici. *Psichiatria e Psicoterapia, 32*(1), 29–44.
Foot, J. (2015). *The man who closed the asylums: Franco Basaglia and the revolution in mental health care*. Verso Books.
Foucault, M. (2006a). *History of madness*. Routledge.
Foucault, M. (2006b). *Psychiatric power: Lectures at the Collège de France, 1973–1974*. Palgrave Macmillan.
Frueh, B. C., Knapp, R. G., Cusack, K. J., Grubaugh, A. L., Sauvageot, J. A., Cousins, V. C., et al. (2005). Special section on seclusion and restraint: Patients' reports of traumatic or harmful experiences within the psychiatric setting. *Psychiatric Services, 56*(9), 1123–1133.
Gansel, Y., & Lézé, S. (2015). Physical constraint as psychological holding: Mental-health treatment for difficult and violent adolescents in France. *Social Science & Medicine, 143*, 329–335.
Gieryn, T. F. (1983). Boundary-work and the demarcation of science from non-science: Strains and interests in professional ideologies of scientists. *American Sociological Review, 48*, 781–795.
Glaser, B. G., & Strauss, A. L. (1965). *Awareness of dying*. Aldine.
Goedhard, L. E., & Heerdink, E. R. (2017). Pharmacological management of aggressive behavior in psychiatric patients. *The Wiley Handbook of Violence and Aggression*, 1–15.
Goethals, S., Dierckx de Casterlé, B., & Gastmans, C. (2012). Nurses' decision-making in cases of physical restraint: A synthesis of qualitative evidence. *Journal of Advanced Nursing, 68*(6), 1198–1210.
Haglund, K., Van Der Meiden, E., von Knorring, L., & von Essen, L. (2007). Psychiatric care behind locked doors. A study regarding the frequency of and the reasons for locked psychiatric wards in Sweden. *Journal of Psychiatric and Mental Health Nursing, 14*(1), 49–54.

Haglund, K., & von Essen, L. (2005). Locked entrance doors at psychiatric wards – Advantages and disadvantages according to voluntarily admitted patients. *Nordic Journal of Psychiatry, 59*(6), 511–515.

Hanji, M. B. (2017). *Meta-analysis in psychiatry research: fundamental and advanced methods*. Apple Academic Press.

Hatling, T., Douzenis, A., & Maguire, J. (2006). Diversity and consistency in the legal management of involuntary admission and treatment across Europe. In D. Richter & R. Whittington (Eds.), *Violence in mental health settings* (pp. 95–109). Springer.

Haugom, E. W., Ruud, T., & Hynnekleiv, T. (2019). Ethical challenges of seclusion in psychiatric inpatient wards: A qualitative study of the experiences of Norwegian mental health professionals. *BMC Health Services Research, 19*(1), 879.

Healy, D. (2000). Some continuities and discontinuities in the pharmacotherapy of nervous conditions before and after chlorpromazine and imipramine. *History of Psychiatry, 11*(44), 393–412.

Hochstrasser, L., Fröhlich, D., Schneeberger, A. R., Borgwardt, S., Lang, U. E., Stieglitz, R. D., & Huber, C. G. (2018). Long-term reduction of seclusion and forced medication on a hospital-wide level: Implementation of an open-door policy over 6 years. *European Psychiatry, 48*(1), 51–57.

Hodgkinson, P. (1985). The use of seclusion. *Medicine, Science and the Law, 25*(3), 215–222.

Hoekstra, T., Lendemeijer, H. H. G. M., & Jansen, M. G. M. J. (2004). Seclusion: The inside story. *Journal of Psychiatric and Mental Health Nursing, 11*(3), 276–283.

Hoge, S. K., Lidz, C. W., Eisenberg, M., Gardner, W., Monahan, J., Mulvey, E., et al. (1997). Perceptions of coercion in the admission of voluntary and involuntary psychiatric patients. *International Journal of Law and Psychiatry, 20*(2), 167–181.

Holmes, D., Kennedy, S. L., & Perron, A. (2004). The mentally ill and social exclusion: A critical examination of the use of seclusion from the patient's perspective. *Issues in Mental Health Nursing, 25*(6), 559–578.

Hotzy, F., & Jaeger, M. (2016). Clinical relevance of informal coercion in psychiatric treatment – A systematic review. *Frontiers in Psychiatry, 7*, 197.

Huber, C. G., Schneeberger, A. R., Kowalinski, E., Fröhlich, D., von Felten, S., Walter, M., et al. (2016). Suicide risk and absconding in psychiatric hospitals with and without open door policies: A 15 year, observational study. *The Lancet Psychiatry, 3*(9), 842–849.

Iversen, K. I., Høyer, G., Sexton, H., & Grønli, O. K. (2002). Perceived coercion among patients admitted to acute wards in Norway. *Nordic Journal of Psychiatry, 56*(6), 433–439.

Jaeger, M., Ketteler, D., Rabenschlag, F., & Theodoridou, A. (2014). Informal coercion in acute inpatient setting – Knowledge and attitudes held by mental health professionals. *Psychiatry Research, 220*(3), 1007–1011.

Johansson, I. M., & Lundman, B. (2002). Patients' experience of involuntary psychiatric care: Good opportunities and great losses. *Journal of Psychiatric and Mental Health Nursing, 9*(6), 639–647.

Kalisova, L., Raboch, J., Nawka, A., Sampogna, G., Cihal, L., Kallert, T. W., et al. (2014). Do patient and ward-related characteristics influence the use of coercive measures? Results from the EUNOMIA international study. *Social Psychiatry and Psychiatric Epidemiology, 49*(10), 1619–1629.

Kallert, T. W., Glöckner, M., Onchev, G., Raboch, J., Karastergiou, A., Solomon, Z., et al. (2005). The EUNOMIA project on coercion in psychiatry: Study design and preliminary data. *World Psychiatry, 4*(3), 168–172.

Kallert, T. W., Katsakou, C., Adamowski, T., Dembinskas, A., Fiorillo, A., Kjellin, L., et al. (2011). Coerced hospital admission and symptom change – A prospective observational multi-centre study. *PloS one, 6*(11), e28191.

Kaltiala-Heino, R., Korkeila, J., Tuohimäki, C., Tuori, T., & Lehtinen, V. (2000). Coercion and restrictions in psychiatric inpatient treatment. *European Psychiatry, 15*(3), 213–219.

Kersting, X. A. K., Hirsch, S., & Steinert, T. (2019). Physical harm and death in the context of coercive measures in psychiatric patients: A systematic review. *Frontiers in Psychiatry, 10*, 400.

King, C., & Voruganti, L. N. (2002). What's in a name? The evolution of the nomenclature of antipsychotic drugs. *Journal of Psychiatry and Neuroscience, 27*(3), 168–175.

Kontio, R., Välimäki, M., Putkonen, H., Kuosmanen, L., Scott, A., & Joffe, G. (2010). Patient restrictions: Are there ethical alternatives to seclusion and restraint? *Nursing Ethics, 17*(1), 65–76.

Lang, U. E., Hartmann, S., Schulz-Hartmann, S., Gudlowski, Y., Ricken, R., Munk, I., et al. (2010). Do locked doors in psychiatric hospitals prevent patients from absconding? *The European Journal of Psychiatry, 24*(4), 199–204.

Lidz, C. W., Mulvey, E. P., Hoge, S. K., Kirsch, B. L., Monahan, J., Eisenberg, M., et al. (1998). Factual sources of psychiatric patients' perceptions of coercion in the hospital admission process. *American Journal of Psychiatry, 155*(9), 1254–1260.

Lincoln, A. (2006). Psychiatric emergency room decision-making, social control and the 'undeserving sick'. *Sociology of Health & Illness, 28*(1), 54–75.

Lind, M., Kaltiala-Heino, R., Suominen, T., Leino-Kilpi, H., & Valimaki, M. (2004). Nurses' ethical perceptions about coercion. *Journal of Psychiatric and Mental Health Nursing, 11*(4), 379–385.

Mason, T. (1994). Seclusion: An international comparison. *Medicine, Science and the Law, 34*(1), 54–60.

Mauceri, S. (Ed.). (2017). "Contenere" la contenzione meccanica in Italia. Primo rapporto sui diritti negati dalla pratica di legare coercitivamente i pazienti psichiatrici nei SPDC. *A Buon Diritto – Quaderni.*

Meehan, T., Vermeer, C., & Windsor, C. (2000). Patients' perceptions of seclusion: A qualitative investigation. *Journal of Advanced Nursing, 31*(2), 370–377.

Menegatto, M., & Zamperini, A. (2018). *Coercizione e disagio psichico. La contenzione tra dignità e sicurezza.* Il Pensiero Scientifico Editore.

Meyer-Gross, W., Slater, E., & Roth, M. (1954). *Clinical Psychiatry.* Cassell and Company Ltd.

Ministry of Health. (2021a). *Rapporto sulla Salute Mentale. Analisi dei dati del Sistema Informativo per la Salute Mentale (SISM), Anno 2019.* Italian document. Retrieved November 26, 2022, from https://www.salute.gov.it/imgs/C_17_pubblicazioni_3081_allegato.pdf

Ministry of Health. (2021b). *Rapporto sulla Salute Mentale. Analisi dei dati del Sistema Informativo per la Salute Mentale (SISM), Anno 2020.* Italian document. Retrieved November 26, 2022, from https://www.salute.gov.it/imgs/C_17_pubblicazioni_3212_allegato.pdf

Muir-Cochrane, E., O'Kane, D., & Oster, C. (2018). Fear and blame in mental health nurses' accounts of restrictive practices: Implications for the elimination of seclusion and restraint. *International Journal of Mental Health Nursing, 27*(5), 1511–1521.

Negroni, A. A. (2017). On the concept of restraint in psychiatry. *The European Journal of Psychiatry, 31*(3), 99–104.

NICE (National Institute for Health and Clinical Excellence). (2005). *Violence. The short term management of disturbed/violent behaviour in in-patient psychiatric settings and emergency departments.*

O'Brien, A. J., & Golding, C. G. (2003). Coercion in mental healthcare: The principle of least coercive care. *Journal of Psychiatric and Mental Health Nursing, 10*(2), 167–173.

O'Donoghue, B., Roche, E., Shannon, S., Lyne, J., Madigan, K., & Feeney, L. (2014). Perceived coercion in voluntary hospital admission. *Psychiatry Research, 215*(1), 120–126.

Olofsson, B., & Jacobsson, L. (2001). A plea for respect: Involuntarily hospitalized psychiatric patients' narratives about being subjected to coercion. *Journal of Psychiatric and Mental Health Nursing, 8*(4), 357–366.

Olsen, D. P. (2003). Influence and coercion: Relational and rights-based ethical approaches to forced psychiatric treatment. *Journal of Psychiatric and Mental Health Nursing, 10*(6), 705–712.

Oster, C., Gerace, A., Thomson, D., & Muir-Cochrane, E. (2016). Seclusion and restraint use in adult inpatient mental health care: An Australian perspective. *Collegian, 23*(2), 183–190.

Perkins, E., Prosser, H., Riley, D., & Whittington, R. (2012). Physical restraint in a therapeutic setting; A necessary evil? *International Journal of Law and Psychiatry, 35*(1), 43–49.

Piccinelli, M. P., Bortolaso, P., & Wilkinson, G. D. (2022). Rethinking hospital psychiatry in Italy in light of COVID-19 experience. *World Journal of Virology, 11*(1), 73.

Pinel, P. (1806). Treatise on mental alienation. In Goshen, C. E. (1967). *Documentary history of psychiatry* (pp. 257–265). Vision Press.

Pollmächer, T., & Steinert, T. (2016). Arbitrary classification of hospital policy regarding open and locked doors. *Lancet Psychiatry, 3*(12), 1103.

Prins, H., Backer-Holst, T., Francis, E., & Keitch, I. (1993). *Report of the committee of inquiry into the death in Broadmoor Hospital of Orville Blackwood and a review of the deaths of two other Afro-Caribbean patients: 'Big, Black and Dangerous?'*. Special Hospitals Service Authority.

Raboch, J., Kališová, L., Kallert, T., et al. (2007). Comparison of the clinical use of individual coercive measures during hospitalization across the EUNOMIA study sites. *BMC Psychiatry, 7*, S31.

Raboch, J., Kališová, L., Nawka, A., Kitzlerová, E., Onchev, G., Karastergiou, A., et al. (2010). Use of coercive measures during involuntary hospitalization: Findings from ten European countries. *Psychiatric Services, 61*(10), 1012–1017.

Rae, M. (2006). Improving safety: Key dilemmas. *The Mental Health Review, 11*(3), 23–26.

Reed, S. C., & Lewis, D. A. (1990). The negotiation of voluntary admission in Chicago's state mental hospitals. *The Journal of Psychiatry & Law, 18*(1–2), 137–163.

Richter, D., & Whittington, R. (2006). *Violence in mental health settings*. Springer.
Rittmannsberger, H., Sartorius, N., Brad, M., Burtea, V., Capraru, N., Cernak, P., et al. (2004). Changing aspects of psychiatric inpatient treatment. *European Psychiatry, 19*(8), 483–488.
Rossero, E. (2022). Covid-19 e sofferenza psichica: reinventare la cura nel contesto pandemico. In A. Maturo & M. Gibin (Eds.), *Malati Sospesi. I pazienti cronici nell'era Covid* (pp. 168–188). FrancoAngeli.
Rossi, S., & Toresini, L. (2015). SPDC aperti e senza contenzioni per i diritti inviolabili della persona, in Rossi S., a cura di, *Il nodo della contenzione: diritto, psichiatria e dignità della persona*, Merano: Edizioni alpha beta Verlag.
Saget, E. (2009). Autisme: le traitement qui choque. L'Express. Retrieved November 26, 2022, from http://www.lexpress.fr/actualite/societe/sante/autisme-le-traitement-qui-choque_768175.html
Salize, H. J., & Dressing, H. (2004). Epidemiology of involuntary placement of mentally ill people across the European Union. *The British Journal of Psychiatry, 184*(2), 163–168.
Sashidharan, S. P., Mezzina, R., & Puras, D. (2019). Reducing coercion in mental healthcare. *Epidemiology and Psychiatric Sciences, 28*(6), 605–612.
Saya, A., Brugnoli, C., Piazzi, G., Liberato, D., Di Ciaccia, G., Niolu, C., & Siracusano, A. (2019). Criteria, procedures, and future prospects of involuntary treatment in psychiatry around the world: A narrative review. *Frontiers in Psychiatry, 10*.
Schneeberger, A. R., Kowalinski, E., Fröhlich, D., Schröder, K., von Felten, S., Zinkler, M., et al. (2017). Aggression and violence in psychiatric hospitals with and without open door policies: A 15-year naturalistic observational study. *Journal of Psychiatric Research, 95*, 189–195.
Shorter, E. (1997). *A history of psychiatry: From the Era of the Asylum to the Age of Prozac*. John Wiley & Sons, Inc.
Simpson, A., Miller, C., & Bowers, L. (2003). The history of the Care Programme Approach in England: Where did it go wrong? *Journal of Mental Health, 12*(5), 489–504.
Sjöström, S. (2006). Invocation of coercion context in compliance communication – Power dynamics in psychiatric care. *International Journal of Law and Psychiatry, 29*(1), 36–47.
Sjöström, S. (2016). Coercion contexts: How compliance is achieved in interaction. In A. Molodynski, J. Rugkåsa, & T. Burns (Eds.), *Coercion in community mental health care: International perspectives* (pp. 131–142). Oxford University Press.

Steinert, T., Lepping, P., Bernhardsgrütter, R., Conca, A., Hatling, T., Janssen, W., et al. (2010). Incidence of seclusion and restraint in psychiatric hospitals: A literature review and survey of international trends. *Social Psychiatry and Psychiatric Epidemiology, 45*(9), 889–897.

Steinert, T., Noorthoorn, E. O., & Mulder, C. L. (2014). The use of coercive interventions in mental health care in Germany and the Netherlands. A comparison of the developments in two neighboring countries. *Frontiers in Public Health, 2*, 141.

Stewart, D., Bowers, L., Simpson, A., Ryan, C., & Tziggili, M. (2009). Manual restraint of adult psychiatric inpatients: A literature review. *Journal of Psychiatric and Mental Health Nursing, 16*(8), 749–757.

Szasz, T. S. (1957). Some observations on the use of tranquilizing drugs. *AMA Archives of Neurology & Psychiatry, 77*(1), 86–92.

Szmukler, G. (2015). Compulsion and "coercion" in mental health care. *World Psychiatry, 14*(3), 259–261.

Szmukler, G. (2017). *Men in white coats: Treatment under coercion*. Oxford University Press.

Szmukler, G., & Appelbaum, P. (2001). Treatment pressures, coercion and compulsion. *Textbook of Community Psychiatry*, 529–544.

Szmukler, G., & Appelbaum, P. S. (2008). Treatment pressures, leverage, coercion, and compulsion in mental health care. *Journal of Mental Health, 17*(3), 233–244.

Takabayashi, A. (2017). Surviving the Lunacy Act of 1890: English psychiatrists and professional development during the early twentieth century. *Medical History, 61*(2), 246–269.

Tone, A. (2015). Mental-health care: Italy's psychiatric renaissance. *Nature, 524*, 290.

Van Der Merwe, M., Bowers, L., Jones, J., Simpson, A., & Haglund, K. (2009). Locked doors in acute inpatient psychiatry: A literature review. *Journal of Psychiatric and Mental Health Nursing, 16*(3), 293–299.

Vedana, K. G. G., da Silva, D. M., Ventura, C. A. A., Giacon, B. C. C., Zanetti, A. C. G., Miasso, A. I., & Borges, T. L. (2018). Physical and mechanical restraint in psychiatric units: Perceptions and experiences of nursing staff. *Archives of Psychiatric Nursing, 32*(3), 367–372.

Whittington, R., Baskind, E., & Paterson, B. (2006). Coercive measures in the management of imminent violence: Restraint, seclusion and enhanced observation. In D. Richter & R. Whittington (Eds.), *Violence in mental health settings* (pp. 145–172). Springer.

Wyder, M., Bland, R., & Crompton, D. (2013). Personal recovery and involuntary mental health admissions: The importance of control, relationships and hope. *Health, 5*, 574–581.
Zhang, S., Mellsop, G., Brink, J., & Wang, X. (2015). Involuntary admission and treatment of patients with mental disorder. *Neuroscience Bulletin, 31*(1), 99–112.

3

A Necessary Evil? Alternatives to Coercive Interventions

Abstract This chapter describes the ethical dilemmas concerning the use of coercive measures in mental healthcare settings, as well as clinical issues raised by the literature on this topic. Then, a historical overview of the attempts to reduce or eliminate coercion, at national and international levels, is provided.

Workplace violence in the entire healthcare sector has been recognized as a primary global problem,[1] which may affect more than half of healthcare workers and specifically nurses (Oud, 2006). Aggressive and violent behaviour in psychiatric settings—which is frequently indicated among the reasons for the use of coercive interventions—is a recurrent event concerning both carers and users and can be categorized as "verbal abuse", "threat", and "physical abuse" (McKenna, 2004). Aggressiveness, which concerns only a minority of people said to have mental disorder, cannot be explained only in terms of diagnostic categories, but it is rather a multi-dimensional phenomenon. Characteristics more frequently

[1] International Labour Office (ILO), International Council of Nurses (ICN), World Health Organization (WHO), and Public Services International (PSI). (2002). *Framework guidelines for addressing workplace violence in the health sector*. Geneva: International Labour Office.

E. Rossero, *Care in a Time of Crisis*, https://doi.org/10.1007/978-3-031-34418-3_3

associated with aggressiveness are clinical (severe diagnosis of schizophrenia or personality disorder, comorbid substance/alcohol abuse), sociodemographic (young age, unemployment, unmarried status), and setting-related (overcrowding, ward climate, staff characteristics and training) (Biancosino et al., 2009). Individual history of previous violent behaviour, as well as number and length of previous hospitalization, are strong predictors of future inpatient violence (Steinert, 2006). Moreover, Richard Whittington and Dirk Richter (2006) shed light on an overlooked aspect, that of interaction. Interpersonal violence happens between a patient and one or more staff members, whose actions are shaped by reciprocal expectations. When the other party does not fulfil the expected role—for example, a nurse treats a patient against his/her will while s/he was expected to be caring, or a patient does not follow nurses' prescriptions—distrust emerges and status asymmetries become evident, potentially leading to an escalation of the conflict and violence. The escalation curve which is usually used to represent progressively hostile behaviour from both parties can be misleading for it suggests a steady increase, whereas in real situations escalation can take from a few seconds to several hours (Richter, 2006). Other elements related to the social system of mental hospital wards, such as psychiatric leadership and authority and predictability of structured activities and schedules, have been found relevant in distinguishing "peaceful" from "violence-prone" wards (Katz & Kirkland, 1990).

The frequency of violent events in psychiatric settings led to the development of many tools to access risk of aggressiveness, both in the form of self-report questionnaires, designed to assess individual tendencies to react in a hostile manner, and aggression observation instruments, which can be incident- and/or period-based scales (Nijman et al., 2006). Nevertheless, risk assessment is an inexact science which ultimately relies on clinical judgement pronounced by a multidisciplinary team and has to take into consideration a number of clinical, environmental, social, and psychological variables (Rocca et al., 2006). As an obvious consequence, not every violent event can be predicted and prevented. Despite this inaccuracy, care in psychiatric settings is grounded in risk aversion, reflecting the conceptualization of people with mental illness as inherently posing risks to self and others (Crowe & Carlyle, 2003). The dominant safety discourse frames risk as pervasive and requiring immediate intervention at the cost of meaningful treatment, legitimizing and promoting ineffective as well as harmful practices (Slemon et al., 2017). An alternative safety culture should instead acknowledge the possibility of risk in the clinical setting and balance it with therapeutic engagement, framing safety as one component of care and not as its paramount aim (ibidem).

Coercive interventions often originate from behaviour that is considered actually or potentially dangerous, within hospital settings or in the community context. Physical techniques have been used by mental health staff to manage violent situations for decades, reinforced by training programmes with a self-defence orientation which teach physical techniques (mechanical/physical restraint, seclusion, martial arts), now generally combined with non-physical (e.g. verbal) ones (Richter, 2006). Their application raises dilemmas for mental healthcare workers, who are expected to provide a safe and, at the same time, therapeutic environment for inpatients while preserving their dignity. Psychiatrists in particular are asked to perform a balancing act between competing demands of society and the best interests of individual patients, which makes dilemma intrinsic to their professional role (Austin et al., 2008). Their double allegiance, Frederic Grunberg (2002) argues, led to dramatic consequences when societal demands persuaded them to abandon Hippocratic principles of beneficence and non-maleficence to patients, such as during mass extermination of the mentally ill in Nazi Germany, or forced hospitalization of political dissidents in the Soviet Union. Today, constraints of a different nature—legal, social, organizational, economic—place mental health professionals in ethically undesirable situations, exposing them to what philosopher Andrew Jameton termed moral distress (1984). Dilemmas do not only pertain to psychiatrists, who generally prescribe coercive interventions such as mechanical restraint, but also to those who usually perform them: nurses (Menegatto & Zamperini, 2018; Marangos-Frost & Wells, 2000). At the same time, nursing staff can represent an additional element of pressure and potential conflict for psychiatrists, sometimes asked to "do something" by means of coercive measures on troublesome patients (Olofsson et al., 1999). During fieldwork, for example, nursing staff has been observed asking for an increase in sedative therapy, consistently with their position of professional group most intensely involved in managing life on the ward (Strauss et al., 1981).

Criticism for the outcomes of coercive psychiatry and the legitimacy of its authoritarianism, expressed by anti-psychiatric movements as well as civil rights movements, gradually led to a shift towards a novel ethical approach, centred around the patient as a person with his/her values, beliefs, and rights to be respected (Abderhalden et al., 2006). These dimensions have been investigated by empirical research on individual accounts of people treated in psychiatric inpatient settings. A specific term, that of "sanctuary harm", was coined to refer to feelings of fear, humiliation, and distress related to abusive actions of the staff, including seclusion and restraint (Frueh et al., 2005). Phenomenological studies of people's experience of being restrained highlighted how, instead of feeling safe or relieved for having external limits to their out-of-control behaviour, they rather felt vulnerable, helpless, and worried about not being able to protect themselves (Johnson, 1998). Anxiety and anger have also been found to be related to witnessing restraint and seclusion, and to anticipating that they are going to take place, sometimes resulting in an escalation of the situation (Stewart et al., 2010). These psychological consequences of coercive interventions only add to the documented physical risks posed both to patients and staff. Mechanical restraint can result in injury (circulatory problems, fractures, bruises, physical deterioration, and consequent increase in falls) and even death (asphyxiation, acute pulmonary oedema, pulmonary embolism, cardiac arrest due to chest compression) (Mohr et al., 2003). This explains why close monitoring of the restrained person is necessary, and why bad practices can lead to tragic consequences (see the case of Mastrogiovanni discussed in the previous chapter). Adverse consequences can also occur for other coercive measures: "takedowns" to the ground of agitated patients can lead to a massive release of adrenal catecholamines that produce malignant cardiac rhythm disturbances (ibidem), while physical restraint is associated with asphyxia by thorax-compression, pneumomediastinum, and cardiac arrest (Kersting et al., 2019). Seclusion has been found to be related to intentional self-harm and suicide, but despite its widespread use, adverse events resulting from it are under-researched (ibidem). Both physical and psychological negative consequences of coercive interventions are not counter-balanced by evidence suggesting that these measures are clinically effective, improve patient safety, or provide better clinical or social outcomes (Chieze et al., 2019; Sashidharan et al., 2019).

Due to these ethical dilemmas as well as clinical issues raised by coercive interventions, their reduction or elimination has been underpinned by national and international initiatives. At the European level, the Working Party on Psychiatry and Human Rights directly addressed the issue stating in its White Paper that "the use of short periods of physical restraint and of seclusion should be in due proportion to the benefits and the risks entailed. Thorough training in techniques of physical restraint should be provided to staff. […] The response to violent behaviour by the patient should be graduated, i.e. staff should initially attempt to respond verbally; thereafter, only in so far as required, by means of manual restraint; and only in a last resort by mechanical restraint" (2000, p. 15).

In 2005, a European Union commission Green Paper proposed to establish an EU strategy on mental health to improve the quality of life of people with mental ill health through social inclusion and the protection of their rights and dignity (European Commission, 2005, p. 8). Difficulty of harmonization of legislation in Europe derives from highly heterogeneous local practices, attitudes, and service funding (Hatling et al., 2006). A survey on European countries legislation and practice of involuntary treatment concluded that national approaches and philosophies concerning the provision of mental healthcare strongly determine the legal framework and the practice of involuntary admission and treatment of mentally ill patients (Salize et al., 2002).

The effort to achieve a less coercive mental healthcare is not entirely new: the history of psychiatry has been characterized by many attempts to abolish coercion, none of which completely and convincingly succeeded in any period or country (Steinert et al., 2014). An international comparative literature study on seclusion seems to be on the same page as it concludes that, when non-coercive interventions fail to treat agitated or aggressive patients, there remain only four things one can do: seclude them, (forcibly) medicate them, restrain them, or transfer them (Mason, 1994, p. 59). Except for seclusion, which is not employed in Italy, all of the other solutions have been observed on the field, in the form of mechanical or other kinds of restraint, forced medication, and transfer (e.g. from community to hospital, or from the psychiatric ward to the Intensive Care Unit) or request for intervention of other agencies (e.g. public force; see Chap. 6 on outsourcing coercion).

In the next paragraph, I provide a historical reconstruction of the non-restraint movement and relative debates, which show difficulties and contradictions of eliminating coercion from psychiatric practice. Then, I describe contemporary alternatives to reduce restraining interventions adopted in different contexts, both in and outside of Italy.

3.1 The No-Restraint Movement: A Historical Overview

The first step towards a humanization of mental healthcare can probably be traced back to 1793, with the removal of chains from psychiatric patients ordered by Philippe Pinel at the Bicêtre Hospital (Abderhalden et al., 2006). This well-known act was not of total liberation, as chains were substituted with two kinds of straitjackets—one for restraining movement in a loose manner and another for punishment by tying arms behind the body and constricting the chest (Pinel & Snaith, 1995). Locking up of patients in darkened rooms was practised as well, for short periods of time, as a form of punishment (Pinel, 1806). Nevertheless, the event symbolizes a change in approach to the treatment of the insane and the beginning of psychiatry as a medical discipline (Steinert et al., 2010).

Moving from France to England a few years later, a house surgeon at Lincoln Lunatic Asylum, Robert Gardiner Hill, published *The Total Abolition of Personal Restraint in the Treatment of the Insane* (1839). The document defined a mode of asylum management which abstained from mechanical restraint, namely the confinement of patients' limbs by means of physical devices: leather straps, straitjackets, muffs, and hobbles (Topp, 2018). The no-restraint system had been successfully instituted at Lincoln Asylum for the previous sixteen months and was lately applied by John Conolly at Hanwell Asylum, in London, marking the birth of the so-called no-restraint movement. The new model received sceptical as well as hostile reactions. Of particular relevance for our purpose is the debate that originated around the topic of seclusion, which at first did not fall within the forms of restraint Hill aimed to abolish. Among his opponents, a rival physician at Lincoln Asylum, William Cookson, and his ally Samuel Hadwen claimed that the abolition of visible restraint had been followed by a hidden form of violence, worse than physical restraint itself. The physicians exemplify their position commenting the case of Miss A., a patient used to be restrained during her violent episodes and then isolated to her room after the introduction of the non-restraint system:

> Here is a difficult, and, under the present system, a wholly unmanageable case of insanity; the unhappy victim of which spends day after day, and night after night, in solitary confinement, in a small, ill-ventilated, ill-lighted, and oppressive apartment; a restraint known to be the most insupportable, and from which the most hardened criminals shrink with dread abhorrence, and, with its additional accompaniments in this instance, a species of restraint infinitely more calculated to convert the sane man into a lunatic, than to restore the lunatic to health. Secluded from the free light of heaven, from the pure air, the bracing exercise essential to health, what chance has this most unfortunate person of obtaining the deliverance from the calamity that made her an inmate of the asylum?

Doubts on the therapeutic effects of seclusion are expressed in the excerpt above (Hadwen in Topp, 2018, p. 759). Hill's successor as house surgeon at Lincoln Asylum, William Smith, moved towards the abolition of seclusion, and in 1841, announces the success of his experiment: isolation can be dispensed by increasing surveillance over attendants—who used to rely on seclusion instead of paying increased attention of problematic patients—and tolerating a degree of "lunatic violence"—which can never be completely suppressed (Topp, 2018).

Criticism of the no-restraint system also tackled the very problem of defining what counts as restraint and what does not. The next quotation is taken from a report on Hanwell Asylum published in 1844 by the Metropolitan Commissioners in Lunacy, charged by the Parliament with inspecting conditions in English asylums (Topp, 2018, pp. 760–761).

> Those who profess the entire disuse of restraint, employ manual force and seclusion as parts of their method of management, maintaining that such measures are consistent with a system of non-restraint. It is said by these persons that when any of the limbs (as the legs or the hands of a patient) are confined by the strait-jacket, the belt, or by straps or gloves, he is under restraint. But in cases where he is held by the hands of attendants, or when he is for any excitement or violence forced by manual strength into a small chamber or cell, and left there, it is said that restraint is not employed, and the method adopted in these cases, is called 'the non-restraint system'. [...] Here restraint of some form or other is manifest; and even in those cases where the patient is forced into a cell by manual strength, and prevented from leaving it until his fit of excitement shall have passed, it is difficult to understand how this also can be reconciled with the profession of abstaining from all restraint whatsoever, so as to be correctly termed 'Non-restraint'. It seems to us that these measures are only particular modes of restraint, the relative advantages of which must depend altogether on the results.

The authors of the report quoted above maintain that mechanical restraint had been just substituted by forced isolation and attendants' use of force, which are still forms of restraint—those we have previously called environmental and physical/manual restraint—coercive and violent as well. They ultimately seem to suggest that no-restraint is but an ideological position (ibidem).

Conolly's subsequent defence of the measure of seclusion is as interesting as its criticism. In his *The Treatment of the Insane Without Mechanical Restraints* (1856), the psychiatrist describes the practice downplaying its coercive aspects and framing it in a scientific discourse, which attributes it a therapeutic value. Negative features, he claims, are associated with the way seclusion is practised rather than the practice itself. To strengthen his argument, Conolly develops a detailed procedure attendants should conform to in order to perform—we might say—"good" seclusion. He described how three or four attendants, with courage and a good temper, should surround the patient, tell him/her that s/he would be much better in his/her own room, and gently induce him/her to walk into it. Although with some loud protests, Conolly argues, the person usually proceeds in that direction. If the patient strikes and kicks them, attendants must act speedily and steadily, even with force, but without resorting to violence (ibidem).

The psychiatrist specifies not only the number of attendants necessary to escort the patient, but how they should approach him/her and escort him/her in the room, which temper they should possess, and how they should dominate their passions and perform what, with Arlie Russell Hochschild (1983), we could call emotional work. To enforce seclusion with anger, neglect or contempt would have reproduced the same evils of mechanical restraint (Hodgkinson, 1985). Similar attention to the way in which coercive measures are practised, rather than on the practices themselves, characterizes both the strategies of proceduralization (concerning how restraint should technically be performed) and that of therapeuticization (pertaining to the emotional work accompanying the measure) of coercion, discussed in Chap. 5.

Terminology is once again relevant, as we saw it is to distinguish between "*contenzione*" and "*contenimento*" (see Chap. 2). The term "seclusion", which Conolly preferred over "isolation" or other nouns, points to its therapeutic and calming effect, as it comes from poetry and is associated with the romantic meaning of a beneficial condition apart from society (Topp, 2018). "Solitary confinement", on the contrary, was opposed by Conolly and used by no-restraint adversaries because it recalled detention and consequently seemed to blur the distinction between the two institutions, asylum and prison (ibidem).

Attention to the characteristics of the space in which the patient was secluded was also part of Conolly's attempt to establish the features of "good" seclusion: the light in the seclusion room should be lightened in order to remove the patient from sensory stimuli, but should never be completely dark. The specification is related to the abuses perpetrated at old Bethlem Asylum in London, which had just been exposed in *The Lancet* by reformers who visited the institution, and which included confinement in dark cells. Seclusion's opponents, on the contrary, argued that the room could rather become a condenser of sensory stimuli, auditory (shouts in a closed space), olfactory (unremoved urine and faeces), and in terms of pain (self-harm through violent contact with the walls or the closed door). These objections led Conolly to admit that a seclusion room did not always provide a suitable solution and to resort to an alternative kind of space for particularly agitated patients: the padded room. The thick mattresses which covered both the floor and the walls, and the absence of furniture prevented the patient from harming him/herself by means of the room without restraining free movement. This novel solution received criticism as well: padded rooms were defined as little more than capacious versions of the straitjackets they were meant to replace, so that they should have been considered in the same category as mechanical restraints (De Young, 2015).

The alternative in the treatment of the mentally ill represented by the no-restraint movement has been discussed and questioned also by Michel Foucault (2006) in his lectures on psychiatric power. The French scholar quotes a letter of the Mother Superior ministering the asylum for women at Lille to her colleague at the asylum of Saint Yon, explaining how they managed to avoid mechanical restraint: "We set to work… taking an agitated woman so as to put her under the supervision of a nun who knew how to impress" (2006, p. 119). Physical restraint, Foucault argues, can easily be removed on condition that an imposing nun is placed beside the agitated patient. The intervention of personnel had just substituted the use of a more eloquent and evident system, that of restraint by means of devices: the choice between the two is deemed superficial and not very serious (Foucault, 2006). This recalls a sort of inversion of the delegation from human to nonhuman agents discussed in Chap. 7 to account for no-restraint aversion to restraining belts and locked doors.

These debates expose the definitional struggles concerning coercive practices, which are constantly brought in or pushed out of the medical discourse by acknowledging or denying their therapeutic value. The definitional issue is not only relevant on a conceptual, abstract level, but in everyday psychiatric practice: actors engage in a definitional work, namely, they perform interpretative practices and social actions involved in providing definitions (Ashmore et al., 1989). Chapter 6 will extensively discuss how care and coercion are practically and discursively held together in the provision of acute mental healthcare in the contexts observed, while Chap. 7 will delve into the issue of preferability between such practices and the values that are enacted through their adoption or rejection.

3.2 Contemporary Attempts to Reduce Coercion in Psychiatric Settings

Despite the increasing recognition of the rights of people with mental health problems and the internationally acknowledged need to reduce coercive practices in psychiatric care, research in this area is little (Sashidharan et al., 2019).

At the national level, laws have been designed to reduce coercion in several countries. In Germany, for example, involuntary interventions were narrowed to life-threatening emergencies only by Germany's Constitutional Court and Federal Supreme Court in 2011 and 2012; nevertheless, this led to adverse effects such as violent incidents and consequent increase in restraint use (Flammer & Steinert, 2015). In Switzerland in 2006, a law authorized psychiatrists only to require compulsory admissions, while previously every physician could do so, resulting in a consequent decrease of this measure (Eytan et al., 2013). Promising legislative changes occurred also in California, Vermont, and in Argentina, where the National Mental Health Law of 2010 introduced interdisciplinary evaluations made by psychiatrists, psychologists, social workers, and lawyers to request civil commitment (Bariffi & Smith, 2013).

Besides top-down processes, local-level leadership has been found relevant in creating and maintaining change (Gooding et al., 2018). Local policies and practices aimed at reducing coercion have adopted both a recovery-oriented approach (focused on the person's ability to overcome crisis and self-determination instead of passive receiving of treatment) and a trauma-oriented approach ("no-force" forms of care to reduce interpersonal violence and possibility of re-traumatization). Evidence is available particularly on hospital-based interventions to reduce seclusion and mechanical restraint.

In 2002, the National Association of State Mental Health Program Directors (USA) articulated the Six Core Strategies model after a thorough literature review, meetings with people who experienced restraint and/or seclusion, and multiple working sessions with experts who have been sustaining coercion reduction in their work settings for years

(Huckshorn, 2006). The six strategies are: (i) active leadership towards organizational change; (ii) using data to inform practice in a non-punitive way; (iii) training the workforce; (iv) using restraint/seclusion prevention tools; (v) actively including consumers, carers, and advocates in the care setting; and (vi) rigorously debriefing restraint/seclusion events after they occur (ibidem). Eight US states were awarded a three-year incentive grant to implement the model. Facilities that had fully implemented the strategies registered more than 70% reduction in hours of seclusion use and more than 50% reduction in hours of restraint use (NASMHPD, 2014). The model has then been taught throughout the USA and in several other countries around the world, which reported additional benefits such as reduced staff turnover, staff injuries, and absenteeism (LeBel et al., 2014).[2]

Another intervention, called Safewards,[3] has been developed in the UK and then evaluated by Bowers et al. (2015) in a randomized controlled trial. Based on the study of staff actions which are known to create potential flashpoints, the Safewards model indicates ten interventions to reduce coercion: (i) mutually agreed and publicized standards of behaviour by and for patients and staff; (ii) short advisory statements (soft words) on handling flashpoints, hung in the nursing office and changed every few days; (iii) a de-escalation model used by the best de-escalator on the staff (elected by the ward) to expand the skills of the ward staff; (iv) a requirement to say something good about each patient at nursing shift handover; (v) scanning for the potential bad news a patient might receive from friends, relatives or staff, and intervening promptly to talk it through; (vi) structured, shared, personal information between staff and

[2] The Six Core Strategies model has been implemented in Finland in 2009, and a randomized controlled study was conducted to verify if restraint/seclusion reduction resulted in increased violence. The team working on the project, led by a psychiatrist-researcher, included a senior nurse and a cultural anthropologist-psychotherapist. Data on coercion and violence were graphed, posted, and discussed with staff on a monthly basis. Individual data on violence and seclusion were used to develop individual crisis plans, revised after each crisis. Daily discussions on violent incidents that occurred on the previous day, as well as restrictions and alternative methods employed, were held between the senior nurse and the cultural anthropologist-psychotherapist. The study registered a reduction in restraint/seclusion use without an increase in violence (Putkonen et al., 2013).

[3] Safewards interventions are freely available on a dedicated website, providing instructional videos, document templates, planning and implementation guidance, and a web-based forum (http://www.safewards.net/, accessed on 26 November 2022).

patients (e.g. music preferences, favourite films and sports) via a "know each other" folder kept in the patients day room; (vii) a regular patient meeting to intensify inter-patient support; (viii) a crate of distraction and sensory modulation tools to use with agitated patients (stress toys, mp3 players with soothing music, textured blankets); (ix) reassuring explanations to all patients following potentially frightening incidents; and (x) a display of positive messages about the ward from discharged patients. The model, tested over a three-month period in thirty-one psychiatric wards around London, was positively evaluated, registering a 15% decrease in conflict events and a 26.4% decrease in containment events (ibidem). The Safewards model has been successfully implemented and evaluated as well in the state of Victoria (Australia), achieving a reduction in the use of seclusion (Fletcher et al., 2017).

Hospital-based interventions to reduce coercion also considered the role played by physical design—such as private space for patients, outdoor space, and replacement of worn-out furniture (Van der Schaaf et al., 2013), staff-to-patient ratio, and male-female staff ratio (Janssen et al., 2007). Non-hospital, community-based interventions to reduce coercion have been explored as well. This is the case of community homes, which host people going through a crisis without resorting to hospitalization, providing fewer beds than in a hospital ward, de-emphasis on medication and a different composition of the staff, usually a mixture of mental healthcare professionals and former service users (Gooding et al., 2018). In Italy, a similar mode of intervention can be found in Community Mental Health Centres in Trieste and a few other cities (including those considered in this study), open twenty-four hours a day and seven days a week, and able to provide day and night support to people in acute crisis avoiding psychiatric hospitalization (Mezzina & Vidoni, 1995). Community-based crisis-intervention programmes can be considered alternatives to coercive practices to the extent that such settings may reduce the likelihood of coercion, even though there is little research available on coercion experienced in community-based services (Gooding et al., 2018).

Evidence-based remedies have been deemed necessary also to balance the "rising tide of compulsory admissions", which have steadily increased over the past two decades in the UK and other countries (Johnson, 2013). Joint care plans are promising tools in avoiding non-consensual treatment, as well as joint crisis plans which involve both professionals and service users in the detailed planning of care in the event of a psychiatric crisis (Thornicroft & Henderson, 2016). Similarly, psychiatric advance directives—in which the patient makes decisions designed to bind him/herself and/or direct others to action during times of crisis—could mitigate the risk of coercive treatments (Swanson et al., 2008). Ethnic minority groups have been found more likely to be compulsorily admitted, so that addressing cultural-specific needs and help-seeking behaviours might be a useful strategy to reduce rates of compulsory admission for these communities (Lawlor et al., 2012). Lastly, dissatisfaction and negative encounters with services can generate fear of coercion, inhibit future help seeking, increase in treatment refusal, and ultimately lead to a heightened risk of coercion (Swartz et al., 2003).

The literature review on alternatives to coercion in mental health setting, commissioned to the Melbourne Social Equity Institute by the United Nations to inform the report of the Special Rapporteur on the Rights of Persons with Disabilities, suggests that besides large-scale quantitative investigation conducted by psychiatrists, phenomenological research could significantly contribute to the knowledge of complex social interventions such as practices to prevent, end or reduce coercion. This derives from the observation that "multiple contested ideas and values are at play" and that "organisational culture was identified as an important site for addressing the use of coercion", and nevertheless "social science disciplines that tend to focus on organisational culture and human behaviour, such as sociology, anthropology and behavioural psychology, were almost entirely absent among the studies" (Gooding et al., 2018). Similarly, Arthur Kleinman (2012) has called for a rebalancing of academic psychiatry, whose research should adopt a more humanistic biosocial framework, strengthening the ties with public health and social sciences.

3.3 Defining the Object: Situated Care and Coercive Practices

This work has as its object of inquiry mental healthcare and coercive practices, specifically mechanical restraint, which represents the most contested practice in contemporary Italian psychiatric context. Before moving to the methodological and then the empirical chapters, I wish to clarify my understanding of the notion of practice, which has been looked at from a variety of perspectives to the point that there is no unified practice approach (Schatzki et al., 2001). Generally speaking, practices can be conceived as arrays of human activities. This definition can then be extended incorporating other elements acknowledged by the majority of practice theorists, such as the dependence of practices on shared understandings and their embodiment (ibidem). The concept of practice that I wish to adopt here is that offered by Silvia Gherardi (2006), who draws from the phenomenological and ethnomethodological traditions to define practice as a socially recognized and relatively stable in time mode of ordering heterogeneous items into a coherent set. If we apply the constituting elements of this definition to care and coercive practices, we can see that exploring them means investigating: how they acquire meaning in a context of situated action; how they are reproduced along time developing a history or tradition (e.g. the no-restraint one); how they become a mode of ordering the world, which both constrain and facilitate action by forbidding some alternatives and privileging others.

Practices produce social bonds between practitioners, constituting a community which has been called community of practices (Lave & Wenger, 1991) or community of practitioners (Gherardi, 2006). Such a community has been defined as an intrinsic condition for the existence of knowledge, providing the interpretative support necessary for making sense of its heritage (Lave & Wenger, 1991, p. 98). Knowledge and learning are not considered mental, individual processes, but social and cultural phenomena: knowledge-in-practice is situated in the historical, cultural, and socio-material contexts in which it occurs (Gherardi & Nicolini, 2000). To become a member of a community of practitioners requires participation to situated activities and acquisition of a professional vision, namely a socially organized way of seeing and understanding (Goodwin, 1994, p. 606). The novice is provided with an ethnography of seeing that instructs him/her on how to look at relevant entities, framing them through a specific coding scheme as objects of knowledge (Goodwin, 1994).

Through clinical practice and hegemonic discourses encountered along their training, clinicians and other mental healthcare workers undergo an apprenticeship in constraint (Henckes, 2014), which also provides them with strategies to justify and contain the ethical dilemmas related to their profession. Indeed, to ethnographically study care practices means to observe what is sought, fostered, or hoped for through their performance (what is performed as good), and what, on the contrary, is avoided or excluded (what is performed as bad) (Mol et al., 2010, p. 12). Notions of "good care" and "bad care" pertain to the ethics of care, which is not a matter of universal principles, but rather of local solutions to specific problems (ibidem). Therefore, the purpose is not to investigate or evaluate normatively described good practices according to specific criteria. Instead, the perspective is that of empirical ethics of care, which allows to empirically approach the ways in which care providers shape goodness in their daily work (Pols, 2015). Since the values at stake and the objects of care are usually multiple, then care practices are intrinsically problematic as they deal with tensions and inconsistencies, in a constant attempt to hold together what does not necessarily hold together (Law, 2010; Mol et al., 2010). Mental healthcare providers regularly experience uncertainty and ambivalence as they have to negotiate between their preferred self-image—that of caring and competent professionals—and the necessity to carry out coercive treatments implying physical force (Brodwin, 2014). In hospital emergency settings, this ambivalence has to be resolved in a short time, and if different orientations between staff members emerge, the tension can possibly block the primary imperative to act (ibidem). Ordinary psychiatric practice indeed has to do with everyday ethics, with making decisions that deal with right and wrong in the ongoing flow of clinical work: decisions that are tied to the legitimacy of professional power (Brodwin, 2013, p. 29).

Perspectives about what counts as coercion and what does not are here considered part of broader professional visions, acquired and reproduced through everyday practice. The restraint and the no-restraint contexts represent as two distinct communities of practitioners, working within the same field of practice, that of acute mental health care. Mechanical restraint is defined beforehand as a bad intervention in the no-restraint context, where alternative (sometimes coercive) practices are performed to deal with acutely disturbed people, mobilizing different discourses and values to argue for their preferability over mechanical restraint (see Chap. 7). In the restraint context, mechanical restraint is not excluded a priori from the category of good care; together with other coercive interventions, mechanical restraint and care are held together whereby practical and discursive strategies (see Chap. 6). In both cases, given the complexities intrinsic to care and specifically mental healthcare, what is good can be ambivalent or difficult to translate into practice, and various relevant goods or values can be at stake at the same time: delivered care therefore depends on tinkering with different "goods" (Mol, 2010). Within each context of care, a specific "mode of doing good" results from a pattern of ideals, routines, and knowledge oriented towards a specific form of good care (Pols, 2003). The ultimate aim of the research that is presented in this book, though, is to explore acute mental health care and coercive practices, investigating situated modes of responding to situations of emergency and how ideas about good care are enacted in daily practice.

References

Abderhalden, C., Hahn, S., Bonner, Y. D., & Galeazzi, G. M. (2006). Users' perceptions and views on violence and coercion in mental health. In *Violence in mental health settings* (pp. 69–92). Springer.

Ashmore, M., Mulkay, M., & Pinch, T. (1989). Definitional work in applied social science: Collaborative analysis in health economics and sociology of science. *Knowledge and Society: Studies in the Sociology of Science, Past and Present, 8*, 27–55.

Austin, W. J., Kagan, L., Rankel, M., & Bergum, V. (2008). The balancing act: Psychiatrists' experience of moral distress. *Medicine, Health Care and Philosophy, 11*(1), 89–97.

Bariffi, F. J., & Smith, M. S. (2013). Same old game but with some new players—Assessing Argentina's National Mental Health Law in light of the rights to liberty and legal capacity under the UN Convention on the Rights of the Persons with Disabilities. *Nordic Journal of Human Rights, 31*(3), 325–342.

Biancosino, B., Delmonte, S., Grassi, L., Santone, G., Preti, A., Miglio, R., & De Girolamo, G. (2009). Violent behavior in acute psychiatric inpatient facilities: A national survey in Italy. *The Journal of Nervous and Mental Disease, 197*(10), 772–782.

Bowers, L., James, K., Quirk, A., Simpson, A., Stewart, D., & Hodsoll, J. (2015). Reducing conflict and containment rates on acute psychiatric wards: The Safewards cluster randomised controlled trial. *International Journal of Nursing Studies, 52*(9), 1412–1422.

Brodwin, P. (2013). *Everyday ethics: Voices from the front line of community psychiatry*. University of California Press.

Brodwin, P. (2014). The ethics of ambivalence and the practice of constraint in us psychiatry. *Culture, Medicine, and Psychiatry, 38*(4), 527–549.

Chieze, M., Hurst, S., Sentissi, O., & Kaiser, S. (2019). Effects of seclusion and restraint in adult psychiatry: A systematic review. *Frontiers in Psychiatry, 10*, 491.

Conolly, J. (1856). *The treatment of the insane without mechanical restraints*. Dawsons of Pall Mall.

Crowe, M., & Carlyle, D. (2003). Deconstructing risk assessment and management in mental health nursing. *Journal of Advanced Nursing, 43*(1), 19–27.

De Young, M. (2015). *Encyclopedia of asylum therapeutics, 1750–1950s*. McFarland.

European Commission. (2005). *Improving the mental health of the population. Towards a strategy on mental health for the European Union*. Green Paper. English document. Retrieved November 26, 2022, from http://ec.europa.eu/health/ph_determinants/life_style/mental/green_paper/mental_gp_en.pdf

Eytan, A., Chatton, A., Safran, E., & Khazaal, Y. (2013). Impact of psychiatrists' qualifications on the rate of compulsory admissions. *Psychiatric Quarterly, 84*(1), 73–80.

Flammer, E., & Steinert, T. (2015). Involuntary medication, seclusion, and restraint in German psychiatric hospitals after the adoption of legislation in 2013. *Frontiers in Psychiatry, 6*, 153.

Fletcher, J., Spittal, M., Brophy, L., Tibble, H., Kinner, S., Elsom, S., & Hamilton, B. (2017). Outcomes of the Victorian Safewards trial in 13 wards: Impact on seclusion rates and fidelity measurement. *International Journal of Mental Health Nursing, 26*(5), 461–471.

Foucault, M. (2006). *Psychiatric power: Lectures at the Collège de France, 1973–1974*. Palgrave Macmillan.
Frueh, B. C., Knapp, R. G., Cusack, K. J., Grubaugh, A. L., Sauvageot, J. A., Cousins, V. C., et al. (2005). Special section on seclusion and restraint: Patients' reports of traumatic or harmful experiences within the psychiatric setting. *Psychiatric Services, 56*(9), 1123–1133.
Gherardi, S. (2006). *Organizational knowledge: The texture of workplace learning*. John Wiley & Sons.
Gherardi, S., & Nicolini, D. (2000). To transfer is to transform: The circulation of safety knowledge. *Organization, 7*(2), 329–348.
Gooding, P., Mc Sherry, B., Roper, C., & Grey, F. (2018). *Alternatives to coercion in mental health settings: A literature review*. Melbourne: Melbourne Social Equity Institute, University of Melbourne.
Goodwin, C. (1994). Professional vision. *American Anthropologist, 96*(3), 606–633.
Grunberg, F. (2002). Patients and society: The double allegiance of psychiatrists. *CPA Bulletin*, 9–11.
Hatling, T., Douzenis, A., & Maguire, J. (2006). Diversity and consistency in the legal management of involuntary admission and treatment across Europe. In D. Richter & R. Whittington (Eds.), *Violence in mental health settings* (pp. 95–109). Springer.
Henckes, N. (2014). Learning constraint. Exploring nurses' narratives of psychiatric work in the early years of French community psychiatry. *Culture, Medicine, and Psychiatry, 38*(4), 597–617.
Hill, R. G. (1839). *Total abolition of personal restraint in the treatment of the insane. A lecture on the management of lunatic asylums, and the treatment of the insane*. W.&B. Brooke Printers.
Hochschild, A. R. (1983). *The managed heart: Commercialization of human feeling*. University of California Press.
Hodgkinson, P. (1985). The use of seclusion. *Medicine, Science and the Law, 25*(3), 215–222.
Huckshorn, K. A. (2006). Re-designing state mental health policy to prevent the use of seclusion and restraint. *Administration and Policy in Mental Health, 33*, 482–491.
Jameton, A. (1984). *Nursing practice: The ethical issues*. Prentice-Hall.
Janssen, W., Noorthoorn, E., van Linge, R., & Lendemeijer, B. (2007). The influence of staffing levels on the use of seclusion. *International Journal of Law and Psychiatry, 30*(2), 118–126.

Johnson, M. E. (1998). Being restrained: A study of power and powerlessness. *Issues in Mental Health Nursing, 19*(3), 191–206.
Johnson, S. (2013). Can we reverse the rising tide of compulsory admissions? *Lancet, 381*(9878), 1603–1604.
Katz, P., & Kirkland, F. R. (1990). Violence and social structure on mental hospital wards. *Psychiatry, 53*(3), 262–277.
Kersting, X. A. K., Hirsch, S., & Steinert, T. (2019). Physical harm and death in the context of coercive measures in psychiatric patients: A systematic review. *Frontiers in Psychiatry, 10*, 400.
Kleinman, A. (2012). Rebalancing academic psychiatry: Why it needs to happen—And soon. *The British Journal of Psychiatry, 201*(6), 421–422.
Lave, J., & Wenger, E. (1991). *Situated learning: Legitimate peripheral participation*. Cambridge University Press.
Law, J. (2010). Care and killing: Tensions in veterinary practice. In A. Mol, I. Moser, & J. Pols (Eds.), *Care in practice: On tinkering in clinics, homes and farms* (Vol. 8, pp. 57–72). transcript Verlag.
Lawlor, C., Johnson, S., Cole, L., & Howard, L. M. (2012). Ethnic variations in pathways to acute care and compulsory detention for women experiencing a mental health crisis. *International Journal of Social Psychiatry, 58*(1), 3–15.
LeBel, J. L., Duxbury, J. A., Putkonen, A., Sprague, T., Rae, C., & Sharpe, J. (2014). Multinational experiences in reducing and preventing the use of restraint and seclusion. *Journal of Psychosocial Nursing and Mental Health Services, 52*(11), 22–29.
Marangos-Frost, S., & Wells, D. (2000). Psychiatric nurses' thoughts and feelings about restraint use: A decision dilemma. *Journal of Advanced Nursing, 31*(2), 362–369.
Mason, T. (1994). Seclusion: An international comparison. *Medicine, Science and the Law, 34*(1), 54–60.
McKenna, K. (2004). Study of work-related violence. *Committee on Workplace Violence. North Eastern Health Board*, Ireland, 1–121.
Menegatto, M., & Zamperini, A. (2018). *Coercizione e disagio psichico. La contenzione tra dignità e sicurezza*. Il Pensiero Scientifico Editore.
Mezzina, R., & Vidoni, D. (1995). Beyond the mental hospital: Crisis intervention and continuity of care in Trieste. A four year follow-up study in a community mental health centre. *International Journal of Social Psychiatry, 41*(1), 1–20.
Mohr, W. K., Petti, T. A., & Mohr, B. D. (2003). Adverse effects associated with physical restraint. *The Canadian Journal of Psychiatry, 48*(5), 330–337.

Mol, A. (2010). Care and its values. Good food in the nursing home. In A. Mol, I. Moser, & J. Pols (Eds.), *Care in practice: On tinkering in clinics, homes and farms* (Vol. 8, pp. 215–234). transcript Verlag.

Mol, A., Moser, I., & Pols, J. (Eds.). (2010). *Care in practice: On tinkering in clinics, homes and farms* (Vol. 8). transcript Verlag.

NASMHPD – National Association of State Mental Health Program Directors (2014). *National executive training institute: A training curriculum for the reduction of seclusion and restraint* (12th ed.). Alexandria, VA: Author.

Nijman, H., Bjørkly, S., Palmstierna, T., & Almvik, R. (2006). Assessing aggression of psychiatric patients: Methods of measurement and its prevalence. In D. Richter & R. Whittington (Eds.), *Violence in mental health settings* (pp. 11–23). Springer.

Olofsson, B., Jacobsson, L., Gilje, F., & Norberg, A. (1999). Being in conflict: Physicians' experience with using coercion in psychiatric care. *Nordic Journal of Psychiatry, 53*(3), 203–210.

Oud, N. E. (2006). Aggression management training programs: Contents, implementation, and organization. In D. Richter & R. Whittington (Eds.), *Violence in mental health settings* (pp. 193–210). Springer.

Pinel, P. (1806). Treatise on mental alienation. In C. E. Goshen (1967), *Documentary history of psychiatry* (pp. 257–265). Vision Press.

Pinel, P., & Snaith, P. (1995). On the removal of chains from the insane. *Psychiatric Bulletin, Royal College of Psychiatrists, 19*, 434–434.

Pols, J. (2003). Enforcing patient rights or improving care? The interference of two modes of doing good in mental health care. *Sociology of Health & Illness, 25*(4), 320–347.

Pols, J. (2015). Towards an empirical ethics in care: Relations with technologies in health care. *Medicine, Health Care and Philosophy, 18*(1), 81–90.

Putkonen, A., Kuivalainen, S., Louheranta, O., Repo-Tiihonen, E., Ryynänen, O.-P., Kautiainen, H., & Tiihonen, J. (2013). Cluster-randomized controlled trial of reducing seclusion and restraint in secured care of men with schizophrenia. *Psychiatric Services, 64*, 850–855.

Richter, D. (2006). Nonphysical conflict management and de-escalation. In D. Richter & R. Whittington (Eds.), *Violence in mental health settings* (pp. 125–144). Springer.

Rocca, P., Villari, V., & Bogetto, F. (2006). Managing the aggressive and violent patient in the psychiatric emergency. *Progress in Neuro-Psychopharmacology and Biological Psychiatry, 30*(4), 586–598.

Salize, H. J., Dreßing, H., & Peitz, M. (2002). Compulsory admission and involuntary treatment of mentally ill patients. Legislation and practice in EU-member states. *Central Institute of Mental Health Research Project Final Report*. Mannheim, Germany.

Sashidharan, S. P., Mezzina, R., & Puras, D. (2019). Reducing coercion in mental healthcare. *Epidemiology and Psychiatric Sciences, 28*(6), 605–612.

Schatzki, T., Cetina, K. K., & von Savigny, E. (Eds.). (2001). *The practice turn in contemporary theory*. Routledge.

Slemon, A., Jenkins, E., & Bungay, V. (2017). Safety in psychiatric inpatient care: The impact of risk management culture on mental health nursing practice. *Nursing Inquiry, 24*(4), e12199.

Steinert, T. (2006). Prediction of violence in inpatient settings. In D. Richter & R. Whittington (Eds.), *Violence in mental health settings* (pp. 111–123). Springer.

Steinert, T., Lepping, P., Bernhardsgrütter, R., Conca, A., Hatling, T., Janssen, W., et al. (2010). Incidence of seclusion and restraint in psychiatric hospitals: A literature review and survey of international trends. *Social Psychiatry and Psychiatric Epidemiology, 45*(9), 889–897.

Steinert, T., Noorthoorn, E. O., & Mulder, C. L. (2014). The use of coercive interventions in mental health care in Germany and the Netherlands. A comparison of the developments in two neighboring countries. *Frontiers in Public Health, 2*, 141.

Stewart, D., Van der Merwe, M., Bowers, L., Simpson, A., & Jones, J. (2010). A review of interventions to reduce mechanical restraint and seclusion among adult psychiatric inpatients. *Issues in Mental Health Nursing, 31*(6), 413–424.

Strauss, A., Schatzman, L., Bucher, R., Ehrlich, D., & Sabshin, M. (1981). *Psychiatric ideologies and institutions*. Transaction.

Swanson, J. W., Swartz, M. S., Elbogen, E. B., Van Dorn, R. A., Wagner, H. R., Moser, L. A., et al. (2008). Psychiatric advance directives and reduction of coercive crisis interventions. *Journal of Mental Health, 17*(3), 255–267.

Swartz, M. S., Swanson, J. W., & Hannon, M. J. (2003). Does fear of coercion keep people away from mental health treatment? Evidence from a survey of persons with schizophrenia and mental health professionals. *Behavioural Sciences & The Law, 21*(4), 459–472.

Thornicroft, G., & Henderson, C. (2016). Joint decision making and reduced need for compulsory psychiatric admission. *JAMA Psychiatry, 73*(7), 647–648.

Topp, L. (2018). Single rooms, seclusion and the non-restraint movement in British asylums, 1838–1844. *Social History of Medicine, 31*(4), 754–773.

Van der Schaaf, P. S., Dusseldorp, E., Keuning, F. M., Janssen, W. A., & Noorthoorn, E. O. (2013). Impact of the physical environment of psychiatric wards on the use of seclusion. *The British Journal of Psychiatry, 202*(2), 142–149.

Whittington, R., & Richter, D. (2006). From the individual to the interpersonal: Environment and interaction in the escalation of violence in mental health settings. In D. Richter & R. Whittington (Eds.), *Violence in mental health settings* (pp. 47–68). Springer.

Working Party on Psychiatry and Human Rights. (2000). *White Paper on the protection of the human rights and dignity of people suffering from mental disorder, especially those placed as involuntary patients in a psychiatric establishment.* Strasbourg.

4

The Empirical Research: Context, Data, and Methods

Abstract This chapter constitutes a reflexive account, necessary to clarify the theoretical assumptions, the researcher's characteristics, and the methods employed. First of all, I will begin by introducing the seminal work of Erving Goffman on asylums, as well as more recent ethnographic contributions on acute mental healthcare. Then, I provide a description of the context in which the empirical study took place, the research design, and the techniques employed. Lastly, I will reflect on the personal implications of being on the field.

4.1 Ethnographic Research on Acute Inpatient Psychiatric Settings: An Introduction

Psychiatric settings, particularly acute ones, have been ethnographically explored from the perspective of various disciplines: sociology, anthropology, and nursing studies.

A key contribution to the understanding of psychiatric care is Erving Goffman's seminal work, *Asylums* (1961). The sociologist conducted one year of fieldwork at the St. Elizabeth Hospital, Washington D.C., which

E. Rossero, *Care in a Time of Crisis*, https://doi.org/10.1007/978-3-031-34418-3_4

hosted over 7000 inmates at that time. The research focused on the social world of hospital inmates as subjectively experienced by them. The total institution in which patients were confined for a considerable period of time was both a place of residence and work, cutting them off from the wider society. Life within the asylum entailed a process which Goffman calls "mortification of the self", whereby the inmates were stripped of their past social roles and took on a purely institutional one. This process began as the new arrival entered the institution, undergoing a number of trimming procedures—such as haircutting, undressing, searching, property dispossession, and assigning of numbers—which allowed the individual to be shaped into an object and fed into the administrative machinery of the asylum (ibidem, p. 16). The loss of one's identity equipment and usual appearance was the first of many acts of degradation and humiliation, such as physical contamination (dirty facilities, unclean food, old clothes worn by other inmates) and attacks to personal safety (beatings, shock therapy). Coercion was part of the asylum life, not only in terms of involuntary institutionalization, but through daily non-consensual practices such as forced medication and forced feeding. Within the walls of the asylum, the inmates carried out their everyday activities—all tightly scheduled according to organizational rather than individual needs—in a situation of forced interpersonal contact with a large number of other patients. Relationships with the staff were characterized by the inmates' need to ask for permission even for minor activities, which in turn allowed the staff to deny, question, and easily put their requests off. The inmate conduct was guided by a set of prescriptions, punishments for rule-breakers, and privileges accessible in return for obedience. Acts of solidarity and collective action were present but limited, in favour of individualistic strategies of adaptation to the ward system. The picture gave by Goffman of the asylum is that of a space where, like in every other total institution (e.g. prisons, monasteries, and concentration camps), the territories of the self are systematically violated, self-determination denied, and freedom of action curtailed. A similar situation emerges from accounts of European asylums of that time, including Italy (Babini, 2009).

The process of deinstitutionalization introduced a profound change in mental health services, markedly in those countries—such as Italy—where asylums have been dismantled and psychiatric care is currently provided within general hospitals and in the community. Even though these processes developed soon after Goffman conducted his research, his model of total institution remains valuable in that it represents an ideal type against which the features of contemporary mental institutions can be compared (Quirk et al., 2006). Moving from his conceptual framework, more recent sociological research on psychiatric institutionalization revealed how personal identity can be preserved and negotiated despite the confinement in a mental hospital (Prior, 1995). Contemporary ethnographic explorations of psychiatric ward life in the United Kingdom developed an alternative model, according to which modern mental health institutions are characterized by greater permeability than older asylums. This is evident in ward membership—which is temporary or revolving—contacts with the outside world (communication and visits from family, friends and social workers, as well as periods of leave), and blurred institutional identities, due to the fact that inpatients are no longer forced to wear standard-issue clothing and their relationship with the staff is characterized by some degree of informality. Because of these relevant changes, a shift from the model of total institution to that of "permeable institution" has been proposed (Quirk & Lelliott, 2004; Quirk et al., 2006).

The work of Michel Foucault on the birth of psychiatry and psychiatric power (2006a, 2006b) inspired ethnographic research as well. Lorna Rhodes' monograph *Emptying Beds* (1991), on the practice of emergency psychiatry in the United States provides us with a rich picture of institutional life within an acute unit, in which she conducted two years of fieldwork. The anthropologist employs the Foucaultian notion of a diffuse, fluid power, to shed light on the relationship between patients and staff, bound together in the same disciplinary space. In her ethnographic account, patients were not passive in the face of power exercised by the institution, and the staff themselves were made subjects of power, to which they attempted to resist through different strategies. Pressure to discharge within a few days was one of the core features of the unit's work, facing daily "disposition problems" due to the shortage of beds, and engaging in a continuous "dispatching process". The ethnography also portrays dilemmas and contradictions inherent to acute psychiatric care, to which participants responded by means of situated knowledge and fragile solutions grounded in the specificities of their contexts. We will see in Chap. 4 the relevance of what I call "circulation work" in current acute psychiatric practice; also, it will show strategies performed by healthcare providers to resist new admissions or foster discharge, and how this contributes to the drawing of boundaries around today's mental health services.

Qualitative research has then specifically addressed the issue of violence in inpatient psychiatric settings. Eileen Morrison (1990) has described the "tradition of toughness" which characterises nursing care in psychiatric units. These contexts are permeated with medical ideology, according to which patients are sick and their behaviour is a symptom of their illness. In this perspective, violent behaviour is a matter of low impulse control, and staff members have as their primary goal to keep patients under control. This is accomplished mainly by using physical restraint, into which new nurses are immediately socialized by peer pressures: if colleagues are called for assistance in a difficult situation by a new staff member who attempts to intervene verbally without resorting to restraint, in future situations they might not be responding to his/her help request. In these settings, some staff members—generally male non-professional staff—take on the role of enforcers, which is accomplished by strategies of policing (the process of carrying out the rules), supermanning (the alleged expert who takes the lead to physically manage dangerous situations), and putting on a show (hiding of abusive behaviour and emphasis on the therapeutic relationship).

Another study on violence in mental hospital wards considered the social mechanisms affecting potentially violent behaviour (Katz & Kirkland, 1990). To illustrate them, the scholars describe two ideal-typical contexts they call "peaceful wards" and "violence-prone wards". In the former, environment is characterized by trust, order, and predictability, provided by regularly scheduled meetings and activities, clearly delineated roles, teamwork, and firm but non-punitive approach towards violent behaviour intended to support patient's effort to enhance self-control. On the contrary, violence-prone wards' main features are uncertainty, confusion, and fear: staff is scared of patients and lacks knowledge on how to handle violent behaviour, responsibilities and roles are unclear, intra-staff communication is poor, and meetings and discussions are occasional. The style adopted by psychiatrists was also crucial and very different between the two contexts: in peaceful wards, the psychiatrist is frequently present, accessible to patients and staff, trustful toward nurses and their professional autonomy, and supportive of their needs. In violence-prone wards, the presence of the psychiatrist is sporadic and unpredictable, s/he does not represent a stable and reliable authority and has little time for interaction with both patients and staff, whose morale is consequently low. The authors conclude that a structured social climate, a competent psychiatric leadership, and the institution of predictable procedures are fundamental elements to provide professionals and inpatients with a sense of spatial, temporal, and psychological security.

More recently, ethnographic fieldwork in psychiatric wards has been conducted from a gender perspective, revealing how hegemonic masculinity is performed and reproduced by hospital security guards (Johnston & Kilty, 2014). Hospital agents are rewarded for their physicality and authority to coerce, control, and intimidate, either verbally or symbolically through their uniformed presence. These hyper-masculine performatives are in tension with health discourses promoting empathy, caring, and compassion, which are specularly constructed as features of femininity. Highly gendered codes of behaviour and relationships between predominantly male security guards, predominantly female nurses, and patients, pose threats to the ward environment, which is supposed to provide a stable and safe context of care to the vulnerable subjects it hosts. Gendered dynamics have been explored as well with respect to mechanical restraint, a practice that embodies a masculine, authoritative psychiatric culture (Jacob et al., 2018).

Besides sociology and anthropology, nursing studies ethnographically investigated acute mental healthcare as well. The issue of power and control has been explored, highlighting how nurses not only exercise it, but are also subject to it. Johansson et al. (2006) describe the healthcare environment in a locked psychiatric ward as overshadowed by control, implying a number of activities, such as door opening and carrying out checks, which negatively impact on the other tasks of the nursing staff. Control is exercised by staff over patients, but in turn, the latter scrutinize and pressure the staff, sometimes resulting in an open struggle for control. The ward, defined as a control-permeated environment, is pervaded by unequal power dynamics, both between patients and nurses, and between nurses when knowledge is asymmetrically distributed (Buus, 2008).

Nurses' micro-therapeutic skills and their invisible work of coordination, facilitation, documentation, as well as knowledge production, have been another topic of research. The use of observation in psychiatric nursing practice has been investigated in a study (Hamilton & Manias, 2007) informed by the Foucaultian notion of clinical gaze. Nurses' specific kind of clinical gaze—the psychiatric nurses' gaze—is not exercised in formal psychiatric interviews but in the social setting of the ward. One feature of this gaze is called "the scan", namely a monitoring activity of the spaces of the unit, informed by sight but also other senses: nurses scan for movements, noises, conversations, tones of voice, as well as emotional elements as potential areas of conflict or distress. Scanning allows nurses to glean valuable information about patients, which is then shared among colleagues and used to determine work priorities and plan more focused work on specific individuals. Besides this peculiar mode of diffuse observation, each nurse focuses on patients assigned to her/his care through different forms of discreet surveillance, looking for evidence as well as absence of symptoms. Discretion is a skilful strategy to assess patients while minimizing confrontation and avoiding probing; nevertheless, it is exactly this silent element of their practice which makes it invisible and readily misunderstood by patients and colleagues as "doing nothing", obscuring nurses' expertise and knowledge which is rich in situated details. Nurses' situated knowledge appeared as crucial in many situations observed on the field, which I will describe in the following chapters (see Chaps. 4 and 5). Sometimes, such knowledge is explicitly acknowledged as valuable by psychiatrists themselves to inform their decisions on discharge, initiation, or termination of restraint, and pharmacological therapy modulation.

What seems to emerge from ethnographic research in acute psychiatric settings is that—besides the relevant insights into contemporary issues of nursing practice in psychiatric settings provided by nursing studies—little is known about how mental healthcare is provided *today* in acute wards (Quirk & Lelliott, 2001). Moreover, most of the available evidence has been produced in the Anglo-Saxon context: United Kingdom, United States, and Australia. Literature on the Italian system is extremely limited, particularly on contexts different than those representing excellence in terms of deinstitutionalization, restraint reduction and recovery, such as the Trieste model (Mezzina, 2014; Oliveira et al., 2018; Okin, 2020). This work contributes to expand the existing knowledge, focusing on care and coercive practices performed by the different professional actors involved in contemporary acute mental healthcare. Ethnographic methods it adopts are specifically suitable in facilitating the exploration of experience within acute psychiatric settings (Quirk & Lelliott, 2001), as they prioritize insider's view of the group under study, without denying its most complex, and at times, contradictory aspects (Griffin & Bengry-Howell, 2017).

4.2 Investigating Coercion

Mental hospitals—according to Goffman—are a type of total institution that care for persons felt to be incapable of looking after themselves and a possible threat to the community (Goffman, 1961). In Italy, the so-called Basaglia Law, approved in May 1978 and then incorporated into the Law n. 833/1978, reformed the Italian psychiatric system, closing down asylums, and replacing them with community-based services. This shift has been conceptual, other than practical: the traditional model saw the mentally ill person as "a danger to him/herself and others", as defined by the psychiatric law of 1904 and in line with Goffman's notion of mental hospital. The new model broke the mental illness-danger association, promoting patients' integration as citizens rather than their isolation. This process of deinstitutionalization gradually led to the creation of local Mental Health Departments, which offer a network of territorial services for prevention, care, and rehabilitation. Within such system, the recourse to hospitalisation is carried out only for acute crisis, and only for a short period. The so-called "*Servizi Psichiatrici di Diagnosi e Cura*" (SPDC) are diagnostic and treatment wards, placed within the general hospitals and hosting a maximum of sixteen inpatients, where people are admitted both voluntarily and compulsorily.

Law 833/1978 states the criteria for which involuntary admission (TSO) is possible: (a) an emergency intervention is needed; (b) the patient refuses treatment; (c) alternative treatment outside of the hospital is not possible. Patients that are coercively admitted to psychiatric wards can be detained for a maximum of seven days, which can be extended if necessary. Among more than 200.000 psychiatric admissions per year, 15% are involuntary (data retrieved on http://dati.istat.it/, the website of the Italian National Institute of Statistics, the main Italian public research organisation).

Besides involuntary treatment, several kinds of restrictive interventions are commonly used within the context of SPDCs (see Chap. 2 for an extensive discussion). Physical or manual restraint (sometimes referred to as holding) implies direct physical contact between mental healthcare providers and patients to prevent or restrict the latter's movements. Mechanical restraint requires specific equipment, such as handcuffs and ties. Pharmacological or chemical restraint entails the use of medication to control someone's behaviour (e.g. forced medication through injections, or regular sedative medication). Environmental restraint consists in the isolation of the patient in a specific area of the ward, away from other patients (e.g. seclusion room, currently not employed in the Italian context), but can also refer to the practice of keeping ward doors locked. The use of different kind of restraints is not limited to involuntarily admitted patient, but also to the voluntary ones.

At the European level, the Working Party on Psychiatry and Human Rights stated that "the use of short periods of physical restraint and of seclusion should be in due proportion to the benefits and the risks entailed. Thorough training in techniques of physical restraint should be provided to staff. […] The response to violent behaviour by the patient should be graduated, i.e. staff should initially attempt to respond verbally; thereafter, only in so far as required, by means of manual restraint; and only in a last resort by mechanical restraint" (2000, p. 15).

Restraining interventions have also been defined by the International Quality Indicator Project as indicators of the poor quality of care provided to hospitalized patients. Nevertheless, the vast majority of Italian psychiatric wards still adopt (or has the possibility to adopt) restrictive interventions, specifically mechanical ones: a study conducted in 2004 by the Italian National Institute of Health on a sample of Italian psychiatric wards showed that 60% of them use mechanical restraint, while more than 70% were provided with the necessary equipment (Dell'Acqua et al., 2007). Almost 80% of the wards keep their doors locked permanently (ibidem). One-fifth of the acute patients are mechanically contained (Ferioli, 2013). Data on the adoption of mechanical restraint are not systematically gathered at a regional or national level, so that the phenomenon cannot be quantified or monitored, but only estimated.

Restraining measures are usually adopted on patients going through acute phases of illness. The expressions "psychiatric crisis" or "acute phase of illness" will be used interchangeably in this work to indicate an acute disturbance of mood, thought, or behaviour which requires an immediate or quick intervention (e.g. hospitalisation, medication). Crisis is sometimes related to a feared outcome, such as harm to self and others; it can be the consequence of a period of non-adherence to the prescribed treatment plan; and it can be detected after the occurrence of actions that endangered the person already (e.g. attempted suicide). Measures to deal with disruptive behaviour a person can show through her crisis can include mechanical restraint, which, as we have seen, is still adopted by the majority of Italian psychiatric wards. An alternative strategy to respond to situations of crisis is represented by a small number of SPDCs which chose to avoid the use of mechanical restraints and to keep the doors of their wards open. In 2006, the association called "Club SPDC No Restraint" has been founded: its underlying logic is that mechanical restraint can be replaced with psychological containment, working on the relation with the single patient and negotiating with him/her the permission to leave the ward (Toresini, 2007). This approach embraces dialectical strategies, and therefore directly challenges the power asymmetry that characterizes the psychiatrist-patient and nurse-patient relationships (Mauceri, 2017). Negotiation and the search for patients' cooperation also represent an attempt to overcome the paternalistic attitude of the staff, which denies the right of self-determination of the inpatients (Di Napoli & Andreatta, 2014). The adoption of such approach requires a profound change in the ward's culture and organization, and the demanding development of new skills and attitudes by the staff that operates in it: a genuine shift of paradigm (Mauceri, 2017).

This short reconstruction shows that, forty years after the psychiatric reform in Italy, two radically different approaches to psychiatric crisis are currently in place: the "restraint" and "no-restraint" one. Clinical differences among acute patients do not justify this heterogeneity. By contrast, organizational and socio-cultural features of each specific context are intertwined and seem to play an important role in the management of psychiatric crises (Di Lorenzo et al., 2012). This intricate interaction between clinical, organizational, and cultural aspects which affects the use of restraining measures has not been adequately investigated within the Italian context from a sociological perspective. Therefore, the purpose here is to provide an analytical description of the complex networks of practices, actors, discourses, and objects that are involved in approaching mental health emergency.

To do so, my aim is to explore care and coercive practices which belong to the two different models, the restraint and no-restraint one. This means to consider representations which are relevant, to begin with, in the definition of mental disorder, its nature, its causes, and the way it should be treated. As a specialty within medicine, psychiatry aims to diagnose sick individuals, predict the prognosis of the disease, speculate about its aetiology, and prescribe a response in the form of treatment (Rogers & Pilgrim, 2014). The biomedical model has been the dominant one and, as a direct consequence of such a framework, physical/pharmaceutical treatments tended to predominate. This has been true for a number of historical reasons as well, such as the opportunity for psychiatry to re-join mainstream medicine offered by the closing of mental hospitals (ibidem). Moreover, physical treatments are suited to psychiatry's dual mandate to control and care for the mentally ill because they can be imposed also without cooperation, while with talking treatments this is hardly possible (ibidem). Despite the dominant biomedical model, psychiatrists vary in their assumptions about mental disorders, their aetiology, and the appropriate treatment, and other approaches have emerged. The bio-psycho-social model, for example, considers the biomedical model to be reductionist, because it only focuses on the organic elements, without taking into consideration the broader psychosocial context the individual is part of (Pilgrim, 2002). While a biological orientation was present in both the restraint and the no-restraint context, it was particularly evident in the hospital settings, while community services acknowledged and had the chance to intervene on several areas of their users' lives through multidisciplinary teams including medical and non-medical figures (e.g. social workers). Such distinction leads us to the second aspect which makes representations relevant, by considering how, within each context, boundaries around (hospital and community) mental healthcare services are drawn. Boundary-work is a classification activity by which groups mobilize who they are, defining and defending themselves against other groups, drawing on cultural repertoires, narratives and traditions that are available and therefore embedded in their environment (Lamont & Molnár, 2002). Representations concerning each service are not intended as mere mental entities, because the product of boundary-work is then enacted through practical activities, including discursive and storytelling practices (Allen, 2001). The drawing of boundaries, as we will see in Chap. 5, is relevant also in shaping everyday practice and relationships between mental health services and in forming conceptions about who should be treated within each service.

A conceptual tool that I considered fruitful to approach the issue of representations within the two contexts is the notion of professional vision introduced by Charles Goodwin (1994). This concept refers to socially organized ways of seeing and understanding events, related to a particular social group. Assuming that every vision is perspectival—so that a farmer and an archaeologist see something different in the same patch of dirt—the anthropologist argues that every phenomenon is coded and transformed into an object of knowledge, highlighting some features that are relevant to the work of a specific profession. Professional visions are reproduced and learnt through discursive practices deployed within specific professional activities, so that those who join a work community are provided with an 'ethnography of seeing' that instructs them on how to look at relevant entities, framing them through a specific coding scheme (see Sect. 6.3.2 in Chap. 6, and specifically Excerpt 5.46 and its discussion concerning the provision of such ethnography of seeing with respect to the body of a restrained person). Therefore, the same domain of scrutiny (i.e. psychiatric crisis, or a specific behaviour) can be understood differently not only from the various professional groups involved in mental health services, but also from professionals working in a 'restraint' or 'no-restraint' context, qualifiable as communities of practice (Lave & Wenger, 1991). Furthermore, it becomes crucial to understand what kind of boundary work (Gieryn, 1983) is in place to draw the line between restraining and non-restraining measures, legitimate and illegitimate coercive interventions, locally good and bad practices. Boundary work is the process and result of a demarcation that distinguishes activities, phenomena, objects, and people (Åkerström, 2002). To explore these underlying definitions may be useful to uncover tacit, uncontested assumptions that are part of everyday work within these contexts.

The focus on care and coercive practices, intended as embodied arrays of human activity organized around shared practical understanding (Cetina et al., 2005), highlights how the body and the material world are involved in the performing of working activities, and how understandings, knowledge and aforementioned representations are embedded in situated practices. Care, in particular, has been described using the metaphor of choreography, in order to invoke its materiality, its performativity, and the co-dependence of setting and performers that it implicates (Cussins, 1996). In order to account for the complexity and effort behind the practice of care, it is important to notice that the objects of care are always multiple (Law, 2010). Psychiatric staff do not only care for the inpatients, but also for themselves, for other members of the staff, for third parties who may be present within the ward (e.g. relatives, volunteers, researchers), even for the society itself. If care is multiple—because different objects are simultaneously being cared for—then practices of care can be in tension, and coherence cannot be ensured. It is precisely the dimension of improvisation and implementation of local solutions that characterizes care practices that allows to handle these tensions, to try to hold together what does not necessarily hold together (ibidem). From the beginning of the design of the research, this appeared as particularly relevant in a controversial context such as that of psychiatric practice, imbued with dilemmas and potentially conflicting purposes. An ethical dimension therefore emerges, related to the different objects being cared for, and the different 'goods' attempted to be enacted in everyday practice. Alternative "modes of doing good" (Pols, 2003), are ultimately the object of inquiry of this contribution. This main question implicates a number of others, more specific queries: how are the dual mandates of care and control held together in everyday practice of mental healthcare workers? which kind of boundary work is in place in the discrimination between acceptable and unacceptable coercive practices? which kind of relations between the different actors and services contribute to shape the framework in which coercive practices take place? how is good care shaped and accomplished locally, through everyday work?

Qualitative research is the best suited to investigate issues concerning the meaning that participants attach to their actions and to grasp how things work in specific contexts (Mason, 2002). The analytical distinction between representations and practices—both of which are objects of this study—lead us to the identification of the more appropriate research techniques, respectively discursive interviews and participant observation.

Participant observation is the characteristic method of ethnographic research, which combines observation and participation to explore a specific social or cultural setting. Through this technique, the ethnographer has a first-hand experience of the studied phenomenon, in which s/he directly observes social action as it takes place in its natural context. Doing participant observation, the researcher is actively involved—though with degrees that can vary, depending also on the overt or covert form of observation adopted—in the social interaction with their participants. This engagement allows her/him to interrogate social actors about the meaning they attach to their actions, to be socialized to the local culture and to test the suitability of her/his own interpretations on the field (Cardano, 2011). Participant observation is appropriate to understand the participants' definition of the situation which guides their action and the tacit knowledge embedded in it. In this sense, the ethnographer has the opportunity to access the practical understanding behind working practices, namely the world of meanings and representations. Her/his presence on the field and the active way in which s/he collects empirical data denotes an intervention in their production—the recourse to interlocution—and determines a degree of perturbation which is mitigated by the temporal extension of the fieldwork (ibidem).

Interviews allow the researcher to ask the interviewees about their experiences, opinions, and beliefs in a more formal setting. The traditional interview entails a face-to-face interaction, which enables interpersonal contact, context sensitivity, and flexibility (Denzin & Lincoln, 2017). The specific form of interview employed for this study is the semi-structured interview, guided by a list of questions intended as issues to be touched, and conducted with interviewees known on the field. This allowed me to directly address topics related to specific situations observed both by them and myself in the ward.

Besides these two research methods, documentary analysis has to be mentioned, even though it held a less prominent role in my research. This technique entails the analysis of naturalistic documents—texts of artefacts—which exist independently of the researcher agency. Within this ethnography, they consist in clinical records, protocols, and texts elaborated in very specific occasions, such as one which anonymously collected the written opinions of nurses about the eventual opening of the doors in the no-restraint ward before it became a standard practice (see Sect. 6.1.2 in Chap. 6). The materiality and architecture of the wards are naturalistic documents subject to analysis as well (see the description of the spaces provided in Sect. 6.1 in Chap. 6).

The research design that is better suited to investigate the issues relevant to our purpose is that of a comparative case study which juxtaposes the "restraint" and the "no-restraint" model. I have chosen to focalize my attention on two composite cases, which include both acute psychiatric wards and mental health centres. In line with the conceptualisation offered by Charles C. Ragin (Ragin & Becker, 1992), I consider a case as a product of a specific research operation, which the sociologist calls "casing": the creation of objects of research made highlighting the theoretically relevant features of empirical units and washing them of their specificity. This operation starts at the beginning of the project, in the phase of research design, but continues and improves in the course of the study, guided by empirical evidence. In this view, cases as such do not exist independently of the investigation process, our orientation, and the general categories—rather mundane or theoretical—in terms of which we identify them (Gomm et al., 2000). The purposeful choice of the cases should answer the question: "what are them a case of?" Not only is this question helpful in distinguishing the phenomenon under scrutiny from the specific case studied, but it introduces us to the issue of generalization (Denzin & Lincoln, 2017). Case study research (and qualitative research more generally) has been often criticized because of its alleged impossibility to generalize its findings. If with the term "generalizability" we mean a nomothetic, context-free, and law-like type of generalization, then it is reasonable to believe that case studies are not able to provide such kind of generalizable findings (ibidem). To dismiss this notion of generalizability does not mean to completely abandon every attempt to extend the scope of our study, though. Argumentation theory provides powerful tools for transferring information from studied to unstudied cases, such as the argument from analogy. In this perspective, cases do not speak for the whole, as the statistical notion of representativeness entails, but for a bigger set of cases with which they share relevant features: they are a diminished version of the synecdoche (Cardano, 2020).

Having clarified this, I now explain what constitutes a case for this study. In order to try to elaborate an answer to my research questions, I knew I had to focus on those institutions that are involved—to different degrees and with different functions—in the treatment of psychiatric crisis, and more generally in the provision of mental healthcare. The observation of acute psychiatric wards (SPDC) is relevant to this purpose because—especially for the "restraint" model, as we will see in the next chapters—they represent the appointed location to host patients going through an acute phase of illness. SPDCs are located in general hospitals and admit both new and already known patients, voluntarily or involuntarily, coming from the Emergency Room or on referral of the territorial psychiatrist. On the other hand, community Mental Health Centres (MHCs) are involved in the prevention of crisis, in the management of the post-crisis phase after the discharge from the hospital, and in the decisions concerning involuntary admissions. In the case of "no-restraint" model, some MHCs also have to opportunity to directly manage crisis by hosting patients in their own facilities, outside of the hospital. This led me to support the inclusion of Mental Health Centres in my study, with the additional aim of understanding the role that these services hold in the two models under consideration.

The concrete empirical contexts that hosted the research, identified as information-rich cases that could function as best examples of the studied phenomenon, are the following. The first case, representing the "restraint" model, comprises an acute psychiatric ward, which I will call the Pine Ward, and a Mental Health Centre I call the Cedar Centre. Both are located in a medium-sized city in Piedmont, capital of that province and centre of management for the local Department of Mental Health. The Pine Ward shares many features of the average Italian psychiatric wards in terms of number of beds, hospital location, and professional figures employed. It is a sixteen-bed unit—with two extra beds for Day Hospital—provided with seven double rooms and two single ones. In line with the 'restraint' model, its doors are permanently locked, and mechanical restraint appears to be routinely adopted to manage specific situations (e.g. psychomotor agitation), both from the quantitative data (collected prior to the beginning of fieldwork) and from the observations on the field. The Cedar Centre is a mental health centre whose characteristics are very typical of the "restraint" model. Like every other centre in Piedmont, it is open from 8 to 18 on weekdays, and from 8 to 13 on Saturdays; on Sundays and holidays it is closed. It does not have the opportunity to host inpatients because it is not provided with any sleeping accommodation. The staff is much less numerous than that of the psychiatric ward, comprising four psychiatrists, five nurses (one of which is working part-time), one nurses-coordinator, and one social worker.

The second case observation represents the "no-restraint" model and consists of one acute psychiatric ward, the Iris Ward, and two mental health centres, the Tulip Centre and the Violet Centre. In this case as well, all of the three services are located in a medium-sized city—this time in the region of Friuli Venezia Giulia—capital of that province and centre of management for the local Department of Mental Health. The Iris Ward is very much similar—and therefore comparable—to the Pine Ward and to other Italian psychiatric wards. It is located in the city general hospital, and it can host up to fifteen inpatients. Besides capacity, the professional figures employed are typical too: psychiatrists, nurses, and healthcare assistants (OSS). The ward is characterized by both of the aspects typical of 'no-restraint' contexts: it does not adopt mechanical restraint, and it is an open-door space (i.e. its doors are open both to exit and to enter the ward twelve hours a day). The Tulip Centre and the Violet Centre are open twenty-four hours per day and seven days a week. Each of them is provided with eight beds to host patients, and they both can admit involuntary patients. The professional figures employed are psychiatrists, nurses, healthcare assistants, social workers, psychologists, and educators. The two centres are situated in the urban context, even though in different parts of the city: respectively the northern and the southern one. This division has direct consequences on the vastness and

Table 4.1 Empirical contexts typology

	SPDC (Acute psychiatric ward)	MHC (Mental Health Centre)
"Restraint" Dep. of Mental Health	Pine Ward	Cedar Centre
"No-Restraint" Dep. of Mental Health	Iris Ward	Tulip Centre Violet Centre

the characteristics of the users, who are assigned to one or the other centre according to the neighbourhood they live in. To consider them both allowed me to cover the entire city, avoiding getting a partial perspective.

Some similarities between the two contexts have been considered fundamental for their comparison. The main one is the size and capacity of the SPDCs. The second, related aspect was that of the proportion between inpatients and staff units at work during a shift. The Iris Ward is similar—with respect to number of beds and staff units per shift—to the Piedmontese wards and, I would add, to the average Italian ones. This similarity represents an important argument for the suitability of my case selection and for preserving the eloquence of my case.

In Table 4.1, I provide a synthetic representation of the empirical contexts which were part of my case study, classified according to the kind of service (psychiatric ward or mental health centre) and the (restraint or no-restraint) model they wish to be eloquent examples of.

4.3 Feeling the Field

The very first contact I have had with mental health and illness was in 2015, when I did a curricular internship on a local association of mental health service users during my Master's degree course. At the beginning, I saw it mostly as an occasion to put into practice what I have learned in the methodological classes: I was eager to conduct my first interview—I remember buying my recorder for the occasion, hoping that it would not be the first and only time to use it for research purposes—and I searched for the perfect notebook in order to prepare for the first day of participant observation. It proved unsuitable—fancy, but definitely too small—after one hour on the field. The association meeting I was attending, on the other hand, was unexpectedly curious and introduced me to a fascinating but delicate world. Few months later, one of the association leaders—and also the first person I have ever interviewed—took his own life after a couple of previous serious attempts. The association parades, music events, and art exhibitions clash in my memories with the pain and the sense of helplessness I felt the day of his funeral, where besides family and friends there were psychiatrists and mental healthcare workers who knew and cared for him. "What does this mean for them? How are they coping with their patients' suicide? What can psychiatry do with so much suffering?", I asked myself. I knew almost nothing about emergency psychiatric wards and mental disorders back then. In that same year, 2015, a man in my city died while being forced onto an ambulance and taken to hospital for mandatory treatment.[1] The tragic event was greatly debated, and during my fieldwork, I found that even outside of Piedmont it is still remembered when asking for cautious police interventions.

Coercive measures which involve the use of force—such as compulsory admission, involuntary treatment, and mechanical/physical/chemical restraint—represent a historically controversial aspect of psychiatric practice and a crucial point that touches upon the very role of psychiatry in our societies. These topics call into question a number of broad sociological issues which have always been of particular interest for me: the definitional mechanisms underlying the notions of health and illness and their evolution over time; the boundary-making of normalcy and deviancy; and the practices through which power and social control are exerted. Then, the opportunity to participate in an interdisciplinary, starting-out research project on mechanical restraint and involuntary treatment represented for me an invaluable opportunity to look into the themes I was passionate about and to grow as a junior researcher.

[1] His name was Andrea Soldi, he was 45 years old, and he suffered from schizophrenia. He died on August 5, 2015, in Turin, after the violent intervention of municipal police officers who were there to execute a mandatory medical treatment ("*Trattamento Sanitario Obbligatorio*", TSO). The police officers and the psychiatrist have been convicted for his death in October 2020, with a sentence (*Corte d'Appello*) of one year and six months.

I entered a psychiatric ward for the first time in December 2018, after the presentation of the preliminary results of the epidemiological study on involuntary treatment and mechanical restraint in Piedmont which took place in a regional hospital. I did not know what to expect, and I was feeling a bit anxious as I waited to get through that closed door and meet the unknown. Also, I was worried that my behaviour could be perceived as inappropriate by the professionals working there and by the patients I was expecting to meet. That first visit was quick—it lasted about ten minutes as a nurse showed me and my colleagues around—and yet some relevant aspects of that space were immediately evident: the closed doors, the empty spaces, the apparent absence of activity in the patients' rooms. A TV screen protected by a thick glass and an empty bookcase caught my attention as I had a look at the living room while walking down the corridor: no one was there. Then, there was silence: none of the confusion, voices, and sounds that are typical of a hospital ward were present. "Is this always so quiet?", I asked myself as I was about to leave the place. As we were approaching the door, a middle-age man came to us, kissing our hands, and insisting to hug one of us. The nurse scolded him—I thought—like he was a little boy used to that kind of behaviour, then asked him to "leave the ladies alone". I felt embarrassed for that act of infantilization and was unsure about the proper reaction. By the way, the visit was over and one minute later, the ward door closed behind our backs.

One month later, together with the Turin research team, I spent four days in two no-restraint psychiatric wards in the Friuli Venezia Giulia region, during a preliminary rapid ethnography meant to help us getting a sense of the organizational features of a no-restraint context. Not only it was my first, prolonged time in an acute psychiatric setting, but it was also my first experience as an ethnographer. I tried to remember everything I had learned about participant observation, and yet I was immediately confronted with the difficulties and doubts specific to that field: was it ok to ask to participate in the clinical interviews? was it appropriate to talk to the inpatients, and how could I explain our presence there properly? would it be better to observe the professionals' activities or to ask as many questions as I could in those few days? I felt weird wandering around the hall, writing notes, making probably the most banal inquiries to the healthcare workers I met. Two elements were determinant in helping me out: the co-presence of my team-mates, and the welcoming ward staff who understood how unfamiliar their world was to me and dedicated time to make me feel more comfortable.

In March 2019, I started my fieldwork in the Pine Ward. On my very first day, I remember feeling a bit more confident because of the short experiences in the previous months, but still I was not sure of what to expect. I guess I entered the field with a slightly naïve approach, for which on my second day of fieldwork I got a reprimand from the ward head as I was sitting in the hall among some inpatients without the supervision of the staff. Fear was not among the feelings I approached that context with, and I experienced it only in few very specific situations I will explore further in the next chapters. I understand, in retrospective, that the ward head's behaviour was probably due to a legitimate concern for having there, for the first time, an inexperienced young female researcher whose safety was under her responsibility. The staff did not know me and did not know what to expect from my presence, just like I did not know them and their world. I was in the first stage of the fieldwork, when the observational roles are reversed and the observer becomes the observed (Cardano, 2011). Day after day, the trust they placed in me gradually grew and I tacitly obtained permission to move freely, unsupervised around the ward.

A dedicated reflection upon my orientation towards mechanical restraint—which I observed in this ward—is needed. I approached this topic without having a clear idea about the concrete features of this practice. Of course, it does not convey particularly positive feelings: it recalls practices that a lay person associates with psychiatric hospitals, abuse and torture. Even today's press deals with this issue only when reporting about terrible outcomes, accidents, or crimes: the death of Francesco Mastrogiovanni is probably the most famous example of this. Most people do not even know that mechanical restraint is still used in most of the Italian psychiatric wards, and I have to say I was one of them: I was not able to quantify the spread of such practice. The encounter with it had a double effect. On one hand, it was certainly disturbing: this was particularly true for those cases I thought could have been managed differently if more human resources were available, for periods of restraining that I considered too prolonged, and for associated humiliating conditions, such as being exposed to the sight of other people, sometimes partially naked, unclean, unable to move. Mechanical restraint exposes the patient to an extreme form of vulnerability which I think is a duty of healthcare workers to minimize as much as possible, considering the acknowledged risks associated with it (Kersting et al., 2019) and the traumatizing experience it can represent for both users and the staff performing it (Bonner et al., 2002). On the other hand, spending time in such contexts allowed me to—at least partially—understand the difficulties and the needs of those who work there. Along their career, they have certainly normalized this practice: I have been exposed to it only for three months and yet sometimes I have found myself considering it part of that routine. Moreover, restraint does not always mean humiliation or lack of relation: attention can be paid to the subjective experience of the restrained person, and acts of practical compassion (Brown et al., 2014) aimed at ameliorating the user's condition are part of the routine too (see Sect. 6.3.3 in Chap. 6). I have seen how relationship can be, and usually is, maintained through tough phases, including restraint. This certainly articulated the opinion I could have had on the topic before this research. Nevertheless, my experience in the no-restraint context showed me that alternative ways to tackle crisis can be possible: they are certainly not free from contradictions and open issues—such as the use and debatable preferability of other forms of restraint, or the question of translation and re-localization of practices to other (culturally and organizationally different) contexts—but they are there. It is necessary, I think, to publicly and critically approach this issue—without demonizing it or downplaying its ethical relevance—in order to improve the kind of mental healthcare that our society is able to offer today.

Moving from the "restraint" to the "no-restraint" case, in the Iris Ward, I was not given any particular limit, maybe because I had already spent a couple days there some months earlier during the rapid ethnography with the Turin research team. I have had the opportunity to participate in clinical interviews from the very first day (exceptions were made for particularly sensitive situations, of course, in both of the wards), and I was never told to avoid talking to patients: instead, I was given the opportunity to ask them questions during medical encounters, and I was encouraged to talk individually to those whose experience was considered "sociologically interesting" by the staff. The eventual presence of inpatients I had to pay special attention to—that is, because they have had unpredictable or aggressive behaviour—was signalled to me every time as I arrived in the ward in the morning. These warnings were similar to the updates that were routinely given to the colleagues of the incoming shift, and even if they implied a protective purpose, I did not perceive them as an attempt to scare me or dissuade me from conducting my observation the way I saw fit. In the Iris Ward, my interaction with the psychiatrists was more intense, because contrary to the Pine Ward they stay for most if not all of their shift inside of the ward, they spend a lot of time working with nurses and they share with them convivial moments such as coffee breaks, which I regularly took part in.

The mental health centres are very different contexts than the psychiatric wards, first of all because they are not located within hospitals. The Cedar Centre is placed in a one-floor building along with other services: the eating disorders department, the administrative offices of the Mental Health Department, and the so-called 'Centro Diurno', a day centre dedicated to patients who can have lunch there, join some activities (such as short trips, afternoons at the local swimming pool, or artistic workshops) or simply spend their days there watching television, reading and enjoying each other company. Most of the time I spent at the Cedar Centre was quite relaxed because we have not been confronted with crisis, and routines are much less frenetic than in the psychiatric ward. This made room for more private and calm conversations with patients and professionals, and supported a peculiar development of relationships with the latter. Downtime between appointments, shared lunches, and car rides toward patients' houses, therapeutic communities or the ward were valuable opportunities for informal exchanges, both around the topic of my study and more personal issues. It was not unusual to extend conversations way beyond the closing time of the centre, assisted by long summer days. It is no coincidence, I guess, that with some people I met at that time I am still in contact, for personal purposes and projects collateral to this research.

The Violet Centre was my first context of observation for the 'no-restraint' model. Their style of working appeared unfamiliar to me the moment I stepped in: the place was much more crowded than the Cedar

Centre, not only because the day centre and the mental health centre are physically undistinguishable and so a lot of patients inhabit that space for different purposes, but also because the opportunity they have to admit up to eight inpatients determines many more professionals at work in every shift. Despite the initial disorientation, I was kindly welcomed by the group of psychiatrists I was first introduced to from the head of the department, and by the nurses I met shortly after. Most of them expressed their interest for the study and willingness to answer the countless questions I had those first days. As for the Iris Ward, my participation in their activities was never precluded; even in potentially dangerous situations—such as a car trip around the city with a psychotic and unpredictable patient—they maintained an open disposition, warned me about the risks and let the decision to join them up to me.[2] Several occasions of informal conversation occurred, especially during lunches in the centre's kitchen, car trips for home visits, and the night shift I joined.

The Tulip Centre was the last mental health centre I visited during my research. The general welcoming I received there felt a bit less friendly and warm than the other contexts, both in the "restraint" and the "no-restrain" model. This can be explained by many factors: the leading figures that usually introduce guests to the other workers were absent (the role of the head of the centre was vacant, while the nurses' coordinator returned from holidays on the penultimate day of my fieldwork); I was not the only "stranger" whom they had to dedicate time and attention to (a resident psychiatrist and a family doctor under training were there as well);[3] nurses and healthcare assistants are very numerous (thirty-five) and I did not have the opportunity to meet most of them for more than two or three times, hindering the development of relationships; the physical structure of the building, which is spread over four floors, does

[2] The not-so-frequently deep and prolonged crisis this boy was undergoing put the Violet Centre's professionals under much pressure. On one hand, this allowed the raising of many crucial issues I had the opportunity to discuss with them as they unfolded in front of my eyes. On the other hand, the time they dedicated to me and my questions despite the challenging situation counts double. For this, I feel deeply grateful to them.

[3] I also had the impression that for some nurses the constant presence of strangers was disturbing. In particular, I remember hearing the following exclamation as I was introduced to a nurse I met for the first time: "oh, so we also have sociologists now?". I understand the problem here was not about me personally, but nevertheless I did not perceive it as a pleasant welcoming.

not promote interaction because workers are usually dispersed, and isolated me as well from the people and activities I was not participating in. My participation to their activities was never precluded (except in cases where another one of the "strangers" was already participating and the presence of too many people was not appropriate, such as in medical encounters). I am not saying I perceived open hostility, but rather coldness and indifference sometimes. Of course, this is not true for every worker I encountered. Two young psychiatrists, an educator, and a couple of nurses have been especially kind and helpful: to them I am particularly thankful, and we have been glad to meet again later as I was conducting my observation in the Iris Ward and they came to visit their patients there. To conclude, no particularly critical situation was in place during the period of my observation, so besides informal conversations with some professionals and some home visits, I spent much time reading clinical records of patients who had been involuntarily admitted and who were indicated to me by their psychiatrists as having potentially interesting histories for the purposes of my study.

The last point I would like to touch in this reflexive account is about my relationship with patients, to whom I owe so much. Some of their experiences and stories touched me so deeply I am not sure how to report about it properly. To begin with, I would say that being confronted with their *sameness* was far more striking than meeting their *otherness*: emotions we are all familiar with sometimes felt just overwhelming, amplified, somehow unfiltered in their behaviours. In some of their stories, I saw myself, or someone I know, or someone I could have become in past moments of my life. I met most of the patients at a time of great vulnerability for them, that of crisis, and I consider myself privileged for having had the chance to listen to them. Of course, empathy was not always a friend of mine along the fieldwork: it happened to me to come home at the end of the day real broken, or sad, or bitter. The hardest moment was the unforeseeable attempted suicide, which had very serious consequences but death, of a twenty-year-old boy I met two weeks earlier, with whom I had discussed social constructionism as he had just graduated at a social sciences high school with a thesis on Berger and Luckmann. The news shocked me, I could not believe it, and I immediately found myself wondering the more stupid and useless question: "Could I have noticed? Is there something that I could have done?". I learned there—through the help and the preparedness of some professionals—about the importance to balance engagement and detachment to survive in such an emotionally challenging setting. On the field, I felt angry after having offered my help to a woman who answered by insulting me; I felt fear when confronted with the violent behaviour of a man; I felt panic when the guy sitting next to me during a medical encounter suddenly stood up and went to the window trying to open it to jump out of it, and I instinctively followed him to stop him. I believe that sharing such tense moments with participants really helped building a sense of strong—though temporary—closeness, of trust, and maybe a partial understanding—through ways that are different from the cognitive ones—of what it means to work in such unique context. I remember some of them saying to me, while recalling some complex situation that was difficult to explain to someone external: "You saw it, you were there, you know what it feels like". I was there, yes. I guess this is the most prosaic thing to say about ethnographic research, and yet this was one of the more intense experiences I will remember for the rest of my life.

References

Åkerström, M. (2002). Slaps, punches, pinches—But not violence: Boundary-work in nursing homes for the elderly. *Symbolic Interaction, 25*(4), 515–536.

Allen, D. (2001). Narrating nursing jurisdiction: "Atrocity stories" and "boundary-work". *Symbolic Interaction, 24*(1), 75–103.

Babini, V. (2009). *Liberi tutti: manicomi e psichiatri in Italia: una storia del Novecento*. il Mulino.

Bonner, G., Lowe, T., Rawcliffe, D., & Wellman, N. (2002). Trauma for all: A pilot study of the subjective experience of physical restraint for mental health inpatients and staff in the UK. *Journal of Psychiatric and Mental Health Nursing, 9*(4), 465–473.

Brown, B., Crawford, P., Gilbert, P., Gilbert, J., & Gale, C. (2014). Practical compassions: Repertoires of practice and compassion talk in acute mental healthcare. *Sociology of Health & Illness, 36*(3), 383–399.

Buus, N. (2008). Negotiating clinical knowledge: A field study of psychiatric nurses' everyday communication. *Nursing Inquiry, 15*(3), 189–198.

Cardano, M. (2011). *La ricerca qualitativa*. il Mulino.

Cardano, M. (2020). *Defending qualitative research: Design, analysis and textualization*. Routledge.
Cetina, K. K., Schatzki, T. R., & Von Savigny, E. (Eds.). (2005). *The practice turn in contemporary theory*. Routledge.
Cussins, C. M. (1996). Ontological choreography: Agency through objectification in infertility clinics. *Social Studies of Science, 26*(3), 575–610.
Dell'Acqua, G., Norcio, B., de Girolamo, G., Barbato, A., Bracco, R., Gaddini, A., Miglio, R., Morosini, P., Picardi, A., Rossi, E., Rucci, P., & Santone, G. (2007). Caratteristiche e attività delle strutture di ricovero per pazienti psichiatrici acuti: i risultati dell'indagine nazionale "Progress Acuti". *Giornale Italiano di Psicopatologia, 13*, 26–39.
Denzin, N. K., & Lincoln, Y. S. (Eds.). (2017). *The Sage handbook of qualitative research*. Sage.
Di Lorenzo, R., Baraldi, S., Ferrara, M., Mimmi, S., & Rigatelli, M. (2012). Physical restraints in an Italian psychiatric ward: Clinical reasons and staff organization problems. *Perspectives in Psychiatric Care, 48*(2), 95–107.
Di Napoli, W., & Andreatta, O. (2014). A "no-restraint" psychiatric department: Operative protocols and outcome data from the "opened-doors experience" in Trento. *Psychiatria Danubina, 26*(1), 138–141.
Ferioli, V. (2013). Contenzione: aspetti clinici, giuridici e psico-dinamici. *Psichiatria e Psicoterapia, 32*(1), 29–44.
Foucault, M. (2006a). *History of madness*. Routledge.
Foucault, M. (2006b). *Psychiatric power: Lectures at the Collège de France, 1973–1974*. Palgrave Macmillan.
Gieryn, T. F. (1983). Boundary-work and the demarcation of science from non-science: Strains and interests in professional ideologies of scientists. *American Sociological Review, 48*, 781–795.
Goffman, E. (1961). *Asylums: Essays on the social situations of mental patients and other inmates*. Anchor Books.
Gomm, R., Hammersley, M., & Foster, P. (Eds.). (2000). *Case study method: Key issues, key texts*. Sage.
Goodwin, C. (1994). Professional vision. *American Anthropologist, 96*(3), 606–633.
Griffin, C., & Bengry-Howell, A. (2017). Ethnography. In C. Willig & W. Sainton Rogers (Eds.), *The SAGE handbook of qualitative research in psychology* (pp. 38–54). SAGE Publications Ltd.
Hamilton, B. E., & Manias, E. (2007). Rethinking nurses' observations: Psychiatric nursing skills and invisibility in an acute inpatient setting. *Social Science & Medicine, 65*(2), 331–343.

Jacob, J. D., Holmes, D., Rioux, D., & Corneau, P. (2018). Patients' perspective on mechanical restraints in acute and emergency psychiatric settings: A post-structural feminist analysis. In J. M. Kilty & E. Dej (Eds.), *Containing madness. Gender and 'psy' in institutional contexts* (pp. 93–117). Palgrave Macmillan.

Johansson, I. M., Skärsäter, I., & Danielson, E. (2006). The health-care environment on a locked psychiatric ward: An ethnographic study. *International Journal of Mental Health Nursing, 15*(4), 242–250.

Johnston, M. S., & Kilty, J. M. (2014). Power, control and coercion: Exploring hyper-masculine performativity by private guards in a psychiatric ward setting. In D. Holmes, A. Perron, & J. D. Jacob (Eds.), *Power and the psychiatric apparatus: Repression, transformation and assistance* (pp. 61–90). Ashgate Publishing, Ltd.

Katz, P., & Kirkland, F. R. (1990). Violence and social structure on mental hospital wards. *Psychiatry, 53*(3), 262–277.

Kersting, X. A. K., Hirsch, S., & Steinert, T. (2019). Physical harm and death in the context of coercive measures in psychiatric patients: A systematic review. *Frontiers in Psychiatry, 10*, 400.

Lamont, M., & Molnár, V. (2002). The study of boundaries in the social sciences. *Annual Review of Sociology, 28*(1), 167–195.

Lave, J., & Wenger, E. (1991). *Situated learning: Legitimate peripheral participation.* Cambridge University Press.

Law, J. (2010). Care and killing: Tensions in veterinary practice. In A. Mol, I. Moser, & J. Pols (Eds.), *Care in practice: On tinkering in clinics, homes and farms* (Vol. 8, pp. 57–72). transcript Verlag.

Mason, J. (2002). *Qualitative Researching*, 2nd Edition. London: Sage Publications.

Mauceri, S. (Ed.). (2017). "Contenere" la contenzione meccanica in Italia. Primo rapporto sui diritti negati dalla pratica di legare coercitivamente i pazienti psichiatrici nei SPDC. *A Buon Diritto—Quaderni.*

Mezzina, R. (2014). Community mental health care in Trieste and beyond: An "Open Door–No Restraint" system of care for recovery and citizenship. *The Journal of Nervous and Mental Disease, 202*(6), 440–445.

Morrison, E. F. (1990). The tradition of toughness: A study of nonprofessional nursing care in psychiatric settings. *Image: The Journal of Nursing Scholarship, 22*(1), 32–38.

Okin, R. (2020). The Trieste model. In T. Burns & J. Foot (Eds.), *Basaglia's international legacy: From asylum to community* (pp. 317–331). Oxford University Press.

Oliveira, T. T. S. D. S., Fabrici, E. P., & Santos, M. A. D. (2018). Structure and functioning of a mental health team of Trieste in its members' perspective: A qualitative study. *Psicologia em Pesquisa, 12*(2), 24–35.

Pilgrim, D. (2002). The biopsychosocial model in Anglo-American psychiatry: Past, present and future? *Journal of Mental Health, 11*(6), 585–594.

Pols, J. (2003). Enforcing patient rights or improving care? The interference of two modes of doing good in mental health care. *Sociology of Health & Illness, 25*(4), 320–347.

Prior, P. M. (1995). Surviving psychiatric institutionalisation: A case study. *Sociology of Health & Illness, 17*(5), 651–667.

Quirk, A., & Lelliott, P. (2001). What do we know about life on acute psychiatric wards in the UK? A review of the research evidence. *Social Science & Medicine, 53*(12), 1565–1574.

Quirk, A., & Lelliott, P. (2004). Users' experiences of inpatient services. In P. Campling, S. Davies, & G. Farquharson (Eds.), *From toxic institutions to therapeutic environments*. Gaskell.

Quirk, A., Lelliott, P., & Seale, C. (2006). The permeable institution: An ethnographic study of three acute psychiatric wards in London. *Social Science & Medicine, 63*(8), 2105–2117.

Ragin, C. C., & Becker, H. S. (Eds.). (1992). *What is a case?: Exploring the foundations of social inquiry*. Cambridge University Press.

Rhodes, L. A. (1991). *Emptying beds: The work of an emergency psychiatric unit*. University of California Press.

Rogers, A., & Pilgrim, D. (2014). *A sociology of mental health and illness*. McGraw-Hill Education UK.

Toresini, L. (2007). SPDC no restraint. La sfida della cura. In AA.VV., *I Servizi Psichiatrici di Diagnosi e Cura. L'utopia della cura in ospedale*. Edizioni Co. Pro.S, Caltagirone.

Working Party on Psychiatry and Human Rights. (2000). *White Paper on the protection of the human rights and dignity of people suffering from mental disorder, especially those placed as involuntary patients in a psychiatric establishment*. Strasbourg.

5

Crisis and Its Places: Boundary-making in and Around Mental Healthcare Services

Abstract The chapter explores the process of boundary-making, which constitutes and continuously redraws the map of today's mental healthcare services. The concept of boundary has become a classic thinking tool for social scientists because of its ability to capture the fundamental social process of relationality between many social phenomena, encompassing topics such as social and collective identity, professions and work, communities and spatial boundaries (Lamont & Molnár, The study of boundaries in the social sciences. *Annual Review of Sociology, 28*(1), 167–195, 2002). Beginning with the definition of the "hospital-community care" dichotomy, which has a long tradition in post-deinstitutionalization mental healthcare, I will then consider the symbolic boundaries drawn around the psychiatric ward as a permeable institution (Quirk et al., The permeable institution: An ethnographic study of three acute psychiatric wards in London. *Social Science & Medicine, 63*(8), 2105–2117, 2006), how its demarcation from the rest of the hospital is performed, and which are the properties and mechanisms concerning its permeability. Lastly, strategies employed to perform circulation work between the different services and to defend the shape (Strauss et al., *Psychiatric ideologies and institutions*. Transaction, 1981) of each of them will be discussed.

E. Rossero, *Care in a Time of Crisis*, https://doi.org/10.1007/978-3-031-34418-3_5

The dynamic nature of boundaries, namely the differentiation between entities, is evident if we think about how our everyday life has changed during the COVID-19 pandemic. Measures introduced to limit the spread of the virus implied a re-organization of our routines, including time, space, and modalities devoted to the domain of work. In particular, many workers saw the blurring of the boundaries of the domestic space, made visible through video calls with colleagues; and we saw the overlapping of areas that used to be clearly separated, such as that of paid work and that of private time spent for other activities. The latter issue resonates with the collapse of spatial and temporal boundaries associated with mobile devices, in particular. messaging apps, which require users to continuously negotiate their availability, drawing the boundaries between different relational contexts (Mols & Pridmore, 2021). This negotiation is called boundary work, a classification activity by which groups mobilize who they are, defining and defending themselves against other groups, drawing on cultural repertoires, narratives, and traditions that are available and therefore embedded in their environment (Lamont & Molnár, 2002). This is not only a mental accomplishment, but it is enacted through practical activities, including discursive and storytelling practices (Allen, 2001). In the present chapter, the boundary work performed around mental health services is articulated, beginning with the Italian reform that changed mental healthcare provision in terms of places and practices.

5.1 The Birth of Community Mental Health Services: A Historical Look at Italian Deinstitutionalization

The process of deinstitutionalization in Italy, which entailed the dismantling of long-stay psychiatric hospitals in favour of community mental health services, began in the early 1960s, with the birth of a radical movement inspired by the psychiatrist Franco Basaglia and some other critical psychiatrists. At that time, asylums' mission was defined in juridical rather than medical terms: dangerous behaviour was a criterion for commitment and the institution had mainly a custodial function aimed at incapacitating a social peril (Donnelly, 1992). In his seminal work, *Asylums* (1961), Erving Goffman described the social world of the American hospital inmates within the total institution: stripped of their previous roles, their lives were scheduled according to organizational needs, their identities mortified through physical as well as social abuse, and their existence confined within a close system with very limited access to the outer world. Similar conditions were detectable in European[1] as well as Italian psychiatric hospitals (Babini, 2009). On the same year of *Asylums*' publication—1961—Basaglia became director of the asylum of Gorizia, which represented the perfect example of the place of isolation described by Goffman: located at the edge of the country, at the border between Italy and Yugoslavia, its architecture consisted of gates, high walls, and locked doors, behind which six hundred patients were contained, many of whom against their will, tied to their beds or even kept in cages (Foot, 2015). In this setting, "therapy" consisted mainly of insulin shock treatment and electroshock, and mental disorders were thought to be chronic conditions requiring long-term care and segregation. In such context, Basaglia and the *équipe* working with him began with making concrete changes, such as the abolition of physical restraints, the use of personal clothes for inmates instead of the standard ones provided by the hospital, and the introduction of cupboards so that they could keep their personal belongings (Donnelly, 1992). By returning their identity equipment to the patients, these changes aimed at restoring the self, mortified as they entered the institution (Goffman, 1961). In fact, the works of both Erving Goffman and Michel Foucault, whose *Madness and Civilization* appeared in 1961 too, inspired Basaglia and provided him with a new lexicon employed to criticize the entire asylum system (Foot, 2014).

The radical reforms implemented in Gorizia transformed the mental hospital into a symbol, attracting activists as well as political and student movements of the 1960s. The work carried out in those years stimulated

[1] The situation within psychiatric hospitals was denounced publicly on the French journal *Esprit*, whose dedicated number titled *Misère de la psychiatrie* (1952) fostered debate throughout Europe (Babini, 2009).

rich discussions and theoretical reflections which, together with vivid accounts of the changes brought to the asylum, were published in two iconic collective books: *Che cos'è la psichiatria?* (Basaglia, 1967) and *L'istituzione negata* (Basaglia, 1968). Such "negated institution" through radically different practices, and the consequent exposure of contradictions concerning the treatment of madness and society as a whole, was the point of departure of a greater revolution: in 1971, Basaglia was offered to become director of the asylum in Trieste, which he and his group managed to downsize and eventually close down along the decade (Foot, 2014). This became a great experimental space, whose revolutionary significance went beyond the hospital's walls and into the city: through artistic and cultural initiatives, as well as communication and media strategies addressing public opinion, the "mad" was taken out among the "normal", in order to engage the external world which Basaglia considered fundamental to overcome the exclusionary nature of psychiatric institutions (Foot, 2015). During the 1960s and 1970s, the movement for the reform of mental healthcare spread elsewhere across the country, inspiring context-specific solutions in Perugia, Arezzo, Parma, and other cities. In 1978, the promulgation of Laws 180 and 833 ended the Italian asylum system and excluded any reference to dangerousness from the criteria for ordering the treatment of the insane, formally purging psychiatry's traditional responsibility of social control (Donnelly, 1992). Beyond its conceptual relevance though, the law was not easily implemented because of heterogeneous situations in terms of resources, staffing, political traditions, and culture across Italy (ibidem). Asylums had to be substituted by small (with a maximum of fifteen beds) inpatient wards located within general hospitals—conceived for the temporary treatment of acute phases of disorder—and community mental health centres dedicated to outpatient and territorial treatment. Nevertheless, continuity of care was not always achieved along this long transition, and the implementation of the reform was geographically uneven, being much influenced by the budget each region allocated to its developing mental health services (Trivelli, 2016). Regional disparities are still visible in terms of quality of care provision, availability of services, and practices employed, which are the product of bottom-up processes and local initiatives, poorly coordinated by the central government

(Jones, 2000). With respect to the management of psychiatric crisis, today the most relevant differences pertain to the techniques adopted—which may or may not entail mechanical means of containment—and the location of acute treatment—the psychiatric ward or, additionally, the mental health centre itself. Few Italian mental health departments have mental health centres open twenty-four hours a day, provided with beds and able to offer a stay alternative to the one at the hospital. Departments which do usually embrace the no-restraint philosophy—inspired by John Conolly (1856) and Franco Basaglia himself—entailing the abolition of mechanical means of restraint and the open-door policy. No-restraint psychiatric wards were twenty-one in 2015 (Rossi & Toresini, 2015) and currently represent 5% of Italian psychiatric wards.[2]

5.2 A Fundamental Dicothomy: *ospedale* Versus *territorio*

The last two decades of the twentieth century, after the international deinstitutionalization process, saw the development of a debate on the relative weight to be accorded to modern hospital care (as opposed to traditional, long-term care provided in former psychiatric institutions) and community care in the new mental healthcare system. Except for extreme positions supporting the exclusive provision of care in community services, systems have historically evolved toward a model of balanced care (Thornicroft & Tansella, 2002), provided as close to the local population as possible in community settings, with the opportunity to quickly resort to short-term hospitalization when necessary.

This model of balanced care has been implemented in Italy as well: legislation (Law 180/1978, article 6) establishes that mental healthcare is normally to be provided by community services outside of the hospital, while conditions requiring hospitalization are to be treated in specific wards called "*Servizi Psichiatrici di Diagnosi e Cura*", which are located in

[2] This information is reported on the online spaces of the association called "Club SPDC no restraint", such as the following: https://180gradi.org/salute-mentale/180gradi/spdc-no-restraint (accessed on 3 December 2022).

general hospitals but are also part of the territorial Mental Health Departments in order to guarantee the continuity of care.

Community care is usually performed by multidisciplinary *équipes* composed of psychiatrists, nurses, social workers, rehabilitation specialists, and psychologists, and organized in territorial, residential, and semi-residential activities. Territorial activities are coordinated by Mental Health Centres (*Centri di Salute Mentale*, CSM) in terms of clinical, preventive, and rehabilitative interventions. Visits, drugs administration, clinical interviews, and other activities are, at the national level, performed in the MHC (75.8%), at patients' homes (8.6%), or elsewhere in the community (prison, general hospital, other facilities) (Ministry of Health, 2021). With respect to residential activities, cases requiring long-stay care can be referred by Mental Health Centres to public or private residential facilities, which provide therapeutic and rehabilitative programs at different levels of specialized staff intensity (twenty-four-hour staffed, day-staffed, or low-staffed residential care). Semi-residential services, such as the so-called "*Centri Diurni*", provide day-time rehabilitative and re-socializing activities carried out by specialized staff, offering the opportunity for people to have lunch, receive medication, or just "hang out".

Hospital care is provided in psychiatric wards with a maximum of 15 beds, as established by law. Such units admit both patients whose hospitalization has been arranged with the Mental Health Centre and people accessing the Emergency Room who may or may not be already in contact with the community services. Admissions can be on a voluntary or involuntary basis, according to the legislation disciplining compulsory treatment (*Trattamento Sanitario Obbligatorio*, TSO).

Using data from the report provided by the Italian Association of Psychiatric Epistemology (Starace & Baccari, 2020),[3] Table 5.1 synthetizes regional data concerning Piedmont and Friuli Venezia Giulia, in terms of community and hospital availability of facilities and number of beds, as well as average length of stay and percentage of patients re-admitted to hospital in 30 days after discharge ("revolving doors").

[3] The report in Italian can be found online: https://siep.it/wp-content/uploads/2020/12/SIEP-QEP-Volume-7.pdf (accessed on 3 December 2022).

Table 5.1 Community and hospital care in Piedmont and Friuli Venezia Giulia in 2018, overview (Starace & Baccari, 2020)

		Piedmont	Friuli Venezia Giulia
N. facilities (per 100,000 inhabitants)	**Territorial**	2.0 (-21.1%)	8.4 (+239.3%)
	Residential	7.0 (+86.9%)	10.0 (+166.8%)
	Semi-residential	1.2 (-29.5%)	14.6 (+789.5%)
N. beds (per 100,000 inhabitants)	**Hospital**	9.7 (+0.1%)	3.5 (-64.1%)
	Residential	97.3 (+90.2%)	37.3 (-27.2%)
	Semi-residential	28.5 (-0.9%)	65.4 (+127.2%)
N. days hospitalization (average)		12.3 (-3.8%)	8.1 (-36.2%)
Re-hospitalization in 30 days ("revolving doors")		14.6% (+5.9%)	11.9% (-13.8%)

Besides each value, the percentage indicates the (positive or negative) deviation from the average national value.

Data show how community care is articulated differently in the regional contexts considered in this study. Piedmont is predominantly oriented toward residential care: its number of residential beds and facilities is significantly higher than territorial and semi-residential ones, and almost double the national value. Friuli Venezia Giulia, on the other hand, prioritizes semi-residential care, which is provided in mental health centres, "*Centri Diurni*" and territorial day hospital: both its semi-residential number of beds and facilities are two to eight times higher than the national value. With respect to hospital care, both regions present a lower number of days of hospitalization than the national one, even if Friuli Venezia Giulia is 32.4 percentage points below Piedmont: the latter seems here to rely on hospital care more than the former. The issue of "revolving doors", namely those patients who need re-hospitalization within 30 days from discharge, seems to be more relevant in Piedmont, where the value is above the national mean value while Friuli Venezia Giulia is below. In a nutshell, we can observe that hospital care seems to have a more prominent role in Piedmont than in Friuli Venezia Giulia and that community care is articulated differently in the two regions, the former being more oriented toward residential care, while the latter consistently invests on semi-residential care.

Given these regional differences, my experience on the field suggests that the dichotomy between hospital care (*ospedale*) and community care (*territorio*) is relevant in both the studied contexts, to the point that they can be (and frequently are) thought of as *two separate social worlds*. The distance between the two is perceived to be so vast by those who inhabit them that a psychiatrist working at the Cedar Centre but previously employed in a hospital psychiatric ward—whom I will call Giorgio—eloquently told me that "they [the occupation at the hospital and that in the community] are almost two different jobs". This is because, he explains, the perspective one can get from working in one of the two settings is extremely partial, due to the different activities they perform and the fact that the hospital context focuses on the acute phase of illness only. Partiality then seems to go hand-in-hand with enduring prejudices on the alleged counterpart: this is the case of frequent admissions and the phenomenon of revolving doors, usually seen by professionals who work in psychiatric wards as the product of poor community care, which fails to prevent crisis and to care for the patient outside of the hospital.

Excerpt 5.1. Giorgio (psychiatrist, Cedar Centre): I began working in a SPDC [in another city] and I always thought I would have worked in that context, so I applied for a job in the SPDC here. [...] Then I was called for a position at the Mental Health Centre, so I said: "ok, I'll try also the other side". While working in the SPDC I was one of those who always thought about the revolving doors, the patients who get in and out of the ward, as a failure of the community services... Than the Dantesque retaliation hit me [he laughs], and I ended up working here [at the Cedar Centre].

Interviewer: What about now, are you happy with this position or...?

Giorgio: I don't know, today I believe that... To polarize professional experiences like that, on one side or the other, maybe, it has some limits, they are almost two different jobs, you know. I think there are circumstances when, I mean, it would be better if everyone did both of the things.

The language adopted by Giorgio reiterates the *separateness* of hospital and community services, described as two opposite sides. They can be conceptualized as two separate, though cooperating, communities of practice (Lave & Wenger, 1991). The negative consequences of the one-sided viewpoint one gets from being a member of either the ward *or* the Mental Health Centre have been acknowledged as well by many participants who have been working in mental health services for more than thirty years, having experienced the organizational unity preceding the creation of two administratively independent health authorities (*Azienda Sanitaria Ospedaliera* and *Azienda Sanitaria Locale*) in the 1990s.[4] Michela, the chief psychiatrist in the Pine Ward, experienced a professional trajectory which is opposite to that of Giorgio, having worked for ten years in community services and then chosen the psychiatric ward to see the "acute side" and get a more complete picture of the mental healthcare system.

> *Excerpt 5.2.* Michela (chief psychiatrist, Pine Ward): I like the SPDC, I like that I have previously worked in the community and that I haven't lost that part as I still do some outpatient [private] activity. Sometimes community work alone seems to me a partial view of the situation, because when the patient is unwell you send him [to the SPDC] and see him later. My colleagues [at the Mental Health Centre] see their patients because they have night shifts here, but somehow there is no taking charge, no decision on therapies, so yes, I liked, I would do it [the transition from community to hospital care] again.

Both Giorgio and Michela acknowledge the partiality of a unilateral perspective and define their transition—respectively from hospital to community care and vice versa—as an opportunity to try or see the "other side", thus reinforcing the *ospedale–territorio* dichotomy. The fact that they have been members of both the communities, though in distinct moments of their professional career, provides them with an insight of the features and logics of the two settings, which is not something that the majority of the healthcare workers I met have experienced.

---

[4] Before that time there was a single professional *équipe* rotating on the different services, both hospital and community ones. Today, healthcare workers of the same mental health department either work in the hospital or in community services, and few of them have moved from one side to the other along their career.

The boundary between the two entities at the Cedar Center and the Pine Ward—representing the "restraint" case study—is discursively drawn as an *institutional boundary* (Kerosuo, 2003), deriving from the reorganization of mental healthcare in 1978 and focusing on the different tasks pursued by the hospital and the community services, the first one being centred around the acute phases of illness. This means that, in this case, the boundaries of the communities of practice are maintained consistently with the institutional boundaries established by the law, which attributes to the ward the domain of acute mental healthcare and to the Mental Health Centre that of non-acute one.[5] The preservation of this boundary is not questioned by the interviewees quoted above and their colleagues, who generally accept the division of labour between the services which followed the de-institutionalization. The permeability of this boundary in terms of professional trajectories, on the other hand, is debated: *équipes* working in one context or the other are distinct, and careers can entirely develop within a single service for both psychiatrists and nurses, potentially resulting in those partial, one-sided views reported by Giorgio and Michela.[6] A colleague of theirs, Carmela, clearly expresses the sense of isolation she feels within the ward, explaining why mental health personnel should work both in hospitals and the community, albeit without questioning the separation of the SPDC, its location in the hospital, and its function in treating acute phases of illness.

> *Excerpt 5.3.* Carmela (psychiatrist, Pine Ward): To be always confined in the hospital sometimes is claustrophobic to me, I mean you always think, because you only see the "inside" and never see the "outside", that the mentally ill, poor thing, will never heal, they will never get better, because you

[5] As we will see further in this chapter, in practice "acuteness" is not so easily determined and allocated, but can be (also strategically) debated, hosted in locations different than the ward, while, on the contrary, non-acute patients can be admitted to the SPDC or their stay at the hospital can be prolonged to the post-acuteness phase if transfer to the community is not promptly feasible.

[6] Besides the different activities performed by hospital and community services, the working activity differs also in terms of shifts: SPDC nursing staff is employed on both day and night shifts (except for individual motivated exceptions) on weekdays and holidays, while MHC nursing staff never works at the night, holidays, and whenever the centre is closed (Saturday afternoons and Sundays). This is partially true for psychiatrists as well, even though community doctors are on-call in the SPDC at night, weekends, and holidays just like their ward's colleagues.

> only see them when they are unwell, you don't see the other side of mental illness that is made of people who work, who have a family, who have fun outside and who—sometimes it happens—have to come "inside". [...] The fact that we are separated between ASO and ASL is a wrong concept for psychiatry, because psychiatry is continuity, continuity with the carer, it's trust, empathy between the patient and the carer, I see you outside and I see you also inside. [...] The SPDC should represent the place of care for acute patients, when I'm not able to manage you outside I lock you in, the terminology is bad but corresponds to reality, I lock you in so that you can recover and then I can let you out again, right? The personnel should do the same, working outside and inside. A single *équipe* rotating [on the two services].

The separation between the two communities, as Michela observes, is mitigated by occasions of interpenetration, such as the night and non-working days shifts that community psychiatrists do in the psychiatric ward. Besides ordinary interactions between hospital and the community (e.g. phone calls or meetings concerning specific patients), this organization of shifts—introduced to respond to an organizational need in terms of resources—allows MHC psychiatrists to have a first-hand experience of the job on the ward, including consultation for people coming to the Emergency Room and the decisions concerning their admission: this aspect, as we will see, is of paramount importance to the management of the ward, and also a typical issue around which conflicts between psychiatrists and nurses tend to emerge. These shifts constitute a practical form of connection and represent an area of overlap between the two (hospital and territorial) communities (Wenger, 1999).

The separateness between a psychiatric ward and a Mental Health Centre is thematized in the "no-restraint" context as well. As I began my fieldwork at the Violet Centre, asking questions about the difference between admitting patients to the SPDC or to the Mental Health Centre, I was immediately corrected about the use of terminology: admission (*ricovero*) was not the proper term to refer to the time patients spent at the Mental Health Centre, which was called accommodation or hosting (*accoglienza, ospitalità*) instead. This terminological choice, as I soon figured out, was not a casual preference but a linguistic act of boundary-making between the centre and the ward, aimed at distancing community services and their practices from hospital language and image.

Separateness is perceived and produced in the SPDC as well. In the following excerpt from the interview with Nadia, nurses' coordinator at the Iris Ward, we can read about past attempts to connect the two realms and the intrinsic difficulty for mental healthcare workers to represent themselves as part of a single community.

> *Excerpt 5.4.* Nadia (nurses' coordinator, Iris Ward): Some time ago we tried this exchange of personnel, nurses only, so we went in the Mental Health Centres and the [nurses working in the] Mental Health Centres came here, and I have to admit that it worked with respect to some tensions and some ideas that every service has about the other, you know? Because we all try to, I mean, we are a bit self-referential, it is not to say that I work better than you but…
>
> **Interviewer: You know better your [part of the job] …**
>
> Nadia: Yes, exactly. Today this exchange would not be feasible, everybody should do it, every worker [of the different professional groups] …
>
> **Interviewer: Do you think that the idea of a common *équipe* or one which rotates [on the different services] would be a good one?**
>
> Nadia: It could be a good idea, but it takes resources, it takes time, it takes a lot of things… It would require a completely different perspective on how services are organized, but instead every time I go to the meetings I see that everyone is firm in their positions, me included. I mean, you tend to carry on what you do, what you believe in, and be absolutely firm, you know? And sometimes we are rightly reminded that we are part of a Department, actually I feel part of a Department. But this is, yes, for many it is something that is difficult to put into practice.

What Nadia describes can be conceived as a boundary practice (Wenger, 1999), which sees SPDC and MHC nurses as regular visitors of one another community, exposing themselves to the reciprocal practices in an attempt to deal with their boundaries and (partially) reconcile their perspectives. Boundary practices do not always succeed in creating connections, and in this case they seem to have worked only to some extent, failing to overcome enduring prejudices and positions tied to each worker's membership of one community or the other.

In the "no-restraint" model, the boundary between hospital and community care is drawn on a prominent *ideological* basis, while the institutional dimension mentioned above and the consequent division of labour between hospital and community services are blurred through everyday care practices. The main challenge to the mainstream model of balanced care is constituted by the opportunity that twenty-four-hour Mental Health Centres have to host people in their acute phase of illness who would have been otherwise hospitalized. Both the Violet and the Tulip Centre have eight beds available for hosting their patients for more or less prolonged periods of time, including involuntary ones who are under TSO. This different organization of care provision is oriented to prioritize community treatment, claiming as its guiding principles those which inspired the reform in 1978 and equating "good care" with minimizing hospitalization and avoiding institutionalization. In fact, deinstitutionalization can be conceived not only as the historical process leading to the closure of psychiatric hospitals, but also as a daily care practice (Muusse et al., 2020). In the context I observed, this translates in the attempt to move patients from the hospital to the community as quickly as possible when clinically appropriate,[7] maintaining contact with the outside world throughout the hospital stay, and increasing the ward's permeability in both directions: patients temporarily leave the ward to attend activities in the community, while community staff enters the ward to build and discuss post-discharge programs.

The attempt to reduce the number of days spent in the hospital is not peculiar to the no-restraint context but is performed according to different logics. SPDCs—both in Piedmont and Friuli—always try to keep the length of the stay under a given number of days. This is due

[7] In specific cases, the hospital environment is deemed clinically more appropriate than the crowded, stimulating setting of the Mental Health Centre (see also Excerpt 6.11 about a community psychiatrist elaborating on this point).

to the managerial goals that physicians are asked to pursue in every hospital ward, according to a logic of productivity which also dictates the range within which the number of inpatients' nights on the ward should be kept (Cardano & Gariglio, 2021). This approach, which sees the influence of relevant company logics in everyday clinical decisions, has been observed in the wider Piedmontese context explored by the team ethnography, "Psychiatric interventions: About TSO and mechanical restraint": if a patient spends less than three nights in the hospital, the ward does not get any economic reward; hospital stays lasting more than twelve nights are equally inconvenient for the organization's managerial target, independently of the patient's clinical condition (ibidem). Consistently with this account, psychiatrist Giorgio (Cedar Centre) described to me how, in the Piedmontese ward where he used to work, their daily practice was influenced by an electronic counter, which displayed real-time average length of stay, forcing them to always keep in mind the ultimate goal to reduce that value. In the no-restraint context, this mechanism is inevitably operating as it is in the general Italian National Health Service (NHS), but the purpose to minimize the length of stay on the ward is rhetorically motivated on a different ground: "the main aim of the SPDC is to reduce as much as possible the stay at the hospital, according to the principle of territoriality of care".[8]

Even though the psychiatric ward is discursively assimilated and claimed to be part of the community, its placement in the general hospital makes it *something different* both from community services and hospital itself. The next paragraph investigates how this dual—but never full—membership of the SPDC is dealt with and reproduced in local mental healthcare workers' practices.

[8] This statement is translated from a poster, hung in the Iris Ward on a wall of the room where clinical interviews and other activities are conducted, which has been produced and exhibited at the national meeting of the "Club SPDC No-Restraint" in 2018. The original, written in bold, states: "*Obiettivo principale dell'SPDC è ridurre il più possibile la durata del ricovero ospedaliero, in linea col principio della territorialità della cura*".

5.3 "We Are in the Hospital, but We Are Not Hospital": A Narrative of "Otherness"

According to the Italian legislation, psychiatric wards are designed as intermediate services, located in hospitals but at the same time part of the territorial mental health departments. This dual membership can be a source of ambiguity and controversy when it comes to practices, rules, or routines, which may be closer to the community rather than the hospital pole (or vice versa) between which the ward lies. The characteristics of the space as well as the clinical conditions of the people it hosts qualify the SPDC as peculiar and somehow different from other hospital wards; but still, being physically and administratively part of the hospital, it is partially governed by norms in force in this organization. This complexity is increased when the hospital responds to a different health authority (called *Azienda Sanitaria Ospedaliera*) than the community services (which belong to the *Azienda Sanitaria Locale*) so that healthcare professionals employed in the same Mental Health Department formally work for two different organizations: this was the case of both the contexts observed in this research.

In the Pine Ward, this intrinsic duality is dealt with by univocally considering the SPDC part of the hospital and unproblematically calling it "*reparto*" (ward) by mental healthcare workers operating in and outside of the unit. Its location in the general hospital is considered an advantage by the psychiatrists who work there, who form a rather homogeneous group in terms of their pharmacological approach to mental illness. The "medical dimension" mentioned by Michela in the following excerpt indicates the biological approach characterizing this context, and the desired integration with other specialties and general mainstream medicine (Rogers & Pilgrim, 2014).

> *Excerpt 5.5.* Michela (chief psychiatrist, Pine Ward): It is definitely an advantage that you feel more in contact, since we are in the general hospital, with other specialties, you have relationships with other colleagues and it seems to have a more medical dimension, and maybe you also know about innovations sooner, especially from the pharmacological point of view.

On the contrary, in the no-restraint context, the SPDC is usually qualified as part of the community, calling into question issues pertaining to organizational identity, feasibility and safety of some practices (e.g. open door policy), and conflicting logics which call for a continuous re-positioning and negotiation of the ward's symbolic boundaries. On our very first visit to the Iris Ward as a team in January 2019, Nadia, nurses' coordinator, and Marzia, her vice-coordinator, introduced their service in the following terms.

> *Excerpt 5.6.* Nadia (nurses' coordinator, Iris Ward): We are part of the Mental Health Department, which is community, right? No, for the hospital health authority [*Azienda Sanitaria Ospedaliera*] and its medical director we are hospital, period. Indeed, if you go seeing our website it calls us SOPDC, "*Servizio Ospedaliero Psichiatrico di Diagnosi e Cura*" [Hospital Psychiatric Service of Diagnosis and Cure/Care], this "O" has been introduced some years ago, it wasn't there, it is a detail but in psychiatry you work with details. […] We have always been considered a fringe of the hospital, but we're not.

This introduction was then followed by a joint account of how, two years before, they have been asked—or, they suggest, forced—to participate with other hospital wards to a validation by the Joint Commission International, aimed at verifying if the hospital met international standards in terms of quality of care and patients' safety. After some initial resistance—they tell—they worked hard to formalize some procedures (e.g. those concerning injuries), update and revise administrative forms, and introduce changes that had been postponed for a long time, such as the integrated medical record, which combines the medical and the nursing observations, once separated.[9] More importantly for the purpose of this study, they used this opportunity to their own advantage, to officially claim their difference from the rest of the hospital, and to make their

[9] This is an important tool which helps integrating the two professional groups working within the ward, while at the same time remarking on the SPDC diversity from other hospital wards: the section of the medical record pertaining to the nursing staff was described as very much discursive, descriptive, and poorly parametrized (contrary to what happens with nursing observations in other medical specialties/wards).

practices visible and known to the outer world. This difference primarily stems from the characteristics of the patient admitted to the SPDC.

> *Excerpt 5.7.* Nadia (nurses' coordinator, Iris Ward): Our patient stands on his feet, wears normal clothes, he's not in his pyjamas, he's not a patient who stays in bed-
>
> Marzia (nurse, Iris Ward): He's not a patient who stays in his room, he's a patient who moves freely.
>
> Nadia: He's a free patient, he eats with the other patients, he doesn't eat alone in his room with a sad tray, but they eat all together in the dining room. These are really different conditions. [...] We benefited from this [evaluation] as we managed to put on paper, while meeting certain criteria, what we wanted to [...], which is part of our way of working and which is functional to the kind of people we host.

What has been described to us can be interpreted as a *practice of accountability*, namely a discursive practice by which this community of practitioners explained and justified their mode of working, making it accountable to other communities (Gherardi, 2006). Prior to that, the procedure entailed a reflexive effort—evident in Nadia words: "we've been able to acknowledge all of the work we already did but was a bit hidden"—and the production of a discourse about the community's pre-reflexive practice and tacit embodied knowledge which made them comprehensible both to themselves and others (ibidem). As the following quotations show, discourses on practices are also strongly tied to the celebration of identity and to the cultural and symbolical production of a community (ibidem).

> *Excerpt 5.8.* Nadia (nurses' coordinator, Iris Ward): There is a document [the evaluation report] which finally states who we are, what we do, that we are part of a Department, that we are no-restraint.
>
> *Excerpt 5.9.* Marzia (nurse, Iris Ward): The daily struggle [for recognition] was all there, on the paper really, in the bureaucracy, in order to say: "I work like this".

The success of this evaluation consists, in their account, less in having met the safety standards required by the Joint Commission International than in having had the chance to resist assimilation to the hospital and to formally assert their specificity and—to some extent—their *otherness* from the organization in which they are located.

> *Excerpt 5.10.* Marzia (nurse, Iris Ward): We have become visible in the hospital company, they didn't know who we are and this definitely distinguished us and our way of working, we managed to create procedures that are specific to us and different from hospital ones, even though they tried so hard to incorporate us into the hospital.

On a pragmatic level, being able to make their practices accountable, producing and providing data on the outcomes of their work, turned out to be a powerful and useful tool to justify their requests (e.g. in terms of human resources needs) and strengthen their position concerning delicate and usually conflictual issues, such as the admission requests coming from the Emergency Room. The admission of patients wearing medical devices (such as CVC and other catheters)—who fall in the category of organic patients—is an interesting example of such problematic questions, which can benefit from arguments rooted in safety discourses and able to account for the rejection of this kind of patient, as Nadia cunningly observes: "I respect safety criteria, and in fact because of those criteria now we can say that safety is not guaranteed for this, this and that reason [and therefore we cannot admit this kind of patient]". Clearly, these qualifications of patients' profiles and priorities can conflict and be debatable: which medical emergency prevails in someone suffering from both an organic and a mental ailment? Answers provided to this question, especially when it is not clinically evident which form of suffering has to be prioritized, are usually the result of conflicts and struggles between the SPDC and the ER professionals, in which strategies pertaining to ward's permeability and the defence of its boundaries are involved (see Paragraph 5.5).

Lastly, having ordered and formalized procedures and practices helps the Iris Ward staff instruct new colleagues, both nurses and psychiatrists, whose activities are now guided by protocols, albeit increasing paperwork as well as introducing a certain degree of rigidity. The rigidity–flexibility dichotomy is another cleavage along which the demarcation between hospital and community is maintained and performed in the no-restraint context. Procedures which are considered to represent a "too much hospital" approach by the Mental Health Department are frequent theatre of conflict. Incident reporting is a good example of this phenomenon: the following excerpts from fieldnotes describe two different but related episodes observed in the Iris Ward.

Excerpt 5.11. I go back to the medical room, where Franco [nurse] is reporting about an adverse event. He explains that this morning he made a mistake as he was administering drugs, giving to one patient the quetiapine he was supposed to give to someone else. The patient has then gone to the Tulip Centre as usual, but came back earlier on a wheelchair, sedated, his legs would not bear him. After having found out about his mistake, Franco fills in the report (it's called "incident reporting", he shows me how it is possible to report near-miss and not only accidents which have actually happened). He explains that this kind of mistakes can happen but can be very dangerous, and constant interruptions during the delicate activity of drugs administration are confusing and make errors more likely to happen. He doesn't seem agitated nor ashamed, he doesn't try to minimize his mistake; instead, he reports about it, saying that in psychiatry it is not a usual procedure: minor assaults, verbal and near-miss aggressions are taken for granted and considered part of the routine in psychiatry, so they are rarely reported. (Iris Ward, fieldnotes)

Excerpt 5.12. During a ward meeting the staff discusses about an audit scheduled in few days after an incident reporting concerning the mistaken administration of methadone to a patient.[10] It seems that the Department's chief psychiatrist disagrees with the incident reporting procedure and would like it to be as infrequent as possible. The procedure, Nadia [nurses' coordinator] observes, is anonymous and voluntary, and the Department director should not even be necessarily informed about it. She continues: "we have a hospital culture that Mental Health Centres and our director do

[10] This incident, occurred a couple of months earlier, was attributed to a lack of communication with the services treating drugs and alcohol addiction (SerD), which did not inform the ward about the service user's interruption of methadone treatment he used to be undergoing.

> not have, they are more naïf/philosophical", and: "we are the usual hybrids accused by the community to be too rigid. I am done going to meetings to play the Department's punching ball just because we are a pain their ass". [...] Franco [nurse] enters the conversation saying that few days ago when he administered the wrong drug he serenely reported it, both for transparency reasons ("there is nothing to hide") and because it can be an occasion to report if something general doesn't work. He adds that in every [medical] discipline, nurses are more inclined to incident reporting, while "medical profession is usually more reluctant because they live it like a questioning [of their job]". Doctors participating to the meeting do not comment. (Iris Ward, fieldnotes)

The first excerpt highlights how psychiatry is traditionally inclined not to report minor accidents because, Franco explains, they are expected to be part of the job. This opinion has been heard in the Pine Ward as well, where I have been told multiple times by different professionals that if they had to report every insult or minor act of violence, as established by the hospital protocols, they would have something to report every day.[11] Incident reporting is a hospital procedure which, Nadia observes, is not part of community culture nor appreciated by the Department. The definition of their service as "the usual hybrids" refers precisely to the dual membership of the SPDC, to its intermediate placement between the hospital and the community, rigidity and flexibility, standardization, and improvisation.[12] The department's pressures to be more flexible despite the hospital framework they work in are negatively commented on in an interview with Elettra, a young nurse working in the Iris Ward for five years.

---

[11] Data on the Pine Ward reported injures tell us that there occurred six in 2016, three in 2017, and three in 2018, all concerning mild to serious events such as thrusts, physical harm, or biological damage. Near-miss incidents can be reported since 2016 but are very rarely reported.

[12] The notion of improvisation does not indicate an unprepared course of action, but rather a skilled application of experience and knowledge to contingent situations requiring a degree of flexibility and creativity (Sparti, 2005, 2013). The concept will be employed and developed in Sect. 6.3.2 in Chap. 6 to indicate the way in which nurses in the Pine Ward approach immobilization and initiation of mechanical restraint of an aggressive person, adapting their tacit and embodied knowledge to the specificities and unpredictability of the situated event.

Excerpt 5.13. Elettra (nurse, Iris Ward): I realized that in my department's viewpoint, SPDC is considered part of the community, it's not hospital, you know?

Interviewer: But this is seen as an advantage as far as I have understood, like "we are physically in the hospital ma we're not hospital, we're community".

Elettra: Sure, it is an advantage, but what I wonder is: an advantage to whom? The patient or the organization, to consider the SPDC as community? It got me thinking, you know, because to be part of a hospital you have to follow certain rules. This is my own interpretation, but what I have noticed in these five years in this Department is that rules are constraints, constraints prevent you from doing many things, but /psychiatry is waiting to be discovered, right?/ [ironic]. It doesn't need rules, which may seem mere obstacles. But if I think of a service which works on the emergency, psychiatric emergency, it has to be located in a hospital, in its organization, it has to be in the hospital! Because patients here take risks that are equal to those of the hospital, so...

Interviewer: And rules here are avoided? Can you give me an example?

Elettra: Yes, sure! We have a big problem here that is drug administration when patients are discharged. [...] The hospital ward is not designated to provide patients with drugs to be taken at home, there are other services, the Mental Health Centre, but if we discharge a new patient who has a medical appointment [some days later at the MHC]-

Interviewer: He's not a patient of theirs yet...

Elettra: [She nods and then cites the MHC] "We do not administer drugs to people we do not know", so the MHC backs out, maybe it's Friday and the general practitioner is not available, the doctor on call...

Interviewer: /He's the doctor on call/ [she laughs].

Elettra: The doctor on call is the doctor on call, so in the end SPDC personnel cuts blisters, therapies. We've been told that all of this can be done, but according to…

Interviewer: The MHD [Mental Health Department].

Elettra: Exactly. If we, if the hospital knew about this, I mean…

Interviewer: You couldn't do this.

Elettra: No, because we have to follow some procedures, some protocols developed to safeguard patient's safety.

Interviewer: So, you're kind of divided in two…

Elettra: Exactly, we are not safe.

Flexibility and improvisation are a leitmotif of the work in the Mental Health Centre. In a recently self-published book I have been gifted with on my first visit to the Department's Direction, which brings together reflections and narrations of different actors who participated in the transformation of local mental healthcare services towards deinstitutionalization, we can read: "we like to think that we work at the margins, in a middle ground without borders, in an open port through which people pass as they look for a place to land, a road along which they can travel, a destination to reach. […] Human relationships go beyond institutional boundaries. To work in a mental health centre sometimes seems like an indefinite work where operative choices are not 'a matter of protocol'". Accounts of how the Violet Centre has been transformed and opened twenty-four hours a day, overcoming initial doubts and fears, revolve around the topic of redrawing boundaries: "We've had a lot of meetings before opening the 24-hours [MHC], we developed regulations, guidelines with well-established limits, such as that users could not be hosted [admitted] during the night, over the weekends, or on Fridays in order to allow the staff to understand the situation better during the week when there was more personnel, but one at a time these limits have been dismantled by healthcare workers themselves". And also: "Flexibility, elasticity, exception, were becoming increasingly common words in our meetings". This complex accomplishment, which combines structure and improvisation, is a fascinating element of community mental healthcare work. Its outline is here provided to represent an additional element of conflict and demarcation between SPDC and the community, which contributes to shaping the positioning of the ward in relation to the rest of the hospital.

To conclude on this topic, I wish to underline how in the Iris Ward, otherness-from-the-hospital is performed also on a linguistic ground—the SPDC is never called "ward" but "service" or, colloquially, *Diagnosi*—and on a symbolic one made immediately visible by the psychiatrists' appearance, as they do not wear the classic white coat but ordinary clothes and a simple ID badge, as I used to do on the field. This is a direction given by the Mental Health Department, which not every healthcare worker agrees with, and which also signals a disparity between medical and nursing figures.

> *Excerpt 5.14.* I go back to the ward corridor with Patrizia, a nurse who spent her whole career working in mental health. A patient walks by, observing that physicians not wearing the white coat can be easily confused with other patients or strangers in the ward if one does not know them already. Patrizia agrees with him saying that we are in a hospital and that physicians should wear the white coat for reasons of clarity, just like nurses wear their uniform. She explains this is a MHD direction, but that she disagrees. (Iris Ward, fieldnotes)

The medical staff, on the contrary, seems to be aligned with the department's position and more aware of the symbolic value of this choice. In a playful conversation between Paolo, a young psychiatrist, and Antonio, a nurse who has been working in the SPDC for a couple of years, the latter observed that the former was not wearing a coat and made fun of him: "What kind of doctor are you?" Paolo promptly replied: "Actually, I haven't yet understood why you're still wearing a uniform!" The psychiatrist does not only agree with the dismissal of the classic medical symbol, but suggests mental healthcare nurses should abandon their uniform too, performing their otherness from fellow hospital nurses. I later discussed this verbal exchange with Emma, chief psychiatrist of the Mental Health Department, who showed to be proud of Paolo's answer and was quite worried about the lack of reflexivity entailed in Antonio's naïve question.

In the Pine Ward, the issue of the white coat takes on a completely different character. Psychiatrists working in the SPDC regularly wear it: they put it on as they enter the ward and take it off as their shift is over and they leave. The medical office outside the ward, where psychiatrists spend most of their time when they are not busy with clinical work, has a coat rack by the door where each doctor's white coat is hung. Community psychiatrists, when they have their night or non-working day shifts, generally wear it even though they do not do it at the Mental Health Centre. This suggests that despite their territorial membership, rules and routines pertaining to hospital setting are acknowledged and uncontested, and that SPDC is not considered as other-than-hospital, but as a fully fledged hospital ward. Also, the figure of the psychiatrist is not performed, at least on a symbolical level, as different from other medical specialists, whose "dress code" is respected. Adherence to hospital routines and symbols emerged also on my arrival at the Pine Ward, when I have been offered a white coat twice: from the nurses' coordinator and from a psychiatrist I met for the first time some days later. The following excerpt describes the former episode.

> *Excerpt 5.15.* As I speak with Carmela [psychiatrist], Angela, the nurses' coordinator, arrives. I introduce myself and the study, Carmela tells her to give me a tour of the ward and introduce me to the rest of the staff. [...] Angela accepts and opens the closet to get me a coat, but I tell her that I have taken my badge and if it is fine for them I would rather use that only. Angela agrees saying that patients could otherwise confused me with a doctor and stop me. I add that it doesn't seem correct to me [as I am not a doctor], Carmela agrees too. (Pine Ward, fieldnotes)

Such symbolic adherence with hospital codes does not mean, though, that the SPDC does not have its rules and practices which differ from a common ward: the possibility for patients to smoke, for example, is an evident exception, whose rationale is accepted both in the restraint and the no-restraint context (see also Sect. 6.1 in Chap. 6 on the role and management of smoke in the wards).

We can synthetize what has been said so far by observing two different strategies to approach SPDC's dual membership and inherent ambiguity. If we image a continuum linking hospital and the community, the restraint context places the SPDC in a position which is closer to the "hospital" pole. It does so by adopting practices and terminology which are typical of the hospital setting, such as the wearing of white coats and uniforms, and the common-use labels "ward", "admission", and "discharge". In the no-restraint context, the SPDC seems to be a site of tougher definitional struggles: while the hospital tries to absorb this unit by pushing it toward local standards and adjusting its name to "SOPDC", the community-oriented department asks for flexibility which is not always unproblematic to adopt. Healthcare workers operating in the Iris Ward are not homogeneously oriented toward one position or the other: while some professionals fought to institutionalize SPDC's otherness within the hospital, but still defend their procedures and practices in front of a department that usually blames them to have a "too much hospital" approach, other professionals question the "ideological" requests posed by the community and support their membership to the hospital in the name of patients' and staff's safety.

5.4 Places of Crisis: Institutional Maps and Wards' Shape

The SPDC's dual membership and the different strategies employed to deal with its specificity in the two cases observed reveal that two different *institutional maps* are in place in the restraint and the no-restraint context.

The notion of institutional map is drawn from Anselm Strauss and colleagues' work *Psychiatric ideologies and institutions* (1981, or. ed. 1964), an investigation on psychiatric ideologies and their daily practice conducted in three mental hospitals in Chicago. This concept was used by the authors to indicate a generally shared conception of a hospital's internal locales—such as the acute and the chronic, female and male, industrial and infirm wards—which guided patients' allocation as they were admitted to the hospital. Here, I adopt the notion of an institutional map to refer to the set of services which constitute a Mental Health Department or collaborate closely with it: psychiatric wards, mental health centres, residential and semi-residential facilities, as well as private clinics operating in agreement with the National Health Service. At different moments and phases of their illness and life trajectory, which is by no means linear nor completely predictable, patients may pass through these different places according to therapeutic pathways planned with their psychiatrist and other professionals. The process of allocation,[13] as I have observed it on the field, is usually a site of conflict and negotiation between the actors working in the different services, both for practical reasons (e.g. lack of resources and shortage of beds) and symbolic ones, pertaining to the functions and purposes attributed to each specific service, which do not necessarily align among the professionals involved.

Indeed, Strauss et al. (1981) further suggest how mental healthcare workers in different positions within the institutional map are likely to see their own and other services differently, so that the allocation of a certain kind of patient may not meet with general approval. Personnel's conceptions and ideas about how their ward is or ought to be, what kind of patients is proper to the ward, which behaviours are appropriate, and what its place is in the institutional map, constitute the *shape* of the ward (ibidem). Shape responds to the staff's need to maintain order and manage the ward successfully despite continuous changes in both patients and personnel, and it influences staff's working strategies as their try to defend their ward from the admission of people who do not belong to it. In this paragraph, I will consider how the specificity of the psychiatric

[13] The term "allocation", used by Strauss et al. (1981), implies a decision on the patient's destination, which is entirely in the psychiatrist's hands. This does not seem to fit current mental healthcare practice because today therapeutic decisions are shared within multidisciplinary teams, negotiated among professionals working in different services, and most importantly discussed with the person concerned. Nevertheless, verbs such as *sending*, *putting*, *placing*, and *selling* patients to the different facilities remain common in everyday professional discourses. I have therefore chosen to use here the term "allocation" to the extent it helps me highlighting the complex and pressing work performed by (especially community) psychiatrists in finding the appropriate—though temporary—place for the patients they care for, but its use does not necessarily imply a unilateral, individually centred decisional process.

ward is determined, defended, and practiced, drawing on Strauss' notions of institutional map and ward's shape.

In the restraint context, the place of the SPDC in the institutional map is that of the setting designated to treat crisis par excellence. The ward admits people coming from the hospital Emergency Room, from residential facilities, nursing homes, and the wider community, and from different wards, whether psychiatric or not. The SPDC is the only service providing beds, assistance, and treatment for twenty four hours, and the only facility where involuntary admissions can be carried out. This entails that people in need of a period of specialized day and night care that does not qualify as an emergency and would not require hospitalization have no opportunity of being hosted elsewhere. In these cases, the community psychiatrist and the wider Mental Health Centre can enhance their assistance, introducing or multiplying home visits, inviting the patient to spend the day at the *Centro Diurno* where they can be assisted in terms of food provision, drug administration, and professional support, and offering medical support (e.g. clinical interviews) on a daily basis if necessary, but this does not always suffice, and it does not cover more than ten hours a day during the week (in the weekends, MHCs are usually open on Saturday mornings only). Hospitalization is then the only feasible solution even when it is not considered by the psychiatrists the more appropriate therapeutic choice—if not a deleterious one—at that moment. Furthermore, this organizational framework places relevant pressures on the SPDCs, which are constantly facing a shortage of beds and, according to what we have observed as a team in different Piedmontese wards, usually exceed their capacity, namely the maximum of patients they are allowed to host.[14] This pressure was once eased by the possibility that Mental Health Centres had to provide day hospital care, and by the activity of "crisis centres", described to me by the psychiatrist Giorgio.

[14] Overbooking is an exceptional solution which needs a special authorization from hospital health authorities, which is routinely granted in those wards where the problem of beds availability is constant.

> *Excerpt 5.16*. Giorgio (psychiatrist, Cedar Centre): There used to be the famous crisis centre [*centro crisi*] [...] which was a sort of pre-, pre-acuteness [centre], so within the system articulated between community-SPDC for those pre-acute situations, not so bad and still interceptable, not requiring coactive interventions, the crisis centre was used, [stay at] the crisis centre didn't have a precise time limit, and it was a lung for the SPDC. In [name of the city] it had ten beds.

The metaphor of the lung, which allowed the psychiatric ward to "breathe" by housing non-acute patients that would have otherwise converged on the SPDC together with actual emergencies, is well representative of the difficulties from which this service is currently suffering.

As I was conducting fieldwork at the Cedar Centre, I had the chance to follow the case of a woman, whom I will call Elsa, who exemplifies these pre-acuteness situations lacking a specific setting and response different than hospitalization. Elsa is a woman in her fifties, mother of a twenty-year-old girl who has recently informed her about the relationship she is having with another girl. To know about her daughter's sexual orientation caused her profound anxiety and inability to concentrate her thoughts on anything else; when I knew her, she had been coming to the Cedar Centre on a daily basis for three months, asking to see her psychiatrist, Giorgio, and insistently requesting extra medication and hospitalization. A consistent amount of time and energy were spent to care for her: Giorgio dedicated several unscheduled clinical interviews to talk to her and discuss the distressing situation, agreeing to administer drugs when dialogue was not sufficient to provide relief, but always encouraging her not to rely on external interventions only: "We could knock you out [with sedative medications] for forty days, but when we stop, if you do not put your effort into this, you are back where you started" (Cedar Centre, fieldnotes). Some nurses at the Cedar Centre were critical toward Giorgio's welcoming approach, which according to them was "spoiling" Elsa and supporting her demanding attitude, but nevertheless they spent time with her and tried hard to help her get through each day. During my fieldwork, nothing seemed to be working, and despite Elsa's request for hospitalization, it was not considered an appropriate or therapeutic solution for her. Giorgio eventually managed to plan a fifteen-day stay at a nearby private clinic that usually hosts patients after the discharge from the SPDC (so called post-acute cases) or admits sub-acute people in need of relief admission (*ricovero di sollievo*) but not hospitalization. Admission was arranged in five days, which she spent at the Cedar Centre in constant agitation, partially relieved by anxiolytics and personnel support, aimed at containing the crisis and preventing Elsa to go to the Emergency Room to be admitted to the SPDC, which would have cost her spot on the waiting list to the clinic.

Cases such as that of Elsa, who are at risk of hospitalization even when it is not the best therapeutic and organizational option, can benefit from a wider range of opportunities in the no-restraint context. There, the SPDC's metaphorical lung is represented by the Mental Health Centres themselves, which can host up to eight patients for longer periods of time than the ward.[15] Across the local institutional map—which includes one SPDC but multiple centres (four within the same department, but more if we consider geographically adjacent departments which do not have a dedicated psychiatric ward at all)—each MHC is evaluated by the ward's staff for its degree of cooperation, its ability to accommodate users who have somehow arrived at the hospital (e.g. by autonomously accessing the Emergency Room), and to provide a discharging plan to get them out of the ward as quickly as possible. As I began my fieldwork, it was immediately clear which reputation each centre had in this respect: among the services I focused on, the Violet Centre was definitely the good one, while the Tulip Centre was ranked among the worst. This opinion was rather homogeneously shared among actors working in different locations across the institutional map. Tulip Centre's workers themselves were aware of their difficulties, though explaining them to me with reasonable arguments, concerning the wider and qualitatively more problematic catchment area of the city they had to cover (95,000 inhabitants—including migrant population—against 65,000 of the Violet Centre, in the face of an equal number of psychiatrists); the structure of the building (which is spread over four floors linked by a spiral staircase, making it very difficult to control and eventually manage and shadow critical patients) and its

[15] In 2019, the average length of stay in the SPDC was of fourteen days, while in the MHC it was thirty-one days (data collected on the field).

location in a residential area (while the Violet Centre is surrounded by a park); and the absence of an official director (who could better coordinate activities and represent their interests in negotiations with the Department).

> *Excerpt 5.17.* Chiara (psychiatrist, Tulip Centre): The catchment area is important because actually marginal areas are practically all on us, and this is one thing, then we have the barrack [a large building currently used as a reception centre for migrants and refugees], I don't think this is what Basaglia meant with "principle of territoriality" [she smiles]. Then the fact that we do not have our own director, and we have the same number of physicians of the Violet Centre even if [it has fewer patients]... And the fact that in our facility we do not have a "*Centro Diurno*", because it breaks my heart to call it [the small space they have] a "*Centro Diurno*". [...] Nice, appropriate spaces are essential.

Notwithstanding the difficulties that specific Mental Health Centres can present, the opportunity they have to host patients and provide assistance twenty four hours a day (in presence, during the day, but also by telephone, day and night) introduces a radical change in the institutional map: the psychiatric ward is not the only place designated to treat crisis. Ideally, SPDC is meant to admit: (i) the "onsets": acute patients who are not known to the community services yet, and therefore need a first clinical (psychiatric and non-psychiatric) assessment; (ii) already known patients who cannot be hosted in the MHCs because of a lack of available beds, incompatibility with already hosted patients, community context deemed inappropriate for the specific patient or organic issues. The Mental Health Centre is expected to support its users while they are in the hospital (e.g. visits from community psychiatrists, psychologists and nurses, or daytime activities at the MHC) and go meeting new ones as soon as possible, in order to plan with the ward's doctors their treatment and their discharge, eventually prosecuting their stay at the centre if a bed is available. Patients who are already known to community services and who have been regularly followed can be directly accessed and be hosted by the Mental Health Centre without passing through the hospital at all. If they need assistance at night (i.e. after 20), when two nurses but no doctors are present to attend only to people already staying at the MHC, they are referred to the Emergency Room (where a psychiatrist is on-call for both the ER and the SPDC), and then interviewed and eventually accommodated the morning after. Generally speaking, cooperation between hospital and community services, and therefore assistance continuity (*continuità assistenziale*) assessed through the promptness with which MHCs respond and take charge of discharged patients (either from hospital or residential facilities), is higher in the no-restraint than in the restraint context: within fourteen days from discharge, 88.9% of patients in Friuli Venezia Giulia receive a psychiatric visit in the community services, while only 38.4% of Piedmontese patients do (Ministry of Health, 2021). Within 30 days from discharge, the trend is confirmed (ibidem).

This different institutional map and the multi-situatedness of crisis management do not dissolve the dichotomy between the hospital and the community, which are described in terms of separated worlds with different viewpoints also from professionals working in the no-restraint context.

> *Excerpt 5.18*. Elia (psychiatrist, Tulip Centre): I think we have a difference in, in viewpoints, you know? Because in the SPDC you, you risk seeing only one part of the story, the most critical one, both for the person but also [for the ward] because in the SPDC, the less the community services work and the more everything is funnelled to the hospital. [...] So [in the SPDC] there is this different, more perspectival vision than here, but the risk is, and I'm being self-critical, to dump on the SPDC all the contradictions, everything that could be managed here, ideally. The SPDC becomes the place where to bring people when you don't have other ideas, it is ok in the moment of crisis, but after that [sometimes] you're not able to discharge them and, and develop a path.

Non-appropriate use of the psychiatric ward described by Elia is crucial to the notion of the *shape* of the SPDC, which is discussed in the following section.

5.4.1 Shape-Preservation Strategies: Circulation Work and Pertinence Permeability

We have seen how the SPDC in the restraint and the no-restraint contexts has different functions according to the institutional map in which it is located. But the Pine Ward and the Iris Ward also differ in terms of shape, namely the conceptions they have about how the ward should be, who it ought to admit, and which strategies are to be performed in order to maintain such shape.

In both contexts, the shape of the ward and the strategies aimed at preserving it are practiced on two grounds: (i) negotiations with the hospital Emergency Room, and (ii) negotiations with community psychiatrists.

To introduce the first kind of negotiation, Table 5.2 provides an overview of the diagnoses of people who access the Emergency Room, which are or may be of psychiatric concern (Ministry of Health, 2021). Data compare Piedmont and Friuli Venezia Giulia, showing no significant differences between the populations: mental retardation, bipolar and personality disorders are the less frequent categories in both contexts, while neurotic and somatoform disorders are the most frequent one. Schizophrenia, alcohol or drug addiction, and depression, appear to be more frequent in Friuli Venezia Giulia, while dementia and organic mental disorders are slightly more common in Piedmont. The residual

Table 5.2 Access to the Emergency Room in 2019 (Ministry of Health, 2021)

Diagnosis	Piedmont		Friuli Venezia Giulia	
Schizophrenia and other functional psychoses	4.117	6.72%	1.049	11.88%
Mania and bipolar disorders	1.514	2.47%	19	0.22%
Depression	3.131	5.11%	697	7.89%
Neurotic and somatoform disorders	29.516	48.21%	4.638	52.51%
Personality disorders	1.802	2.94%	118	1.34%
Alcohol or drug addiction	6.275	10.25%	1.455	16.47%
Dementia and organic mental disorders	5.676	9.27%	751	8.50%
Mental retardation	59	0.10%	5	0.06%
Other psychiatric disorders	9.340	15.25%	100	1.13%
	61.230	100	8.832	100

category called "other psychiatric disorders" is less straightforward to interpret. It also includes people whose definitive diagnosis is unsure or has not been provided yet. The habit of indicating "other" for new patients whose diagnostic process is not yet completed has been observed on the field at the Cedar Centre and could explain the higher percentage registered by Piedmont, while Friuli Venezia Giulia is probably more inclined to indicate a tentative diagnosis than resorting to the residual category.

It is important to stress that these data do not describe the profile of the population admitted to the SPDCs but that which access the ER and which ward's psychiatrists called for consultation and possible admission are asked to select and filter.

Despite the apparently similar landscape which psychiatrists are confronted with in the ER, the populations admitted to the Pine Ward and to the Iris Ward are quite different, both in terms of numerousness and profile.

With respect to *numerousness*, both the wards have a similar capacity: sixteen beds in the Pine Ward, fifteen beds in the Iris Ward. Nevertheless, the former usually exceeds its capacity and tolerates overcrowding better than the latter. The following excerpt from my fieldnotes exemplifies this attitude, as the Pine Ward's chief psychiatrist defines thirteen patients as "a handful of people" despite the number being close to the maximum of available beds.

> *Excerpt 5.19.* Around 9.20 a.m. Michela [chief psychiatrist] enters the ward and starts the morning briefing with Angela [nurses' coordinator], Sara and Simona [nurses]. Michela observes: "we don't have much to say, there is just a handful of people". Patients are 13 with a maximum of 16 beds, but to her they are few since there are frequently up to 18–21 patients. (Pine Ward, fieldnotes)

Overcrowding is common in the Pine Ward to the point that the big white board on which inpatients are listed includes, besides sixteen slots corresponding to the regular beds, spots dedicated to extra-beds, called "bis" and one "TV room" spot. Additional beds are available to the ward, and they are routinely placed in double rooms which are spacious enough to introduce a third bed, in the space which is assigned to day hospital (which is used for administration of depot therapies whose clinical risks are not manageable in the Mental Health Centre, outside of the hospital setting), and even in the shared TV room. Well-known and frequently implemented strategies to locate extra beds denote a normalization of the overcrowding phenomenon, which appears to be part of the Pine Ward's routine.

Situations of considerable or persistent overcrowding—sometimes due to external obstacles to the discharge of patients who are not in their acute phase of illness anymore (e.g. waiting to be admitted to a clinic for post-acuteness recovery), which impede the admission of other patients in a situation of emergency—require the ability to discharge or send patients to other places, using the network of relationships with other wards and facilities which can increase the chances of succeeding in negotiations. In the Pine Ward, the most skilful psychiatrist in this respect was Carmela, admired by the unit's staff for this crucial ability.

> *Excerpt 5.20*. When Michela arrives, the briefing begins. There is the need to discharge someone, because there are 18 patients, a man in the hallway sitting in a wheelchair waiting for consultation who might require admission, a girl in another SPDC waiting to be transferred here [she was out of town and has been temporality admitted elsewhere], and the ward is already overcrowded. One patient is expected to be discharged tomorrow, but no one else seems ready to go. They hypothesize to discharge a woman, then call her family to discuss about it, but the relatives observe they have visited her yesterday and she was still very confused. Michela comments: "actually she is still confused"; the discharge would have not been proposed under normal circumstances, it has been proposed only to try to clear one bed. The staff then suggests moving some patient to another SPDC. Two wards belong to the same Mental Health Department: the first already hosts the young girl, the second refuses to take any patient as Michela calls them to ask. After some hesitation, Carmela [psychiatrist] decides to ask the first ward despite it is already hosting one of their patients, and, after a friendly phone call with a colleague and the promise to send "the meekest patient on the ward", she gets an unexpected "yes". [...] When Carmela hangs up, triumphant, Maria [healthcare assistant] comments: "I love her for this!": she is the most skilled at emptying the ward when necessary. (Pine Ward, fieldnotes)

The need to perform what I will call here *circulation work*, namely to constantly keep patients moving across the institutional map from one service to the other, derives on one hand from new admissions lining up because of the limited bed space (Wilson, 1983) and on the other hand from the goal pursued by mental health legislation to discharge patients back on the community as quickly as possible, minimizing their stay in the hospital. As observed by Lorna Rhodes in her work on American emergency psychiatry *Emptying beds* (1991), today's acute psychiatric wards are not managing the stable, chronic population which was typical of the asylum, but an ever-changing set of patients: they are *managing movement*, making the SPDC a space of transition.

From the SPDC personnel's point of view, circulation work is crucial also to maintain the ward's shape, which depends on the numerousness as well as on the profile of the inpatients. This is well represented by the statement of this Iris Ward nurse, Marzia, observing how a single difficult patient—Pietro—can influence the manageability of the whole unit: "fourteen patients are too many if one of them is Pietro". In the no-restraint context, overcrowding is far from being normalized: in fact, the legal capacity is never exceeded. The term "overcrowding" is alternatively used by the staff to refer to those situations where the legal capacity is almost or actually reached, but not exceeded, and it is related to personnel's difficulties of appropriately controlling and managing the inpatient population if it gets numerous.

> *Excerpt 5.21.* I stay in the doctors' office with Marzia [nurse], who complaints about the ward's overcrowding [15 patients]: "this morning I am not able to work as I should, I don't like it, I can't keep an eye on the ward". Lorenzo [nurse] agrees and adds: "yesterday afternoon was the same, with this background buzz I don't like at all". He then tells me that buzz makes everyone raise their voices and it stresses people out. The more patients they have, the less nurses feel like they are in control of the ward. [...] A phone call from the ER announces that there is a person to be examined for attempted suicide. The ward is full, so if she required hospitalization other regional SPDCs should be asked to admit her as an off-site. This is a hardly ever occurring event, and transfers between wards are rare, probably because of the network of the MHCs (in the Pine Ward exchanges with other SPDCs were frequent). (Iris Ward, fieldnotes)

Circulation work in the Iris Ward hardly ever involves other SPDCs, which are not operationally part of the institutional map which mental healthcare workers rely on to allocate patients after discharge. As observed in the fieldnotes above, this is probably due to the network of Mental Health Centres, which can host discharged patients even in their acute phase of illness, working as the SPDC metaphorical lung discussed earlier. When MHCs do not promptly perform this relieving function, conflicts arise between community and the ward, but also among members of the SPDC's staff.

> *Excerpt 5.22.* The ward has almost reached its maximum capacity (14 inpatients, one patient in the ER waiting to be admitted, and a TSO expected in the afternoon). During the daily meeting, Luana [psychiatrist] announced that Emma [Department's chief psychiatrist] opened up to the possibility of hosting extra-patients during the weekend. She then observes that the ward physically has 15 beds only, so that to admit extra-patients they should first get additional beds. This information triggers Marzia's reaction, who raises her voice saying: "I do not get additional beds because I do not do the asylum!". She then adds in an aggressive tone that every time the ward has been full, something bad happened (e.g., a patient hung himself some years ago) because nurses cannot provide assistance for too many inpatients. Luana stands up for herself saying that she is doing what she can, and that according to her they could get one extra bed for possible emergencies. Marzia, supported by her colleagues, disagrees: emergencies do not exist, if the sixteenth person arrives at night s/he can spend it in the ER. Moreover, if on Saturday mornings there are 14 or 15 patients, discharges should be made like Tania [former ward's director] used to do, to free up space for the weekend. Marzia adds: "I will accept extra-patients when all of the inpatients will be acute ones!". This is a jab aimed at Luana, who, according to the nurses, could discharge some patients, manageable in community MHC. (Iris Ward, fieldnotes)

The last excerpt shows that, contrary to what happens in the Pine Ward, overcrowding in the Iris Ward is not normalized. Instead, it is an exceptional event which needs to be managed as soon as possible, and which can never translate into the exceeding of ward's legal capacity, a materially impossible occurrence due to the lack of additional beds. To equip themselves with those, in Marzia's words, would somehow make the SPDC similar to the old, crowded asylum, and the option is not taken into consideration despite the psychiatrist's opinion about its utility in case of emergency.[16] The discussion, and the polarization between the doctor and the nurses (more directly involved in keeping order within the unit), exemplifies the tensions concerning the number of inpatients deemed appropriate to a manageable ward. These conflicts are present but far less explicit in the Pine Ward, partly because of the normalization of overcrowding, and also because of a nursing disposition which hardly ever challenges the medical group openly. On the contrary, in the Iris Ward nurses tenaciously defend their ward's shape, contesting and taking position against the admission of specific kinds of patients when they believe they do not "fit" (Strauss et al., 1981).

This last point is evident when we look at negotiations around the *profile* of the admissible patient. Pertinence is judged when the Emergency Department asks the SPDC for a consultation for a patient belonging to one or more categories listed in Table 5.2, or who shows symptoms (such as hallucinations, agitation, or behavioural issues) requiring a mental health assessment. The categories in which one patient can fall, as I have drawn from my observation on the field, are the following: the *pure psychiatric patient* (a person suffering from a mental disorder in its acute phase), the *hybrid patient* (the so-called dual diagnosis: a mental health issue and a drug or alcohol addiction), the *organic patient* (suffering from organic conditions which may alter his/her behaviour), the *non-acute psychiatric patient* (psychiatric patient in a sub- or non-acute phase of illness), and the *non-psychiatric patient* (encompassing situations related to homelessness, criminality, drug/alcohol addiction without psychiatric comorbidity, and so-called social cases). Such categories are common among acute mental healthcare, in both the restraint and the no-restraint context. Differences concern the degree of permeability—which I call here *pertinence permeability*—that each context, and specifically each

[16] In the no-restraint context, references to the former psychiatric hospital are frequent to signal trends toward undesired situations, such as a prolonged stay at the hospital or an increased number of beds. During a one-day visit in a third MHC of a different Department in Friuli, the following sentence was pronounced by a psychiatrist as she described a residential facility with fifteen beds: "they are too much, it becomes an asylum".

SPDC, shows for each type of patient, which strategies it adopts to decide upon their admission, and the bargaining power it has as it negotiates with the Emergency Department or the community psychiatrists.

With respect to pertinence permeability, boundaries around the Pine Ward appear to be looser, while in the Iris Ward they are less porous. This means that in the former case, every type of patient is potentially admissible after s/he accesses the Emergency Room: during fieldwork, I have met inpatients suffering from the most diverse conditions, including alcohol abuse, mental retardation, and dementia. These are usually problematic categories, requiring relevant efforts of the SPDC staff to assist them as they can show physical agitation, confusion, wandering, and age-related issues. Significantly, many of these cases get mechanically restrained on their arrival to the ward, later during their stay, or regularly at night, because the assistance they need exceeds ward's resources or is deemed to be not manageable otherwise (see Chap. 5). Within the hospital institutional map, the SPDC is nevertheless the designated place to host them, at least temporarily.

For the most problematic cases, such as those who belong to multiple categories (e.g. alcohol abuse, organic disorder, aggressive behaviour, and criminal background), the decision to place them in the SPDC is not uncontested, but it can nevertheless succeed for short periods of time, such as during the night. In this respect, an eloquent episode has been narrated by Davide, psychiatrist at the Cedar Centre, during a meeting I attended.

> *Excerpt 5.23.* Davide [psychiatrist], on-call on the night between Saturday and Sunday, sees a patient who accessed the ER after alcohol abuse, sent to the SPDC for a night in observation.[17] He defines him "an animal", as he arrives to the SPDC restrained and sedated with the usual Midazolam, which has a brief effect, and soon wakes up, very agitated, and manages to tear the IV needle out of his arm. They would like to tighten his belts but there are not enough magnets [closing mechanism] and no one feels like untying him to tie him more firmly. Davide: "the most natural thing we could think of was to keep a pillow on his face, but then you risk suffocat-

[17] Observation (*osservazione breve*) is a forty-eight-hour maximum status in which patients can be kept within the hospital, waiting for a decision to be made about their admission or discharge.

ing him. I tried to keep his head down on the mattress, but he was so sweaty it slipped away under my hands. He was so agitated and loosely tied that he would sit if we didn't keep him down". According to Davide, the patient, still intoxicated and with a problem of epilepsy, should not even have entered the SPDC, because it was too dangerous to be managed there: "we gave him one Entumin, one En, and I was there praying that nothing happened". He shows us his fingers crossed as he talks. He says that such a patient should be provided with intensive care and be constantly monitored in an adequately equipped ward. (Cedar Centre, fieldnotes)

This account reveals not only a problematic patient in terms of behaviour management but also a clinically challenging one because of the co-occurrence of a state of intoxication and a neurological disorder such as epilepsy. The psychiatrist suggests he should be treated in an Intensive Care Unit for reasons of clinical safety, but this is not part of the hospital routine, which tends to attribute hostile, agitated, and confused patients to the psychiatric ward regardless of their behaviour's underlying causes. Gaia, a nurse at the Pine Ward with a long professional experience in the psychiatric context, observes how this has not always been true.

Excerpt 5.24. Gaia (nurse, Pine Ward): We [in the past] used to take the pure psychiatric patient, stop. Now it seems that everything can be put in the cauldron of psychiatry, so we have alcoholism, drug addiction, the antisocial, adjustment disorders […] everything ends up in psychiatry, eating disorders […]. When I began working here [30 years before] alcohol-related issues used to be treated in the gastroenterological unit or the ER, they were kept there in observation and then admitted if necessary. […] We used to have the pure psychiatric patient, there were four or five diagnoses and if you didn't fit in one of those you were not admitted to the psychiatric ward, period. So much so that sometimes we might have maybe nine, eight, eleven patients, when we had sixteen we were packed. Now we are packed when we have twenty-one [patients].

Gaia's account describes how not only routines and hospital practices have changed over time, but perceptions too: SPDC's staff used to consider the ward overcrowded when they reached sixteen inpatients, just like it still happens in the Iris Ward, while today the range extended up to twenty-one, even if the official legal capacity of the unit never changed. This conveys the image of the ward's shape as an elastic, dynamic set of conceptions, which influence practices but at the same time are influenced by them, in a process of mutual shaping evolving over time. Moreover, Gaia suggests a connection between the inpatient population's numerousness and its increasingly heterogeneous profile, a link which is supported by the Mental Health Department's chief psychiatrist as well, Riccardo.

> *Excerpt 5.25*. Riccardo (Department's chief psychiatrist): Every behavioural problem ends up in the SPDC, actually I always tell our directors that the hospital's more important ward is Psychiatry, [because] all of the problematic cases end up there. Even a patient with brain cancer who's a bit confused ends up in the SPDC, because Neurology cannot admit him as it is an organic disease, so in fact psychiatric wards are full because 70% [of their inpatients] are not appropriate patients. And then there is the social dimension, people you cannot discharge, you don't know where to send them, you don't know what to do, there is no family, or families don't have money, the population is old and cannot afford 1500 euros per month to pay for a nursing home. These are all social care problems.

If the extensive definition of the Pine Ward's shape blurs its boundaries and exposes it to overcrowding and an increasingly heterogeneous population, the Iris Ward shows more rigid boundaries, whose permeability is governed by stricter criteria. In this context, relationships with the Emergency Department are generally good, and routines have been slowly developed over time through negotiations about the treatment and management of people accessing the ER with a possible psychiatric disorder. Although not formalized through protocols, these routines entail that medical examinations are conducted before the psychiatrist is called for consultation, including basic blood tests, toxicological screening, electrocardiogram and, if necessary, CT scan and other exams to detect serious organic conditions. This allows the psychiatrist to conduct his/her assessment knowing about the patients' general health status and potential non-psychiatric causes for their behaviour. If a neurological or otherwise organic pathology is found, the patient is not admitted to the

SPDC but treated accordingly to the emerging condition, while a positive toxicological screening results in a period in the ER or the Intensive Care Unit to get over the intoxication within a monitored and clinically safe environment. This means that patients like those described by the psychiatrist Davide in the Pine Ward would hardly be admitted to the Iris Ward. A colleague of his operating in the no-restraint context, Paolo, discusses these routines and how they have gradually shaped ER doctors' conceptions about symptoms and behaviours that might be, but do not necessarily are, of psychiatric concern.[18]

> *Excerpt 5.26.* Paolo (psychiatrist, Iris Ward): To filter means that when a case arrives and he is hallucinated, they [the colleagues working in the ER] do not necessarily expect it to be an absolutely acute and absolutely psychiatric problem, and they conduct all of the examinations required before we go there for a consultation, because if it takes an hour and a half and I go down without a clue what can I do? There are also physical reasons for people to have [psychiatric] symptoms, so how can I rule out the possibility that for example a woman has cancer? I can't say anything to my [ER] colleagues because I don't know what happened, they may have admitted her with a lot of medical troubles, so we expect them to filter, and we have to filter too.
>
> **Interviewer: As far as I have noticed, [SPDC] nurses also ask you to...**
>
> Paolo: They would like the patient to be blonde, tall, blue-eyed, only psychotic, kind, likeable and with a good character. /And who goes away at the right time/ [smiling], who takes all medications, they, yes, they do not want any hassles.

Paolo's ironic words about nurses' preferred patient—the best version of the pure psychiatric patient outlined above—reveal an important site

[18] Routines do not prevent ER doctors, on specific situations, from occasionally trying to expedite or force a patient's admission, suggesting a constant and everlasting struggle around permeability and circulation work between the ER and the SPDC. The following excerpt provides an example of an ER successful manoeuvre: After ten minutes, [ER] calls the ward to inform us that the patient will be sent here tonight. [Paolo] did not manage to avoid his admission, he says something like: "they [ER] screwed us again"» (Iris Ward, fieldnotes).

of conflict between psychiatrists and the nursing staff, whose visions about the shape of the ward and the appropriateness of the admission of a patient do not always align. In everyday practice, nurses exert relevant pressure on doctors every time they are called for a consultation in the ER, and recommendations are made until they leave the ward: "don't take him if he's positive [to drugs]!" or "let him sober up down there [in the ER]!" Moreover, strategic categorization of patients is performed in order to sustain the inappropriateness of their admission and ask for their discharge. This was the case of Mattia, a 40-year-old man with a history of substance abuse, who accessed the Emergency Room after having destroyed his apartment in a moment of intense agitation. During the clinical interview in the ER, he shows me and Paolo some self-inflicted cuts on his arms and he tells us about the voices he has heard for some time, which lead him to drink and use heroin and cocaine to try to silence them. When Paolo asks him about recent suicidal thoughts, the man denies, but as we go back to the ER waiting room after the interview, he tells me that two days ago he searched on Google for the highest building in town which he could throw himself off. Lately, I report this piece of information to Paolo, who thanks me and tells me that he intends to admit him, believing he might be a dual diagnosis. Then, he adds: "nurses won't be happy with this admission and will say he's an addict, but whatever". In this case, the strategic categorization aimed at claiming the inappropriateness of the admission consists in a shift from "hybrid patient" (dual diagnosis, entitled to stay in the SPDC) to "non-psychiatric patient" (drug addiction without any psychiatric disorder, who does not fit in the SPDC). This strategy of reframing is a very common one in the Iris Ward, usefully employed to discourage psychiatrists from admitting drug-addicted patients and to press for their discharge ascribing responsibilities to the services treating addictions (SerD).[19]

Ability to filter inappropriate patients is expected from community psychiatrists too, who work in the ward during the weekends or night shifts. Sonia, psychiatrist at the Violet Centre, recounts: "they [the

[19] SerD does not have dedicated spaces in or outside the hospital to admit its service users, but only has rehabilitation clinics hosting people pursuing detoxification for prolonged periods of time. This means that intoxicated people accessing the ER cannot be referred to any specific acute service.

SPDC's nurses] are very sensitive to this, oh my god, when you're on-call you have to be the best for them, I mean you have to filter everything, but this is not always easy". Her words are consistent with other accounts collected on the field, describing a general tendency of ER doctors to consider and treat as psychiatric what is non-psychiatric. The issue of the psychiatrization of difference and the socially deviant is not a recent phenomenon: psychiatry always had to negotiate its boundaries with other disciplines concerned with the maintenance of social order (Castel et al., 1979). The following quotations highlight how psychiatry redraws its disciplinary boundaries through daily practice, every time that mental healthcare workers are demanded to defend the jurisdiction of their discipline in front of other agencies asking for their intervention.

Excerpt 5.27. Alice (nurses' coordinator, Cedar Centre): It's coming back, this idea that psychiatry has to deal with social control. [...] We continuously receive requests, if they have to evict someone, /psychiatry has to be there/ [she laughs], if there is a patient who throws rocks at the kids we have to go. Not a patient, a person [without a psychiatric diagnosis]! When someone commits a crime, they take him to the ER and then to psychiatry! [...] Or the prosecutor writes to us because, I don't know, there is a vagabond who sleeps in front of the city hall. Like we could solve every problem and restore public order.

Excerpt 5.28. [At the weekly meeting] Giorgio recounts that on Saturday afternoon the 118 doctor asked him (who was on-call in the SPDC) to admit a man involuntarily, validating his TSO proposal motivated on the basis of dangerousness only. Giorgio refuses to validate it, asking the colleague to present a new proposal based on the three legal criteria for TSO, if they are met (this is not the case, and the second proposal never came). The man spends the night at the hospital in observation and when he leaves in the morning Giorgio informs the police that he has been threatening to kill his own partner and son. On Sunday evening the partner is assaulted by him and calls the police, who violently stops the man and breaks his nose. An ambulance is called and the man is taken to the ER for his broken nose, but once he gets there the ER doctors call Davide, who is on-call in the SPDC, to ask him to admit the man for the night (again). He categorically refuses to take him. Half an hour later, Davide is informed that the man is being taken to the prison: he did not suffer from psychiatric disorders but has a criminal record and an expulsion order from Caserta for violent behaviour and stalking of his ex-wife. The staff criticize the tendency to psychiatrize and dump on the SPDC cases like this, who are more on the criminal side than on the illness one. (Cedar Centre, fieldnotes)

In this context of heterogeneous requests of admission, the role of the psychiatrist is that of the gatekeeper of the SPDC, who controls access to the ward and is expected to defend its shape from inappropriate use. The physician does not act in a vacuum but within a set of routines and non-formalized practices developed over time among hospital departments. Nevertheless, even in those contexts where the SPDC seems to benefit from less permeable boundaries, such as the Iris Ward, routines are never permanent and can never be taken for granted. In a situation of permanent negotiation, lack of resources and beds, and power struggle, ER colleagues can always try to bypass consolidated practices if they need to, as the psychiatrist Paolo puts it: "We don't have a bad relationship, sometimes they screw us but, I mean, it's part of the game".

Personnel's worries about the admission of improper patients are not equally distributed but depend on the degree of trust they have in the specific psychiatrist's ability to filter inappropriate requests. At the beginning of each night shift, nurses' reactions as they read the name of the psychiatrist who is on-call on that night are very telling: they can feel relatively relaxed because they know that the ward's shape will not be threatened, or they can hope that no calls for consultations will come from the ER because the doctor on duty is "one who takes [admits] them all". While in the Iris Ward trust is generally higher for SPDC's psychiatrists, in the Pine Ward the opposite is true: community psychiatrists have built stronger relationships with the nursing staff because of the quality and amount of time they spend together at nights and weekend shifts, as the nurse Gaia observes.

Excerpt 5.29. Gaia (nurse, Pine Ward): With the doctors of our ward we do not have a great relationship, maybe we have more familiarity and, I don't say friendship but complicity, with community doctors than with our ward's ones. [...] When a community doctor is on duty, he spends a lot of time here, in the ward /with us/ [emphasized], not in the external medical office. So we developed a closer collaboration, because clearly if you spend the entire Sunday afternoon in here, with your colleagues and the doctor, it's four people who are constantly working together.

The area of overlap (Wenger, 1999) between the hospital and the territorial community of practices, represented by the shifts that MHC psychiatrists have in the Pine Ward, seems to be more successful in strengthening relationships across the two communities than the boundary practices performed in the no-restraint context with the explicit aim of connecting the ward and the centres (see paragraph 5.2).

In fact, the second stage on which negotiations about admissions and general circulation work are performed, besides the ER, is that between SPDC and community psychiatrists. In this case, the objects of negotiation are not only admissions but also discharge and the transfer of patients to other facilities (residential or semi-residential ones, clinics for post-acute assistance). Since community psychiatrists are in charge of planning post-discharge trajectories for their hospitalized patients, as well as for new ones (the "onsets"), they are actively collaborating with the psychiatric ward in the performance of circulation work. Conflicts around these issues are attributed to the difference in perspective intrinsic of the two communities working in the field of mental healthcare, which provide different definitions of "acuteness" and therefore express conflicting opinions about the need for hospitalization.

Excerpt 5.30. Giorgio (psychiatrist, Cedar Centre): [Conflicts generally arise] because of a discrepancy in the evaluation of the actual need for admission. If one usually has to do with urgencies, the emergency/urgency dimension holds a different connotation for those who work in the community with a different perspective. And mutually it is possible that they [SPDC colleagues] are critical about our choice to keep [not discharge] or to admit someone, this is the thing, because of a different perspective [of the two services].

In the MHC view, the need for hospitalization is not necessarily motivated by an emergency as those who work in the ward intend it but can be meant to overcome a moment of mild crisis or pre-acute phase (for which the restraint context does not provide dedicated spaces outside of hospital), so that admission can be thought of as a preventive action aimed at avoiding severe crisis. These definitional discrepancies are understood as part of different perspectives on mental illness and its treatment, and they are accompanied by radically different working experiences. Work in the ward entails the management of situations requiring readiness and the taking of quick decisions, sometimes individually (e.g. as the psychiatrist is deciding upon admission in the ER), and relationships with the patients are defined as difficult and emotionally charged (anxiety, fear, uncertainty have been mentioned). Work in the community, on the contrary, is a collective enterprise, carried out with the support of the *équipe* and made of "small achievements distributed over time" (Giorgio, psychiatrist at the Cedar Centre).

> *Excerpt 5.31*. Arturo (nurse, Cedar Centre): The ward hosts acute patients, when they arrive they are in their acute phase, so it's difficult to relate to them and you generally develop relations that are very symmetrical, very much based on blackmail also [...] you are constantly bargaining, negotiating, you know? It is a ward where people, psychotics, have no awareness of their illness, or they are bipolar so, dialogue is very difficult and, and very limited in time, as soon as they start to get better they are discharged, also because of the shortage of beds, while here in the community you see patients also when they feel better, not in their acute phase, you can know them in their everyday environment and acquire many more tools to understand them and plan interventions, it is a job based on networking with the social services, general practitioners, it's a bit more gratifying [than working in the ward].

For these two apparently incompatible worlds to cooperate requires the development of strategies, specifically by the psychiatric ward which needs to protect its shape and filter hospitalization requests which always exceed its capacity. A common justification SPDC's psychiatrists use to refuse their community colleagues' requests of admission, or to demand them to organize the discharge to empty some spots, is the shortage of beds. This objective problem can be exploited or even *pretended* as a strategy to avoid the admission of problematic or unwanted patients. In the

Pine Ward, this has been observed on multiple occasions. The episode I selected to illustrate this strategy was observed at the Cedar Centre, where a woman in her sixties, Ada, arrives in the middle of a hot summer day after having walked for miles under the sun. She is a patient already known by the centre, and I have met her already in the Pine Ward when she had been admitted three months before as she was suffering from persecutory delusions. Persuaded that somebody was trying to poison her by contaminating food in her fridge, she developed bad relationships with her neighbours; kids living in the same building began mocking her for her unusual behaviour, and she reacted by throwing cans at them and cutting their bicycles' wheels. The judge ordered her to stay in the SPDC as investigations and official psychiatric evaluations by the court were made, and then approved her returning home though indicating her to follow a therapeutic program with the community services (*obbligo di cura*). Ada did not modify her behaviour, continuing to spend most of the day outside, wandering around the city despite the heat. When she arrives at the Cedar Centre, she seems very tired and debilitated, but also upset and hostile toward the personnel: she refuses to be accompanied back home by car, and also to spend the following days at the *Centro Diurno* nearby, with staff picking her up and taking her back daily to avoid her walking in the sun. She insists returning home on her feet but at the same time she feels unwell, so she does not leave the centre. Giorgio negotiates with her for almost one hour, while gently taking her blood pressure and convincing her to drink some water, until she accepts being admitted for some days to the ward, where she can recover. The fieldnotes which follow describe the phone call the psychiatrist made to arrange her hospitalization.

> *Excerpt 5.32.* Giorgio doesn't feel like letting her go home, she's physically debilitated, so he calls the Pine Ward [to ask if they can admit her], but they tell him they're full (I can tell from his facial expression that he is very sceptical, like he doesn't believe them) and invite him to try another SPDC. He reluctantly calls another SPDC [in another city], but the nurse who answers the phone tells him that psychiatrists are not in the ward at the moment, so she cannot give him an answer. He decides to call the Pine Ward again, I understand he's talking to Carmela, who accepts to admit the

> woman. [...] We go back to Giorgio's office, joking around the fact that the Pine Ward has magically found a place for her in less than ten minutes. (Cedar Centre, fieldnotes)

We can observe how Giorgio's first attempt with the Pine Ward fails, as they tell him that no beds are available for Ada (a patient already known to the ward). The doctor does not believe his colleagues' words, because—he explains later—this is a common strategy they use to try to avoid an admission by referring the patient to another SPDC. The fact that he calls the Pine Ward back, after also the second ward refuses to provide an answer, shows that he did not believe that no beds were available in the first place. His ward's colleague Carmela does not insist that the ward is full after she is called back, and immediately accepts to admit Ada: she tried *diverting* the patient somewhere else, and if the other SPDC had taken her, the Pine Ward would have succeeded in its strategy to avoid a new admission.

A variation of this strategy consists in negotiating with a different SPDC the transfer (or, more rarely, the exchange) of a patient, *manipulating* or *omitting information* that would make the success of the operation less likely. This has been observed with respect to Aldo, a "historic patient" of the Pine Ward, known for thirty years and frequently hospitalized. His psychiatrist, Giorgio, tried to find a place for him in several residential facilities, none of which succeeded in hosting the man for more than a few days: they send him back to the ward as soon as he shows signs of aggressiveness and then refuse to host him again, forcing Giorgio to look for another facility and wait for a bed to be available. For this reason, Aldo spent nearly a month in the Pine Ward, where he has been frequently mechanically restrained because of his aggressive behaviour toward Iris, a young patient suffering from borderline disorder who was seven months pregnant (see Sect. 6.3.4 in Chap. 6). Because of sedation and the prolonged time spent in bed, Aldo is non-autonomous and unable to walk on his own legs: he sits on a wheelchair, barely talking, covered with a sheet which works as a giant bib for his intense sialorrhea. The intensive assistance he needs, along with ward's overcrowding and worries that he can harm Iris and her baby, lead the chief psychiatrist, Michela, to arrange Aldo's transfer to another SPDC. His demanding conditions will be omitted in negotiations with the recipient ward because they would have probably made the patient unacceptable.

> *Excerpt 5.33*. Michela calls Giorgio on the phone to discuss about Aldo, a patient of his. She says: "tomorrow I'll try a sleight of hand to send Aldo to [another SPDC], I don't know if they'll take him, here we have to keep him restrained because of Iris [a pregnant patient]". [...] After some phone calls, Aldo's transfer is planned for tomorrow at 14.30, even if nurses comment they have never seen him in such pitiful conditions and they are afraid that the other SPDC will send him back as they see him (his conditions have not been described to the colleagues on the phone). [...] The day after, before I leave the ward, the phone rings: it's a doctor of the SPDC where Aldo has been transferred. Dennis [OSS] answers, then hands the phone to Sandra [psychiatrist] and goes to his colleagues to inform them about the call, laughing: they bet that Aldo will be sent back tomorrow already, because the SPDC did not expect to receive a patient in such a bad shape. (Pine Ward, fieldnotes)

These excerpts from fieldnotes show how opacity in negotiations is considered a legitimate conduct in the strategic performance of circulation work, normalized both within the ward (where the staff seems to express amusement and some pride for the successful move) and with the community psychiatrist informed of this cunning "sleight of hand". Stratagems like this are part of routine interactions between SPDCs, which in turn can be recipients of what is colloquially called a "scam" (*pacco*), namely a problematic and difficult-to-discharge patient.

In the no-restraint context, strategies concerning the reaching of the ward's capacity cannot be performed with community psychiatrists because Mental Health Centres receive the list of the patients hosted in the SPDC every morning. The document reports each inpatient's name, date of birth, city, MHC and psychiatrist of reference, date of admission, and voluntariness (or involuntariness) of the stay.[20] The sharing of this list

[20] A similar tool had been recently introduced in the restrain context while we were doing fieldwork, even if it was meant to be shared among the psychiatric wards and the medical emergency support (118), which could know in advance about free beds when it had to decide on where to take patients in need for admission. Nevertheless, many SPDCs did not use to update their list, or they did by performing some strategies, such as waiting to discharge patients after the daily communication of their bed availability.

represents a coordinating mechanism between the two communities of practices—the ward and each centre—which connects the activities of the two and which can be thought of as a boundary object (Star & Griesemer, 1989). This notion refers to objects intersecting different social worlds, which are both recognizable in order to work as means of translation, but at the same time have different meanings in the different sites employing them (ibidem). As Wenger observes (1999), boundary objects can enable coordination without necessarily creating a bridge between the two worlds' perspectives and meanings. Within each community, the boundary object—in this case, the inpatient list—is interpreted and adapted to local needs, thus it is employed differently. In the Mental Health Centre, the document provides a detailed overview of the ward's situation in terms of saturation and profile of the inpatient population, helping professionals to have a map of the available options if they need to hospitalize someone or, conversely, discharge some of their patients. Its relevance is evident in the fact that in both the Violet and the Tulip Centre it is printed daily, placed on the main desk and consulted by psychiatrists as they arrive, together with the notebook (*quaderno delle consegne*) where salient events of each shift are written down by the staff. This daily rite offers relevant information not only about the situation in the MHC but also in the ward, providing them with a general frame of the extended context in which they are going to operate. Additionally, the inpatients list reveals the degree of the ward's use of each MHC, namely the quota of patients that every centre has hospitalized at that moment. For centres which usually have many patients admitted to the ward, such as the Tulip Centre, this works both as a reminder—they cannot "forget" who and how many of their patients are currently in the SPDC—and as an organizing tool, which they use to plan visits in the ward, prioritize activities and discharges, and allocate beds in their centre as they return available.

In the SPDC, the document is employed with a double purpose. On one hand, it allows the staff to easily observe the time each patient has already spent in the ward, because the date of admission is indicated. On the other hand, information about each patient's MHC of reference represents a tool they can use to solicit discharges or transfers to those centres which appear poorly collaborative. Negotiations with community colleagues usually revolve around these two elements, resulting in discharge requests which typically take on the following forms: "the patient has been in hospital for many days" or "you [as a centre] have N patients here, would you take *at least* one of them?" These negotiations occur by phone but also face to face, when community psychiatrists visit the SPDC to have clinical interviews with their patients or discuss post-discharge plans with their colleagues. If the Iris Ward benefits from more defined boundaries which allow it to defend itself against improper admission requests in the ER, it has lower bargaining power when it comes to Mental Health Centres. The following extracts describe two episodes which represent the ward's impossibility to resist an admission decided by community psychiatrists, despite the staff's opinion about its appropriateness.

> *Excerpt 5.34.* In the morning, Tatiana has talked to her psychiatrist (Tulip Centre). Tatiana refuses the depot therapy. Her psychiatrist said she is not ready for discharge e the centre has no available beds to host her, so she is going to stay in the ward at least until Monday [four days later], because according to the doctor she is on the verge of a crisis. I perceive ward's staff dissatisfaction with this decision: they have known Tatiana for years and they are sure she is not near decompensation. (Iris Ward, fieldnotes)

> *Excerpt 5.35.* We are waiting for a patient named Pino, to whom the Tulip Centre psychiatrists have decided to do an ASO [mandatory health assessment] followed by hospitalization (voluntarily or under TSO). Franco [nurse] bursts out laughing as he hears the news, because Pino is a dual diagnosis patient very well known to the services, who has always lived in precarious conditions. Marzia [nurse] later describes him as a "super chronic [patient]" (*cronicone*). All the staff considers the ASO and the admission inappropriate to the difficult time the ward is going through, without any apparent urgency. With Pino we will have 14 inpatients, including a minor, 10 of which are Tulip Centre's patients. (Iris Ward, fieldnotes)

Besides ordinary negotiations between ward and community psychiatrists, the SPDC cannot refuse to admit patients from the centres if it has available beds, and cannot discharge people who are not about to be hosted in the centres, in other facilities, or deemed ready to go home by their community doctors. This situation is considered to be unbalanced because while the Mental Health Centres can read their inpatient list daily, the ward has no access to information about people hosted in the centres besides that which is provided directly by the community psychiatrists. When ward's staff is told that the centre has no availability of beds, and cannot send anybody home to free some, it has no opportunity to verify this information, while it perceives itself completely exposed to MHCs surveillance. On one hand, this apparently uneven distribution of information is rational because Mental Health Centres coordinate patients' trajectories and have to know if they can rely on the ward when they have to manage a crisis. Moreover, each patient's situation is complex and could never be summarized nor discussed in detail with the ward's staff in order to decide collectively—assuming that this would make any sense—about his/her actual need to "occupy a bed" in the Mental Health Centre. On the other hand, the ward's worries that opaque strategies can be performed by the centres (especially the apparently less cooperative ones) are understandable. Nevertheless, as far as I have observed on the field while I was there, no explicit lies have been told about bed availability—which, as we have seen, cannot be said for the Pine Ward—and community psychiatrists can decide to make their choices more transparent to the staff's ward by describing the situation of their centre, offering full collaboration and reassuring about the forthcoming discharge of their patients when not immediately feasible.

5.5 Conclusion

The present chapter has provided an overview of mental health services as they have evolved along the de-institutionalization process. Within each observed context, the model of balanced care (Thornicroft & Tansella, 2002), which combines hospital and community services, developed differently according to local resources and sensibilities. In the Piedmontese context, hospital care seems to have a more prominent role and community care is more oriented toward residential care. On the contrary, Friuli Venezia Giulia invests on community services and specifically on semi-residential care, provided in twenty-four-hour Mental Health Centres.

In both cases, the "hospital" and the "community" components are defined and practiced as two different social worlds, where working experiences, perceptions of time, and relationships with patients acquire different features and meanings. If in the restraint context the *ospedale–erritorio* dichotomy is sustained on an institutional basis, deriving from Law 833/1978 and the division of labour among mental health services it established, in the no-restraint context the dichotomy assumes ideological traits, stemming from the principles which inspired the reform and which prioritize the community over the hospital. This results in two different institutional maps (Strauss et al., 1981), on which the psychiatric ward (SPDC) performs a different function: it can be the only place designated to treat crisis (restraint context) or it can be one among other places which treat specific cases (e.g. the "onsets") in a context of multi-situated crisis management.

Beyond this ideal division of labour between the services, in everyday practice conflicts arise around the allocation of patients because professionals working in different locations can see the institutional map differently. Each service acquires its own shape, constituted by staff's conceptions about how it should be, who it should treat, and which are the conditions necessary to proper work (ibidem). Here I have discussed the shape of the ward, focussing on the two most debated issues in everyday practice: numerousness and profile of the admitted population. With respect to numerousness, despite the similar maximum capacity of the Pine (sixteen beds) and the Iris Ward (fifteen beds), we have observed a tendency to normalize overcrowding in the first context (which hosted up to twenty-one inpatients during my fieldwork), and to reconceptualize it, equating it with an almost full or particularly problematic ward, in the second context. With respect to the patients' profile, the Pine Ward shows more permeable boundaries to many categories of people, both psychiatric (pure or with concurrent organic pathologies or addictions, acute or not) and non-psychiatric. This is clearly related to overcrowding and it produces staff's general discontent for the ward's misuse by colleagues and other agencies, which attribute heterogeneous behavioural problems to psychiatry. On the contrary, the Iris Ward's boundaries seem less porous, and pertinence of admission more severely evaluated: intoxication from alcohol or substances is treated in the Emergency Department, organic conditions (especially those requiring medical devices) are not allowed in the ward for safety reasons, and non-acute patients are generally treated by Mental Health Centres.

When it comes to deciding upon admission, the categorization of patients is not always straightforward, and negotiations become crucial. They are performed on two main grounds: in consultations in the Emergency Room and with community psychiatrists and other colleagues outside of the hospital who ask to admit one of their patients. In the ER, the shape of the ward has to be defended by the consultant psychiatrist, who works as the SPDC gatekeeper and is asked to filter inappropriate requests of admission. The doctor's decision does not necessarily meet with nursing staff's approval, and can be contested operating a re-categorization of the admitted patient so that s/he can be deemed inappropriate (e.g. from hybrid patient to drug addicted only, and therefore a non-psychiatric patient). Community psychiatrists actively cooperate with SPDC's colleagues to perform circulation work, namely that set of operations (admissions, discharges, transfers, and exchanges with other services) which allow patients to circulate and the ward not to be overcrowded, reduce the average length of stay, and make beds available to new emergencies. Strategies employed in negotiations differ according to the context: in the Pine Ward, they consist in pretending the ward is full, diverting patients to other SPDC, or omitting information which may hinder transfer requests; in the Iris Ward, the invocation of each MHC's load on the unit is a useful strategy to solicit discharges or trade a new admission with a discharge or transfer. In both cases, strategies are supported respectively by personal "allocation skills" and relationships with the colleagues and by the inpatient list which works as a boundary object connecting the ward and the community. This document undermines the bargaining power of the SPDC because it makes it transparent in terms of bed availability: while the Iris Ward has better chances in negotiating with the Emergency Room because of routines and informal agreement between departments, the Pine Ward is more skilful in negotiations with community psychiatrists and other facilities (e.g. other SPDCs) when it comes to admission, but more exposed to delays in discharges.

Table 5.3 provides a synthetic overview of this chapter's content.

Table 5.3 SPDC's profile and practices in the restraint and the no-restraint contexts

		Restraint context	No-restraint context
SPDC's position on the institutional map		Place of crisis	One among other places of crisis
SPDC's shape	***Inpatients numerousness***	Overcrowding normalized	Overcrowding re-conceptualized as near-fullness
	Inpatients profile (pertinence permeability)	Pure, Hybrid, Organic, Non-acute, Non-psychiatric patient	Pure, Hybrid (detoxification in ER or ICU), Post-acute patient
Nurses' strategies to defend SPDC's shape		–	Re-framing of patient's profile
Circulation work strategies (with community psychiatrists and other agencies, e.g. other SPDCs)		Pretending ward's fullness Diverting patients to other SPDCs Omitting information	Invoking near-fullness Invoking MHC's load on the SPDC
Resources supporting circulation work strategies		Personal "allocation skills"' Relationships with colleagues	Inpatient list
Bargaining power	***With ER doctors***	Low	High
	With community psychiatrists	High (admission) Low (discharge, transfer)	Low

References

Allen, D. (2001). Narrating nursing jurisdiction: "Atrocity stories" and "boundary-work". *Symbolic Interaction, 24*(1), 75–103.

Babini, V. (2009). *Liberi tutti: manicomi e psichiatri in Italia: una storia del Novecento*. il Mulino.

Basaglia, F. (Ed.). (1967). *Che cos'è la psichiatria?* Amministrazione Provinciale di Parma.

Basaglia, F. (Ed.). (1968). *L'istituzione negata*. Einaudi.

Cardano, M., & Gariglio, L. (2021). The neoliberal politics of otherness in Italian psychiatric care: Notes on a team ethnography in six acute psychiatric wards. In J. Gabe, M. Cardano, & A. Genova (Eds.), *Health and illness in the neoliberal era in Europe*. Emerald Publishing.

Castel, F., Castel, R., & Lovell, A. (1979). The psychiatrization of difference. *International Journal of Law and Psychiatry, 2*(2), 235–247.

Conolly, J. (1856). *The treatment of the insane without mechanical restraints*. Dawsons of Pall Mall.

Donnelly, M. (1992). *The politics of mental health in Italy*. Routledge.

Foot, J. (2014). Franco Basaglia and the radical psychiatry movement in Italy, 1961–78. *Critical and Radical Social Work, 2*(2), 235–249.

Foot, J. (2015). *The man who closed the asylums: Franco Basaglia and the revolution in mental health care*. Verso Books.

Gherardi, S. (2006). *Organizational knowledge: The texture of workplace learning*. John Wiley & Sons.

Goffman, E. (1961). *Asylums. Essays on the social situation of mental patients and other inmates*. Anchor Books.

Jones, J. (2000). Mental health care reforms in Britain and Italy since 1950: A cross-national comparative study. *Health & Place, 6*(3), 171–187.

Kerosuo, H. (2003). Boundaries in health care discussions: An activity theoretical approach to the analysis of boundaries. In N. Paulsen & T. Hernes (Eds.), *Managing boundaries in organizations: Multiple perspectives* (pp. 169–187). Palgrave Macmillan.

Lamont, M., & Molnár, V. (2002). The study of boundaries in the social sciences. *Annual Review of Sociology, 28*(1), 167–195.

Lave, J., & Wenger, E. (1991). *Situated learning: Legitimate peripheral participation*. Cambridge University Press.

Ministry of Health. (2021). *Rapporto sulla Salute Mentale. Analisi dei dati del Sistema Informativo per la Salute Mentale (SISM), Anno 2019*. Italian document. Retrieved November 26, 2022, from https://www.salute.gov.it/imgs/C_17_pubblicazioni_3081_allegato.pdf

Mols, A., & Pridmore, J. (2021). Always available via WhatsApp: Mapping everyday boundary work practices and privacy negotiations. *Mobile Media & Communication, 9*(3), 422–440.

Muusse, C., Kroon, H., Mulder, N., & Pols, J. (2020). Working on and with relationships: Relational work and spatial understandings of good care in community mental healthcare in Trieste. *Culture, Medicine and Psychiatry, 44*(4), 544–564.

Quirk, A., Lelliott, P., & Seale, C. (2006). The permeable institution: An ethnographic study of three acute psychiatric wards in London. *Social Science & Medicine, 63*(8), 2105–2117.

Rhodes, L. A. (1991). *Emptying beds: The work of an emergency psychiatric unit*. University of California Press.

Rogers, A., & Pilgrim, D. (2014). *A sociology of mental health and illness*. McGraw-Hill Education UK.

Rossi, S., & Toresini, L. (2015). SPDC aperti e senza contenzioni per i diritti inviolabili della persona. In S. Rossi (a cura di), *Il nodo della contenzione: diritto, psichiatria e dignità della persona*. Edizioni alpha beta Verlag.

Sparti, D. (2005). *Suoni inauditi. L'improvvisazione nel jazz e nella vita quotidiana*. il Mulino.

Sparti, D. (2013). On the edge. A frame analysis for improvisation. In G. Lewis & B. Piekut (Eds.), *The Oxford handbook of critical improvisation studies* (Vol. 1, pp. 182–201). Oxford University Press.

Star, S. L., & Griesemer, J. R. (1989). Institutional ecology, translations' and boundary objects: Amateurs and professionals in Berkeley's Museum of Vertebrate Zoology, 1907–39. *Social Studies of Science, 19*(3), 387–420.

Starace, F., & Baccari, F. (2020). La Salute Mentale nelle Regioni. Disuguaglianze di sistema. *SIEP. Quaderni di epidemiologia psichiatria*, 7/2019.

Strauss, A., Schatzman, L., Bucher, R., Ehrlich, D., & Sabshin, M. (1981). *Psychiatric ideologies and institutions*. Transaction.

Thornicroft, G., & Tansella, M. (2002). Balancing community-based and hospital-based mental health care. *World Psychiatry, 1*(2), 84–90.

Trivelli, E. (2016). The Basaglian legacy in Italian psychiatry: Remembering, myth-making and crystallising. In D. Kritsotaki, V. Long, & M. Smith (Eds.), *Deinstitutionalisation and after: Post-war psychiatry in the Western world* (pp. 217–239). Palgrave Macmillan.

Wenger, E. (1999). *Communities of practice: Learning, meaning, and identity*. Cambridge University Press.

Wilson, H. S. (1983). Usual hospital treatment in the United States' community mental health system: A dispatching process. *International Journal of Nursing Studies, 20*(2), 75–82.

6

Combining Healthcare, Compassion, and Coercion Repertoires and Strategies to Provide (Good) Care in Acute Psychiatric Settings

Abstract Care and coercion are held together in everyday clinical practice, in a combination that is not unproblematic for the actors involved: the adoption of coercive means can pose ethical issues debated within the professional teams, as well as produce negative personal feelings and threats to professional identity as carers. This chapter presents how the coercive dimension of psychiatric practice, when acknowledged as such—either because it seems evident in interventions implying the use of force, or made explicit in the discussion, such as during interviews—is dealt with by mental healthcare workers and practically made compatible with the provision of good care.

In describing how the training of mental health professionals entails both the empathic connection with experiences and emotions of vulnerable people and the performance of non-injurious methods of restraining and coercively treating violent patients, psychologist Joseph D. Calabrese (2011) observes that psychiatric treatment is a combination of compassion and coercion. Indeed, the coercive dimension he refers to points to the most controversial problem of psychiatric institutions (Steinert et al., 2014). The use of coercive tools—whether physical, pharmacological, or

E. Rossero, *Care in a Time of Crisis*, https://doi.org/10.1007/978-3-031-34418-3_6

environmental—within the clinical context of mental health services contributes to the "therapy *versus* custody" dilemma, which has been acknowledged in other controversial fields, such as prison nursing (Willmott, 1997) and forensic psychiatry, described as moral minefields (Austin et al., 2009). As Calabrese (2011) suggests, the inherent risk of focusing on coercive interventions is such settings is that of obscuring the compassionate and caring dimension of mental healthcare, reducing psychiatric treatment to an instrument of social control and overlooking the complexities intrinsic to everyday clinical work. Such work is particularly arduous when patients are so ill and self-destructive that they evaluate everything negatively, including the prospect of a continuing existence (Calabrese, 2011). The aim of this chapter is to account for how care and coercion are held together in everyday clinical practice. These two dimensions can be so entangled to become practically undistinguished by professionals themselves. The following excerpt from the interview with Paolo, psychiatrist in the Iris Ward, provides an example of how, in the everyday prescription of pharmacological therapy, mandates to cure and control behaviour are pursued simultaneously, in this case by using drugs having a double—curative and sedative—effect, or by combining different drugs which make harder to draw the line between such purposes.

Excerpt 6.1. **Interviewer: Without environmental restraint, such as the locking of the doors, or mechanical restraint, the available tools you have are both relational and pharmacological, right?**

Paolo (psychiatrist, Iris Ward): Yes.

Interviewer: If I got it right, the pharmacological tool seems to have a double dimension: therapy administration as needed, and the regular sedative therapy. Do you think this is a correct interpretation?

Paolo: I think it is an interpretation which is more nuanced. [...] For example, the man who just got agitated, we gave him therapy as needed to contain this temporary verbal aggression, this agitation, but we can also change his [usual] therapy, so I changed it and prescribed both a therapy which will have a curative effect over the days, and a more sedative one.

Interviewer: Ok. So the distinction between a curative and a sedative dimension of therapy makes sense?

Paolo: Not always, I mean, usually therapy includes both of the things. [...] We usually administer them both [a curative and a sedative therapy]. [...] It [therapy] has a double function.

Interviewer: When you give En [delorazepam] to Giulia [a young inpatient who used to try to harm herself], is it also meant to cure, to reduce her anguish [besides controlling her behaviour]?

Paolo: This is difficult to say.

Interviewer: Yes, it is difficult for me to understand.

Paolo: It is difficult for me as well, I never thought so much about it, we give both sedative drugs and drugs which influence the structural dimensions of delusions for example, of hallucinations.

Interviewer: Such as antipsychotics?

Paolo: Usually sedative drugs are antipsychotics too. I mean, there are antipsychotics which make you very drowsy, but also facilitate sleeping and the restoration of normal sleep patterns, and there are antipsychotics which simply affect hallucinations. We use them both.

Interviewer: [...] But when nurses ask you to increase sedation, are there /specific drugs/?

Paolo: /Particular drugs/, yes, which only play that part, such as promazine, Talofen, or Entumin [clotiapine] when promazine is not enough. [...] On the other side, Haloperidol affects delusions, over the days it potentially turns hallucinations off [besides having a sedative effect].

This excerpt shows that not only can coercive and curative purposes become undistinguished in everyday clinical practice, but that they can overlap and invest different temporal frames: control of behaviour whereby medical means (i.e. pharmacological therapy) may be relevant either to manage and contain situations in the short term or to perform a prolonged effect, usually as long as the curative medication takes to show its efficacy (e.g. to turn off those hallucinations which make the person agitated or aggressive). This also relates to the exploitation of sedative effects antipsychotics can have in the short term, despite their prescription for treatment purposes over time: we have called such sedation a *deliberate collateral effect* of the administration (see Sect. 2.3.3). The routine combination of sedative and curative medication, however, does not prevent professionals from intervening on one of the two dimensions only, if they wish to: the administration of promazine, as Paolo explains, pursues the aim of controlling a patient's behaviour, of disciplining it. It is no coincidence that requests in this sense usually come from nurses, who are the professional group more concerned with the management of life in the ward (Strauss et al., 1981). When stimulated by the questions asked in the interview, the psychiatrist acknowledges the controlling (sedative) purpose of a specific medication, which is nevertheless accompanied by other therapeutic elements, both pharmacological and relational. Either within a single intervention (e.g. the administration of a sedative and curative dose of antipsychotic) or a combination of them, care and control seem to go hand-in-hand in everyday psychiatric practice.

The complex entanglement between situated, temporary goals in treating acute patients—and ultimately between the purposes of psychiatric treatment—can be practically solved by two repertoires: the first one I will call *outsourcing coercion*, which consists of excluding coercion from practices and discourses of care and attribute it to different actors, and the second one I will call *embedding coercion*, entailing the performing of coercion as (good) care. Repertoires convey different notions of good mental healthcare and result in different attempts to realize it in practice, for they consider both ideals and their performance or enactments (Pols, 2003; Mol, 2002). The following paragraphs present pure, ideal-typical versions of these repertoires I separated for my analysis: in the real world, they are not exclusive of one or another mental healthcare context considered (e.g. they do not belong either to the "restraint" or to the "no restraint" context), but instead they are adopted transversally, combined, or contaminated with spurious local elements. Moreover, they are employed to talk about different coercive interventions, whether mechanical, chemical, or manual restraint, but also involuntary treatment and forced medication. Besides the description of each pure repertoire—and the presentation of empirical data from both contexts in which they are rooted—residual aspects, deviations, and controversial elements will be discussed.

6.1 Managing Crisis in and Outside the Hospital

Before analysing coercive practices and strategies which practically and discursively hold them in a registry of (good) care, I will provide them with context by describing the services in which fieldwork has been conducted. I will consider here services where acute patients have been hosted during my period of observation: the Pine and the Iris Wards, but also the Violet Centre which usually hosts people alternatively to hospitalization. Since no acute phases of illness or involuntary treatments have been observed there, the relevant aspects of the Tulip Centre—common to other twenty-four-hour MHCs—will be mentioned in the paragraph dedicated to the Violet Centre. Spaces, routines, door policies, professional groups involved, and an outline of practices performed to care for acute patients, will be considered for each context.

6.1.1 The Pine Ward and the Iris Ward

The Pine Ward is a sixteen-bed unit, provided with seven double bedrooms and two single ones, located on the ground floor of the local general hospital. Two doors separate the ward from the crowded corridor connecting the main entrance, the café, and the other units. The first door encountered when walking towards the ward is usually open[1]: only in situations of elevated risk of absconding (i.e. the patient may leave the ward without having arranged a temporary exit or discharge with the staff), the door is locked to introduce a second barrier, should the patient manage to pass the main door. The closing of this door is an exceptional measure—which we could call *reinforced environmental restraint*—I have observed twice on the field, for a period of time limited to a few hours only. This represents also a warning sign to the members of the ward's staff who begin their shift, indicating that the situation behind the door(s)

[1] By "open" I mean wide open, held open by a wedge or other mechanism. Other door states are: "closed" (the door is not wide open but is not locked, so that anyone can open it) and "locked" (the door cannot be opened without a key or a security code).

is probably tense[2]: "After few minutes, Michela [chief psychiatrist] arrives, and fears the worst as she sees the double doors locked. I have my keys at hand, and as I open the first door I explain this is a precautionary measure for Ms. Rossi [a patient the staff believes could try to leave the ward]" (Excerpt 6.2, Pine Ward, fieldnotes).

Beyond this first door, there are four rooms: the chief psychiatrist's office; a shared medical office, where psychiatrists spend most of their time when not busy in clinical work to carry on administrative work, receive colleagues or inpatients' relatives; the nurses' coordinator's office; and a small room with a bed which is used at night by doctors on-call. This spatial configuration allows psychiatrists to work outside of the ward to perform activities which do not require contact with inpatients, being called on the phone by nurses in case of need. As a consequence, the time spent working with the nursing staff is perceived by the latter to be limited, resulting in more superficial relationships between the two professional groups.

> *Excerpt 6.5.* Cristian (nurse, Pine Ward): With the doctors we [nurses] have a relation which is less close if compared to other wards, I think. This is maybe the aspect I find more deficient. There's a reason for it because in Heart Surgery you work closely together, you share activities, treatment administration, urgency, you work side by side, there is this complicity you develop day after day in these operations where the nurse is with the doctor, there is more collaboration, more interaction. Here, the doctor does his job, which is diagnosis, therapy [prescription] and prognosis, while we administer medication and manage life on the ward. Moments of real

[2] Analogies about this "warning sign" can be drawn with the Iris Ward too. When the open-door policy was not yet implemented, the ward occasionally had the main door's glass broken and repaired with adhesive tape. This image has been described to me by staff members as the consequence of a closed-door policy, which increased tensions within the unit and sometimes resulted in patients' violent attempts to leave by hitting the door, injuring themselves and the personnel who tried to stop them. Anxiety resulting from being "welcomed" by such view as they reached their workplace was employed in nurses' discourses to sustain that danger and fear resulting from keeping patients locked in should not be part of a mental healthcare worker's job. Quotations from fieldnotes include Patrizia stating that "those who say that we should close our doors have never come here to work and found the glass with the tape, giving you gooseflesh as you were about to enter the lions' den". (*Excerpt 6.3*) and also Elettra: "I come to work in a hospital, not in Vietnam!" (*Excerpt 6.4*).

interaction are fewer, so at the beginning this is something which surprised me, and I think it should be improved.

Excerpt 6.6. Gaia (nurse, Pine Ward): With the doctors of our ward we do not have a great relationship, maybe we have more familiarity and, I don't say friendship but complicity with community doctors than with our ward's ones. [...] When a community doctor is on duty, he spends a lot of time here, in the ward /with us/ [emphasized], not in the external medical office.

The consequence of this partial exclusion from life on the ward is acknowledged by both psychiatrists and nurses: the latter know the patients better because of the time they spend with them, and this knowledge is considered and valued by doctors in the decisional process concerning discharge, suspension, or renovation of mandatory treatment, but also initiation and termination of mechanical restraint.[3] In the following excerpts from the interviews with Sandra, a psychiatrist, and Gino, an experienced nurse at the Pine Ward, we can observe how knowledge produced by nurses through observation and their daily relationship with inpatients represents a useful element for decisions concerning the performance of circulation work (see Chap. 5) and also of coercive practices (notably mechanical restraint and involuntary treatment).

Excerpt 6.7. Sandra (psychiatrist, Pine Ward): They [nurses] tell us how the patient is doing, I mean, how he behaves, if his behaviour is adequate, if when they administer medication the patient accepts it regularly and easily, if he has a good behaviour, a good attitude towards them, the ward and the other patients, because obviously they are daily in contact and they can notice the smallest hints that can emerge along the different moments of the day.

[3] The Italian verbs for these operations, "*contenere*" and "*scontenere*", will be translated as "restraining" (or "initiating mechanical restraint" to focus on the physical manoeuvre of tying the patient to the bed) and "unrestraining" (or "ending/terminating restraint" to indicate the act of untying the patient). Nouns "*contenzione*" and "*scontenzione*" will be respectively rendered as "restraint" and "unrestraining". Unless otherwise specified, the notion of restraint refers to mechanical restraint, the adjective being not repeated to make the text easier to read.

Excerpt 6.8. Gino (nurse, Pine Ward): Let's say that restraint ... is signed by the doctor. If in a situation of need the doctor is not in the ward, we [nurses] can initiate it, if it's 2 in the morning and the doctor is not here, or it's 8 in the evening and the doctor is not here and the patient goes into crisis, if we believe it is the right thing we can restrain the patient, then you inform the doctor, but we can do it. Termination of restraint as well is decided by nurses and doctors. This morning it happened with Aldo [restrained patient]. I entered the ward and Ernesto [nurse] told me: "look, he's calmer, I would unrestrain him", I said: "alright". Sandra [psychiatrist] has just arrived, she was in the external office doing some things, so I called her on the phone and I told her: "look, we were thinking of unrestraining Aldo because he looks more calm", she said: "yes, it's ok, go on", and later she came to the ward and formalized the operation, but there is this trust between the two members of the équipe, you know? [...] Usually we suggest, "we think that ...", because yes, doctors see them [the patients], they come and see them in THAT moment, right? Because when we say: "he could be unrestrained", they come and assess it, we ask them to come visiting the person. But in the end, it's us who see the patients 24 hours a day, because we have them here all the time, so even if during the visit the patient seems well, but we have seen him agitated all day long, doctors take us into consideration and say: "no, we do not unrestrain him".

The emphasis that Sandra places on behaviours, and the description provided by Gino, resonates with the relevance of nurses' observation work discussed in previous literature (Hamilton & Manias, 2007). While doctors' knowledge of patients is produced mainly in the context of formal psychiatric interviews, nurses' clinical gaze provides an account of *mental states in action*, produced through both probing and discreet observation of patients' everyday activities (ibidem). Such knowledge is rich in situated details and rooted in the social life of the ward, which nurses both observe from a distance (e.g. interactions between patients) and participate in (e.g. by interacting with patients while administering drugs, assisting with meals, or playing cards with them in the living room). This virtually continuous observation, annotation, and codification of each patient's behaviour in the clinical record is also a disciplinary tool, which produces a permanent dossier (Foucault, 2006) accessible to every member of the organization at any time, useful to inform decisions about discharge, restraint, exit permissions, and need for involuntary treatment.

Time on the ward is regulated according to a specific routine, providing temporal regularity to both patients and the staff. This constitutes what Eviatar Zerubavel has called a *clockwork environment* (1979), namely a social setting whose daily life is structured according to fairly rigid schedules. At the time of admission, a booklet is supplied to patients and their families which synthetizes daily activities organization and rules on the ward. Similarly to other hospital wards, meals are scheduled at specific times (breakfast at 8, lunch at 12, a snack at 16.30, and dinner at 19), and so is the administration of medication (after breakfast, at 15, and at 22) and relatives' visits (between 13 and 14.30 and between 19.30 and 20.30). In the afternoon, on weekdays only, rehabilitation activities such as art- and music-therapy are carried out by an OSS who is independently trained in this field: participation is open to inpatients, both individually or in groups, and occasionally to people who wish to continue with their individual therapy for some time after discharge.

With respect to the ward's rules, there are a number of objects which are not allowed for safety reasons (e.g. lighters, scissors, belts, drugs), while others are withdrawn for the night (e.g. phone chargers) or kept by the staff and provided on request for specific activities and in rationed amounts (e.g. cigarettes, money, shampoo, and shower gel). Patients can generally have their own cell phones and personal computers, but these can be kept by the staff if their use is deemed inappropriate or dangerous (e.g. frequent calls to the police, uncontrolled online shopping, and money wastage). For people whose phones have been withdrawn or who do not possess one, calling is allowed using the ward's telephones, which nevertheless allows the staff to exert some control over patients' communications.

Smoking is regulated as part of the ward routine—being allowed once per hour, at half past, from 6 in the morning to 23—so that a few minutes before the established time patients come to the nurses' room or go to the ward's terrace waiting to receive a cigarette. These timed smoke breaks have been introduced by the staff to avoid continuous interruptions by patients asking to smoke, but also to prevent them from smoking too many cigarettes a day and running out of them quickly.[4] Coffee consumption is regulated as well, being allowed twice a day, once in the morning and once after lunch. Coffees are brought to the ward by a member of the staff, who collects the requests of patients and the money from their personal drawers controlled by the personnel and goes to the coffee makers outside the unit with a small trolley to transport the cups. Patients can temporarily leave the ward to go to the coffee makers or the hospital's café if accompanied by a member of the staff, and only if their exit is deemed appropriate by the personnel. Decisions upon the appropriateness of "taking a patient out" can be made by nurses themselves, but some of them do not wish to take on responsibilities and prefer to ask psychiatrists about it, sometimes generating tensions around an evaluation which doctors consider falling within nurses' competencies. This attitude is related to a more general defensive approach, which intensified over the years, progressively reducing the number of activities and completely suppressing exits and walks outside the hospital, which were once allowed. Initiatives and flexibility about rules are now left to individual staff members or to group decisions in the single shift, sometimes resulting in internal discussions with "too permissive" colleagues and tensions with patients who may feel disoriented or complain about differentiated treatment depending on the nurses on duty.

Working shifts are organized in three intervals: the morning shift (from 7 to 14), the afternoon shift (from 14 to 21), and the night shift (from 21 to 7). During the week, four among nurses and OSS are on duty in the daily shift, three in the night; in the weekend, staffing in the daily shifts is reduced to three units. At every shift change, a short meeting called handover (*passaggio di consegne*) is held, involving one nurse of the previous shift and all of the colleagues of the following one. The average

[4] Provisions of cigarettes appeared to be a fundamental element in both the studied contexts: rates of smoking among people with mental disorders are generally higher than the general population (Lawn et al., 2002), and hospital's smoking ban is considered both risky (it would make patients nervous because of nicotine dependency) and unfair (a couple of nurses in the Pine Ward have observed how patients in other wards are free to exit the ward to smoke, while SPDC hosts cannot). Literature on this topic highlights how control over patients' access to smoking is both a mechanism of social control and a health protection measure, even though a smoking routine such as that observed in the Pine Ward might lead to increased levels of consumption, by making it a focus of the day in a context characterized by boredom and few other activities (Wood et al., 2013).

duration ranges from fifteen to thirty minutes, during which each inpatient's case is synthetically described, together with significant recent events, expected admissions or discharges, and any other information relevant to the ward activity. Nurses coordinator is occasionally present, while psychiatrists never attend these meetings: they are present only on the morning briefing which precedes clinical visits, and which is mostly useful to orient activities and perform circulation work (see Chap. 5) by evaluating and organizing discharges and transfers.[5] Psychiatrists are on duty from 8 to 20 on the weekdays, from 8 to 14 on Saturdays, and they are on-call on Saturday afternoons, Sundays, and nights. Their presence on the ward is not fixed in terms of number, and due to a chronic shortage of human resources, it was not infrequent, during fieldwork, to observe only one doctor on duty on a weekday shift.

CCTV surveillance is present on the ward in the single bedrooms, in the communal spaces (i.e. living room, terrace, hall and dining room), and by both sides of the main door. Screens showing CCTV camera images are placed in the nurses' room and are looked at by the staff routinely during the day and more carefully at night.

The Iris Ward has fifteen beds available distributed in ten bedrooms, which are used as single bedrooms when there are up to ten inpatients, or as double ones when needed. This frequently allows to provide patients with single bedrooms, avoiding conflicts and difficulties which might emerge in specific situations between roommates; on the contrary, due to overcrowding, in the Pine Ward patients have one if not two roommates most of the time.

The Iris Ward is located on the second floor of a general hospital. It is the only ward on the floor: by using either the stairs or the lift, a big hallway is reached, and the ward entrance can be found on the left. Right outside the ward's main door, there are a couple of medical offices—one for the chief psychiatrist and another which is used for meetings with

[5] As we will see in the following paragraphs, this is not true for the no-restraint context. In the Iris Ward, a meeting involving nurses, psychiatrists, and OSS is held in the morning, while the *équipe* meeting in the afternoon sees again the participation of all the professional figures, of both the morning and the afternoon shifts. The only meeting psychiatrists do not attend is the one preceding the night shift, because no doctor is present at night but only available on-call. The same applies to the Violet and the Tulip MHCs.

community mental healthcare workers and patients' relatives when the offices within the ward are not available or too small for the number of visitors—a coffee maker and a couple of plastic chairs.

The ward's door is wide open twelve hours a day, from 8 to 20. This is a relatively recent measure, introduced in 2015 by the former chief psychiatrist, and achieved gradually by opening the door from a few to several hours per day. The staff explained to me that it would be sufficient for them to keep the door closed (unlocked), so that everyone could open it freely, but due to the automatic, magnetic mechanism which locks the door as soon as it is closed (so that a code known only to the staff has to be typed on the keypad next to the door to unlock it), they have to keep it wide open.[6] This policy change has been accompanied by the introduction of a box where staff could anonymously deposit their written thoughts on the opening of the door. These have been copied into a file I had the opportunity to read and print for the purpose of this study. Topics addressed by these texts concern the reduction of tensions and patients' aggression resulting from opening the door, and the blurring of the boundary between the "inside" and the "outside", but also the perceived reduction of patients' privacy who may wander around the ward in their underwear and be visible from outside the ward, and the demanding task of discreetly monitoring the hall (e.g. while being seated and chatting with patients), which is sometimes mistaken by visitors as negligence. Indeed, the open-door policy requires the constant presence of at least one member of the staff in the hall, in order to observe who enters the ward and who might attempt to leave. Inpatients are free to go to the coffee maker beyond the ward's door, and to walk in the hallway as they drink their coffee or chat with some visitor, but they cannot take the stairs or the lift unaccompanied. Walks in the yard, to the hospital's café or chapel, are allowed with a member of the staff if the exit permission is deemed clinically appropriate, and temporary leaves of several hours can be arranged with relatives or with community professionals if activities outside the hospital have been planned and agreed with ward's

[6] Was it actually impossible to find alternatives (e.g. by asking the hospital to replace the door mechanism) in these five years, or does this solution perform other (expressive) necessities as well?

psychiatrists.[7] In this respect, the ward's (and, more generally, hospital's) boundaries are more permeable than in the Pine Ward, in both directions: not only exits are more frequent and can cross the hospital's perimeter, but also external visitors are allowed to stay in the ward outside of predetermined spans of time.

With respect to the ward's rules, patients can generally keep their money and cigarettes, though they can deposit them in a personal drawer in a dedicated locked room with other personal effects if they wish. Potentially dangerous belongings—such as lighters, drugs, and sharp objects—are not allowed in the Iris Ward either. Smoking is possible around the clock, in the smoking room or on a small balcony used by the staff as well, but patients have to rely on personnel to light their cigarettes.

Working shifts are organized on three intervals: the morning, the afternoon and the night shift, which is longer than in the Pine Ward (from 19 to 7). Five between nurses and OSS are on duty in the morning shift, four in the afternoon and three at night. Psychiatrists are on duty from 8 to 20 in the weekdays, from 8 to 14 on Saturdays, and they are on-call on Saturday afternoons, Sundays, and nights. Shortage of human resources was so severe when I conducted fieldwork that there was usually one doctor for each shift, except for occasions of overlapping in the central hours of the day: the morning doctor usually had to leave the ward later to finish clinical and administrative work s/he was not able to complete in the morning, especially if consultations had been required from the ER or critical situations occurred.

Between one shift and the other, a short meeting is held to synthetically communicate information about relevant events, involving one nurse of the previous shift and all of the colleagues of the following one. Each morning, around 9, a meeting involving nurses and psychiatrists is held to organize the activities of the day and discuss each inpatient's situation. Between the morning and the afternoon shift (h. 13–14) an *équipe*

[7] Temporary leaves and walks in the surrounding of the hospital were once allowed in the Pine Ward as well but have been gradually reduced to the point of suspending them due to an increasingly defensive attitude after an accident (the self-inflicted death of a patient who had received a temporary permission to go home). Today, when deemed clinically appropriate, patients are at best accompanied by the staff to the hospital café—50 meters away from the ward door—for short periods of time. Critiques to this risk-aversive approach have been expressed by both the nursing staff of the ward and external figures of the MHD (e.g. Cedar Centre's nurses coordinator).

meeting takes place involving all of the nurses and OSS of the two shifts, the nurses coordinator, psychiatrists, and nursing or psychiatry students when present.[8] This *équipe* meeting hosts discussions between the different professionals about each inpatient, incorporating debate on concrete issues and reflection on ward's practices in everyday work. To the purposes of this study, this activity—to which I have had daily access—represented a privileged occasion to observe discursive practices addressing conflicts and contradictions inherent to mental healthcare, how staff collectively shaped the rightness or wrongness of a specific decision or act of constraint, and how they combined it with notions of good care (Brodwin, 2014; Mol, 2010). Occasionally, the discussion can open to professionals external to the ward, such as community psychiatrists, extending the discussion to issues concerning broader mental healthcare services, called into question by specific cases. For the other shift changes (i.e. at the beginning and the end of the night shift, namely at 7 and at 19), a shorter meeting is held to synthetically communicate information about relevant events, involving one nurse of the previous shift and all of the colleagues of the following one.

6.1.2 The Violet and the Tulip Mental Health Centres

The Violet Centre is located in a wide and beautiful park, quiet, well-tended, and rich in biodiversity. In order to prevent its identification, I will refer to it as the Peaceful Park, because of the feeling of calmness I got from walking along its trails in those warm, late September days of fieldwork. The park, located in a peripheral area of the city, used to host the former psychiatric hospital, and its name is still associated by many inhabitants with the old institution. The past is not only embedded in the local language, memories, and common sense, but visible, even readable: the very name of the bus stop I used twice a day with many patients and service users—because the park also hosts the local SerD (drugs and other

[8] A member of the staff—usually an OSS—does not participate in the meeting to remain in the hall and provide assistance to people in the ward. S/he also protects the meeting by asking patients or visitors to wait for it to be over and answering the ward's phone so that non-urgent calls do not interrupt the discussion.

addictions service) and several administrative health facilities—still reports "psychiatric hospital" right after the name of the park. The immediate association between the place and mental health can represent an obstacle to the treatment of new people, who might prefer being admitted to the neutral general hospital instead.

> *Excerpt 6.9.* Sonia (psychiatrist, Violet Centre): This Mental Health Centre rests in an area that is the same as the former asylum, so the patient can live it like: "I'm not coming to the Peaceful Park because it's a place-, because it's for those of the asylum, because there was the asylum, I'd rather go to the hospital because it's more socially acceptable to be admitted to the hospital without saying where [in which ward]".

The organization of a whole new model of mental healthcare after the dismantling of the asylum entailed also a re-signification of the place, in an attempt to overcome the stigma and related feelings of shame linked with frequenting and staying in that area. This is accomplished through a complex set of mnemonic products and practices (Olick, 2008), such as books, stories, and the recalling of specific episodes, but also buildings and the names they are identified with, which tell us something about their past and—more crucially—about their transition to the present and the very process of deinstitutionalization. In the following excerpt Cecilia, nurse at the Violet Centre, explains to me why a residential facility near the MHC is still called "the Director's House".

> *Excerpt 6.10.* [Cecilia] tells me about one of these [residential] facilities, called The Director's House ['*la Casa del Direttore*'], focusing on its name: it was the facility which hosted the director of the former psychiatric hospital, right outside of its walls. When, at the beginning of the 90s, the first [asylum] wards began to be closed, change was so profound for people who had spent their life in the asylum, that they moved to that facility with some mental healthcare workers, literally just outside the asylum's gate. Nowadays, the residential facility maintains this name in order to remember what it had been, which is something Cecilia considers of fundamental importance. (Violet Centre, fieldnotes)

From a spatial point of view, the Violet Centre is a single-floor building, provided with three entrances on three sides. It can host up to eight people in four double bedrooms. User population of the centre is heterogeneous and generally numerous: besides up to eight patients hosted in the twenty-four hours, people can come to the centre to have lunch, collect medication, have medical interviews with their psychiatrist, spend the day at the centre, or walk in freely to seek help if they are not known by the service yet. Visitors are allowed in the communal spaces and generally in the bedroom area as well (under staff's supervision if deemed necessary), and some patients come to the centre with a relative or a caregiver. In a typical weekday shift, the staff on duty at the centre includes four psychiatrists, a psychologist, a social worker, a rehabilitation specialist, an average of six between nurses and OSS, and the nurses coordinator, none of whom wears a uniform, white coat, or identifiable clothing.[9] Some staff members continuously leave and return to the centre for home visits and other activities (e.g. visiting patients admitted to the SPDC). Contrary to the more static ward setting, the MHC context is much more dynamic, dispersed, and difficult to observe globally: multiple activities are performed simultaneously around (and outside of) the centre, involving several people, and including also an intense telephonic activity with other services but mostly with patients, who receive day and night support also by phone. These organizations and *équipe* are typical of the Tulip Centre as well. As a consequence, the Mental Health Centres are deemed inappropriate for specific types or phases of illness which benefit from relaxed, less crowded environments, such as the SPDC.

> *Excerpt 6.11.* Chiara (psychiatrist, Tulip Centre): [A patient is admitted to the SPDC] if he requires less stimuli, because if the person is in a frank, flourishing, psychotic phase, here [in the MHC] there is too much chaos, there are false recognitions [the person can confuse those she meets with

[9] This is consistent with the approach of Basaglia and the professionals working with him, who contested their own power as psychiatrists by stripping themselves of its symbols, such as white coats (Foot, 2015). In the no-restraint context, references to Basaglia are frequent in many discourses, practices, and in the material environment (e.g. a poster hung on the wall of the office of Violet Mental Health Centre's director).

> someone else], while there [in the SPDC] the environment is more protected. Also, for manic episodes it can be useful, it is related to the [ward's] routine, its tidy spaces, which sometimes are experienced more easily than MHC, at the beginning. It's more hospital.

In MHC busy environment, the management of crisis entails a reconfiguration and prioritization of the activities around the patient's needs: one or more healthcare workers can be designated to follow him/her around and outside the centre (a practice which is called "*affiancamento*"), accompany him/her for a walk in the park or to the nearby coffee bar, administer extra medication (also coercively) and prevent the patient from leaving the centre by temporarily locking the exits or, if s/he is outside, by obstructing his/her way and physically stopping him/her (only when the person is under compulsory treatment, TSO). Show of force, through the gathering of an elevated number of staff members from different professional groups, is usually performed to dissuade escalation of the patient's behaviour. No mechanical means of restraint are present at this and other centres, while the (oral or intramuscular) administration medication with the purpose to control patient's behaviour should be limited—to some extent—by the impossibility for the centre to monitor severe health conditions (MHCs cannot perform emergency blood tests, nor electrocardiogram).[10] A medical assessment in a hospital environment is performed prior to hosting patients who are not known or who have not maintained contact with the service for a long time.

In the Tulip Centre, the situation is complicated by an undesirable spatial configuration: the building develops over four floors connected by a spiral staircase, and the area dedicated to the "*Centro Diurno*" is small, provided with a little garden, lacking the wide and safe spaces surrounding the Violet Centre. Crises requiring "*affiancamento*" are very

[10] In the only case of involuntary treatment observed in a Mental Health Centre (the Violet Centre) during fieldwork, the patient—Santiago—was treated with different drugs (quetiapine, olanzapine, promazine, biperiden, valproate, and delorazepam altogether), at dosages that the medical staff considered very high but collectively decided to administer daily. A nurse, for example, commented: "it's impressive to read his therapy and know that he breaths autonomously" (i.e. that he is not mechanically ventilated in an ICU). Chapter 6 will further discuss on this point comparatively with other practices and their preferability according to our participants.

demanding for the staff, which has to follow the person up and down the different floors, or in small areas which are usually crowded (e.g. the first floor where users wait to receive medication, the "*Centro Diurno*" populated by both external and admitted patients). Nevertheless, when beds are available and the MHC is deemed appropriate for the patient and the phase of illness s/he is going through, the Tulip Centre hosts crises as well, including compulsory treatments, and despite the efforts required to involuntarily treat patients in an open environment such as a Mental Health Centre.

Due to the open and heterogeneously populated environment of Mental Health Centres, control over patients' belongings is a bit looser than in the hospital. After a previous agreement with their psychiatrist, users hosted on the twenty-four hours can leave the centre alone or with relatives and friends, and searches are not performed once they go back to the centre. Surveillance over dangerous objects and drugs is performed by the staff in a more informal and discreet modality than the ward, through enhanced observation and with regular interactions with users. Patients can generally keep their money and cigarettes, unless this is considered problematic for specific reasons (e.g. the person may lose or waste money, or run out of cigarettes quickly). Smoking is possible around the clock, in the area outside of the centres or, at night, in a dedicated space within the building. Specific rooms are locked because they are not accessible to the patients unsupervised, due to the inherent risks of the spaces or objects stored in there (e.g. pharmacy, kitchen, and dining room).

Working shifts in the MHCs are organized in three intervals: the morning (7–14), the afternoon (13–20), and the night shift (from 19 to 7). Overlapping portions of shifts are dedicated to handovers or extended *équipe* meetings (from 13 to 14 or more), which take place daily with the participation of all professional groups. Once a week, in the Violet Centre, the *équipe* splits in two segregated meetings (psychiatrists/psychologist and nurses/OSS) to discuss intra-professional issues (e.g. the doctors read the record of new service users and assign them to a psychiatrist who will take charge of that case).[11] Psychiatrists are on duty from 8 to 20 on the weekdays, from 8 to 14 on Saturdays, and they are on-call on Saturday afternoons, Sundays, and nights. In case of critical situations (such as that of Santiago, involuntarily treated at the Violet Centre) psychiatrists, nurses and nurses coordinator have been observed to be available to prolong their shift over its official ending, or be telephonically reached at nights or weekends even when not formally on-call.

6.2 Outsourcing Coercion: Segregating Care and Coercion

The first repertoire observed in both contexts to hold together care and coercion operates by segregating the two and attributing them to different actors: respectively mental healthcare workers and law enforcement agencies (police forces, but also hospital's security guards). This strategy faces a number of problematic issues, concerning both the definition of what counts as coercion, and its practical separation—which, as we have seen (Excerpt 6.1), is not straightforward—from ordinary care practices. Moreover, it provides a tentative—and not always agreed upon—answer to a question which appeared to be crucial to our participants: which interventions are expected from (mental) healthcare workers? Which fall under their jurisdiction, and which do not?

Even though different actors may draw the boundary between healthcare-related and non-healthcare-related differently—by including as legitimate practices which other contexts exclude and vice versa—the strategy of outsourcing (specific forms of) coercion emerges transversally,

[11] Attribution of the psychiatrist to a new patient is here performed through a discussion: the record of the unknown person (written by a nurse who has met her for a first assessment and information gathering) is read aloud, and doctors can express their will to "take" the case, in a generally smooth (sometimes described as "natural") distribution. In the Cedar Centre, new contacts are not met by nurses beforehand, and therefore no information prior to the first medical encounter is available. Attribution follows a casual order (doctors are listed and patients are assigned according to the order of the requests) to avoid disagreement emerged in the past when other criteria, deemed non-neutral, where applied (e.g. territorial competence penalized the psychiatrist associated with more problematic areas in terms of population, extension, and accessibility).

in both community and hospital settings. This paragraph addresses this operation of exclusion of coercion from the realm of healthcare, while the following ones, pertaining to the repertoire of embedding coercion, will consider how coercive interventions can be retained in that realm and performed as acts of (good) care.

The issue of separating healthcare from non-healthcare practices when it comes to intervening on a patient in crisis appeared plastically with respect to the case of Pietro, a patient involuntarily admitted to the Iris Ward after having assaulted his general practitioner (the man, after three months without medication, was delusional, believing in a conspiracy against him between the GP and the mental health services). Pietro is already known in the ward: he has been admitted before and has already shown aggressiveness, especially toward other inpatients (he once assaulted a Black woman for racial reasons, causing her serious injuries). He is a man in his forties, in good physical shape, and a former paratrooper: his admission causes some tension in the ward because of his reputation and the aggressive response to delusions he has just showed by assaulting his doctor. On his arrival, he is coercively treated with the most commonly used forced medication (Raboch et al., 2010), namely sedative and antipsychotic drugs (delorazepam, promazine, zuclopenthixol, and haloperidol). Like for every inpatient, therapy is administered three times a day, but Pietro does not accept treatment from the ward's staff alone: he demands the presence of police officers.

The issue of treatment refusal and forced medication on involuntarily admitted people has emerged transversally across my field: episodes of forcibly medicated acute patients have been observed both in the restraint (Pine Ward) and the no-restraint (Violet Centre) contexts, generally performed by the healthcare staff itself. On such occasions, the person is held and manually restrained (on the floor, on the bed, or in a standing position) by two or more members of the staff for a few seconds, while another nurse administers medication through injection. In the Iris Ward, forced medication is practically *decomposed* into its constitutive parts: the coercive dimension (the "forced" act of restraining the person refusing treatment) and the medical dimension (medication itself, namely the act of injecting therapy). The two elements are attributed to different figures—respectively the police (or equivalent agencies) and the healthcare staff—which need to be contemporarily present and cooperating to perform forced medication. Since police officers are not routinely present in the ward (even though the hospital has two dedicated officers intervening in the different wards), they have to be called on purpose in situations of need. In the case of Pietro, who regularly refuses therapy, police have to be called three times a day for regular therapy administration, as well as for extraordinary episodes (e.g. should the patient leave the ward or assault someone). Such frequent requests for police intervention are not easily accepted by officers, which do intervene but question the appropriateness of their presence for medical purposes (i.e. to administer pharmacological therapy within a hospital setting). The following excerpt reports fieldnotes covering a whole day with Pietro, synthesizing events and discourses around the issue of police intervention for therapy administration.

> *Excerpt 6.12.* At 10 Pietro is awake but still in bed. Rosa [nurse] calls 112 to ask for police intervention for therapy administration, but when she hangs up she tells us they have been unkind: they told her they have more important things to do, and that the *SPDC has enough doctors and nurses to intervene without them.* Marzia [nurse] calls the internal [hospital] police. The officer says he will come, and he will contact the external police if necessary. He arrives a few minutes later and they [officer, nurses and doctor] go to Pietro's room. I observe from the doorway. Nurses measure his blood pressure and other parameters, then he let them administer IM therapy without complaining (En, Talofen, acuphase, Clopixol depot). We return to the medical office. The officer stays in the hall with us for a while, talking with me and Marzia, whom he knows well. When discussing about who should intervene in cases like this, Marzia says *they [nurses] are only healthcare workers.* The officer agrees but replies that the internal police is entitled to intervene only if something happened (e.g. an aggression), so their presence now is almost a personal favor, because they know the ward and its situations. The same cannot be expected from external police which does not know/understand the ward. [...] It's almost 14, when afternoon therapy has to be administered. Elettra [nurse] tries to call the internal police to ask for an officer to come, but nobody answers the phone. Luana [psychiatrist] calls 112, explaining that hospital police is not available. After fifteen minutes, two [Carabinieri] officers arrive. Pietro is in the TV

room. Lorenzo [nurse] approaches him, telling him that he should do En and Talofen. Pietro replies: "I do them but not aripiprazole" (Abilify). Lorenzo reassures him [and Abilify will not be administered]. Pietro goes to his room, followed by Lorenzo (who brings ready syringes, cotton wool and gloves), the two officers and me. The man lays on his bed and let Lorenzo inject medication without batting an eyelid. We go back to the medical office. The officers, both young, seem perplexed, like they did not understand the need for their presence for such a calm patient. One of them kindly tells nurses that *police cannot intervene for a simple therapy administration*, that they are not allowed to put their hands on anyone within the hospital [...] and that they can only operate outside, to bring the involuntary admitted patient to the hospital for admission or if he leaves the ward, or if the patient smashes something or hurts somebody. [...] [On the following day, during a staff meeting] Elettra [nurse] says: "yesterday an officer told me that we [nurses] are allowed to put our hands on patients, and that they [police] come only as a favor". [...] Franco [nurse]: "when I worked in [another service] there used to be a great relationship with the police, *they knew who had to intervene when a patient had to be immobilized.* Today nobody wants to raise their hands and intervene anymore". (Iris Ward, fieldnotes)

As we can read from the excerpt, the segregation of the coercive dimension from medical elements of forced medication, and its attribution to a third figure (police officers), is not straightforward. While the ward's staff underlines its own healthcare role, maintaining that coercion should be performed by other (designated) figures, police officers prioritize the medical setting and purpose of the intervention (therapy administration), contesting the pertinence of their involvement.[12] This situation reveals a general lack of formal agreements between the different organizations—mental health services and the police forces—which leaves the

[12] Questioning of the appropriateness of the police intervention has been observed also in the Violet Centre: "Clarissa [nurse] speaks about yesterday evening's intervention of the police officers, who used their physicality to persuade Santiago to take medication [show of force]. After the successful intervention they complaint with nurses, saying that for similar cases they should call the doctor on-call or the ambulance, because they [police officers] are officers of justice and *they are not comfortable in intervening to convince a patient to accept therapy*. Clarissa says that they replied claiming that Santiago was in involuntary treatment, so it was legitimate to call the police" (Excerpt 6.13., Violet Centre, fieldnotes).

management of contextual situations to informal routines, relationships developed over time between the actors, and personal dispositions of nurses and individual officers (e.g. the hospital police which intervenes "as a personal favour" to the nurses they have known from a long time).[13] Police officers internal to the hospital are generally more available than external police forces because they know and—to some extent—they share the ward's perspective and practices, but nevertheless do find frequent interventions demanding. Police willingness to intervene on mental health service users is also influenced by additional elements, such as limited resources (external police has only two patrols covering the whole city, and interventions in the ward or the MHC usually take some time), and a general defensive attitude (highlighted also by Franco in the excerpt above) influenced by recent serious accidents (e.g. the death of Andrea Soldi in Turin after a violent police intervention to perform a TSO). Police intervention does not necessarily translate into the use of force, either because their sole presence is sufficient to persuade a patient to cooperate or because some officers have developed relational skills useful to gain patients' trust and convince them to accept medication or admission. In the case of Pietro, medication is not materially forced on him: coercion is due to the involuntary treatment, and in front of the police officers he allows nurses to inject therapy. What I wish to focus on here, though, is the repertoire adopted by SPDC mental healthcare workers, who discursively (i.e. by maintaining their healthcare role) and practically (i.e. by calling the police) separate coercion from care, even when the two are entangled in the performance of a single intervention (i.e. involuntary therapy administration). Exclusion of coercion from ward's practice has been maintained also with respect to other coercive interventions, such as the prevention of patients' absconding through environmental restraint (temporary locking of the doors) or physical restraint: "the only place when you can be sure that a person does not escape is prison. We are healthcare workers, security is a police matter, and that's all!" (Franco, nurse in the Iris Ward).

[13] Lack of formal agreements between mental health services and police forces is present (and potentially problematic) in both the restraint and the no-restraint context. Relationships between the two are then fluctuant over time and space, depending on the position of the local police leadership.

Outsourcing of coercion and the issue of involving the police in tense situations with patients has been observed also with respect to another interesting case, that of Santiago. Santiago is a Bolivian young man going through a profound psychotic crisis, involuntarily treated in the SPDC and then transferred to the Violet Centre few days before my arrival. At the beginning of September 2019, he starts to show signs of worsening psychic decompensation and he accepts to be admitted to the SPDC. In the following days, community psychiatrists and nurses go to the hospital to visit and talk to him, and despite his voluntary admission, he attempts to leave the ward on several occasions. He eventually manages to leave twice: on the first time, he arrives at the Violet Centre at night, where he is hosted and then accompanied back to the ward in the morning; the second time, police are called to find him and take him back to the hospital. His voluntary admission is transformed into an involuntary one. The Violet Centre staff will talk to me about these days as very difficult ones, criticizing the ward's staff for letting Santiago go away too easily. According to the community professionals, besides relational and pharmacological therapy, SPDC staff should have physically stopped the man to prevent him from leaving. Ward's staff, on the other hand, maintains that such measure (*atterramento*) does not belong to their practices and refuses to perform it.

> *Excerpt 6.14.* [Paolo, psychiatrist] tells me what happened when Santiago tried to leave the ward. In the first place, the staff went after him, trying to convince him to go back. If he exited the hospital perimeter, an ambulance and the police were called. According to Paolo, *it would have not been ethically correct to force him to the floor* [as the Violet Centre suggested], especially *because there was no effective therapy they could administer.* He maintains that on those occasions the Violet Centre refused to send some of its staff, blamed the ward for Santiago's leavings, and called Paolo on the phone to tell him what to do (force Santiago to the floor). Paolo seems offended by this unfair and rude behaviour, interpreted as an attack to his work and a form of interference. (Iris Ward, fieldnotes)

Emphasized text in the excerpt above describes how, according to Paolo, the measure of forcing a patient to the floor is a coercive intervention they are not willing to perform, especially because, he observes, no pharmacological therapy could be effectively administered afterward. In this case, the measure called into question (*atterramento*) does not even include a medical dimension: it performs a function of mere control, aimed at preventing the patient from leaving the ward, and therefore it is excluded from the ward's practices. In his interview, Paolo will further explain that Santiago's attempts to leave were not motivated by suicidal (or otherwise dangerous) intentions which might constitute a "state of necessity" and call for an imminent response to prevent him from leaving by whatever means, so they saw the coercive intervention as further unmotivated. On the other hand, the psychiatrist discusses about (healthcare-related) interventions they have legitimately performed to deal with Santiago's frequent attempts to leave the ward. Besides pharmacological therapy, which was administered at elevated dosages and nevertheless seemed not to show any relevant effect, relationship was prioritized, together with non-coercive attempts and strategies to convince the patient to return to the hospital.

> *Excerpt 6.15.* Paolo (psychiatrist, Iris Ward): Santiago escaped several times and we always went after him. It's not that if you administer therapy then you don't invest on relationality: you administer therapy and you stay with people. I mean, with Santiago we laughed, and we joked around, we went with him to take a coffee also in paradoxical conditions, you know? [...] Once I ran after him, I mean, I went after him with someone [ward's nurse], and while he was leaving, I asked him: "would you like to have some coffee?"—I tried even though nobody would expect him to say yes—but he said yes, so we went in [a café outside of the hospital], then the ambulance arrived and he accepted to get in [and go back to the ward].

Since Santiago was under TSO, police were called every time he attempted to leave the ward, remarking upon the different functions expected to be performed by healthcare workers (dialogue, persuasion, therapy administration) and by police officers (show of force, physical restraining of non-compliant patients, if necessary).

In the restraint context, specifically at the Cedar Centre, a similar segregation of functions has been described to me during the interviews by both psychiatrists and nurses. In tense situations, such as a (repeated) patient's refusal to take medication, the staff working within the MHC relies mainly on relational tools, consisting of de-escalation techniques and involvement of the different personalities and approaches (more reassuring, firmer, depending on what might be effective in the specific case) composing the *équipe*. Police forces are called to represent (more frequently than to enact) the possibility to resort to a forced intervention, which is usually sufficient to persuade the person to cooperate.

Excerpt 6.16. Giorgio (psychiatrist, Cedar Centre): It recently happened with a boy, he would not accept depot medication, we had to call the police because, the presence of the police when you do not have other [relational] tools anymore, it gives substance … It's symbolic.

Excerpt 6.17. Cesare (nurse, Cedar Centre): Police forces are useful as a deterrent, for their uniform. If [a patient] raises his voice, we manage to contain a bit, you have to attenuate, calm him down, de-escalation and everything. If we see that the situation keeps escalating, we call the police and usually the uniform, most of the times to see the police, to see the uniform is effective.

Interestingly, the same coercive intervention which the Iris Ward refused to perform (*atterramento*) is not necessarily excluded from practices adopted by another service within the same no-restraint context: the Violet Centre. As we can read in Excerpt 6.14, the community psychiatrist calls the ward asking them to force Santiago to the floor should he attempt to leave the ward again. When the boy is transferred to the MHC, still under involuntary treatment, his most serious behaviours (e.g. aggressiveness, or serious attempts to leave the centre) that could not be solved through non-coercive measures (dialogue, persuasion, show of force) are actually dealt with through the performance of *atterramento* by MHC's personnel, either to forcibly administer medication or to prevent him from leaving and coercively bring him back to the centre. The measure is physically demanding and potentially risky for healthcare workers involved in its performance: during a staff meeting, nurses complain about the previous Sunday afternoon, when they had to force Santiago to the floor in the park. Once they managed to take the boy back to the MHC, they called the police and the psychiatrist on-call. The following excerpt reports the psychiatrist's reply to their complaints.

> *Excerpt 6.18.* Claudio [psychiatrist] maintains that *having to intervene like last Sunday (forcing Santiago to the floor in the park surrounding the MHC) is part of their job* and it is something which can happen. Terms used to refer to the intervention are: "containment" (the act of obstructing the way to prevent a patient from leaving) and "physical containment" (the act of physically stopping the person by grabbing him or, like Sunday, forcing him on the floor). Then, Claudio underlines that in case of need the first figure to call is the *healthcare* one (he emphasizes this word), namely the doctor on-call, and that police officers are only ancillary figures. (Violet Centre, fieldnotes)

The words of Claudio retain the coercive intervention in the registry of care, claiming it to be part of their job (as healthcare providers) which sometimes is necessary to perform. The psychiatrist's last indication—to preferably call the doctor on-call rather than (or at least before) the police in difficult situations—shows a general inclination to avoid involving the public force and solve the emergent problem within the realm of the healthcare setting. This point is further developed during her interview by another psychiatrist of the MHC, Sonia.

> *Excerpt 6.19.* Sonia (psychiatrist, Violet Centre): We resort to the police as an extrema ratio, it has been done at night, it is understandable because it is a risky moment, there are only two nurses per shift, or there can be situations when other people in the centre have to be protected, so it can make sense [to call the police], otherwise … it seems like a defect in our work, like *we are delegating to a uniform something which maybe could be solved through the relationship with the patient*, it may take some time but maybe you can do it without asking for a [police] intervention. […] This is something that sometimes is questioned by the nursing staff, like we should work only in critical-but-not-too-critical situations. Like: "until this point yes, then no". I think that sometimes, it is not the norm, sometimes we can

go beyond, it's not usual, it's occasional, but we can be asked to do things which are not very nice, which we don't like, which we limit and attempt to limit to few and rare cases, but … it can happen.

Such *autarchic approach*—which avoids resorting to external, non-medical forces, also if this means that healthcare workers have to perform coercive interventions—takes us to the second repertoire, that of embedding coercion in the medical setting, and to the strategies employed to perform coercive acts as acts of (good) care. The different orientation toward one repertoire or the other seems related to structural aspects, such as the Iris Ward's location in a protected setting—that of the hospital, surrounded by a wide and circumscribed inner yard and other hospital annexes—and the availability of police officers internal to the organization and syntonic with SPDC approach. Community services cannot rely on any similar resource, but only on external police forces that are not always immediately available, nor necessarily aware and supportive of Mental Health Centres' practices and orientation. Moreover, MHCs' placement in a park near a country road (Violet Centre) or residential neighbourhood (Tulip Centre) can imply more immediate risks for unwell patients walking away, and require a prompter intervention necessarily performed by the staff itself. In the restraint context, the SPDC is located in a secondary hospital building about three kilometres away from the main one and it does not usually rely on internal security guards (I never saw them in the ward, nor heard about episodes implying their involvement), but only on external police forces which have been described as reluctant to intervene within the hospital unless serious accidents have occurred. These structural aspects which hinder the outsourcing of coercion facilitate the development and shaping of both practices and discourses that frame the healthcare staff as independent and "autarchic" also with respect to coercive interventions, which are attempted to be included in a healthcare framework and embedded in the therapeutic relationship through different strategies presented in the following section.

6.3 Embedding Coercion: Performing Coercion as (Good) Care

The second repertoire operates by embedding coercion in everyday practices and discourses, which allow to legitimize it and perform it as good care. To this extent, four strategies have been identified: (i) therapeuticization of coercion, performed by maintaining the beneficial effects of the coercive intervention; (ii) proceduralization of coercion, which frames the coercive act as safe, controlled, correct, even scientific; (iii) relationalization of coercion, implying the combination of coercion with relational elements of trust, honesty, dialogue and compassion; and (iv) multiplication of the objects of care, which justifies the coercive measure on the basis of others' (inpatients, staff, family, society itself) best interest. In what follows, I will consider coercion in its multiplicity of manifestations: mechanical and other forms of restraint, but also enforced medication, and involuntary admission and treatment. These measures are characterized by different degrees of coercion (see also Sect. 2.1.1) and imply differentiated attempts of persuasion and negotiation to be avoided, even though the eventually achieved patient's consent does not necessarily indicate genuine voluntariness: medication or hospitalization can be accepted consequently to an explicit verbal threat (e.g. "either you accept admission or we will hospitalize you coercively"), a physically performed one (e.g. show of force), or the general "coercive shadow" that looms over mental healthcare, pushing service users to accept an intervention to avoid fear, stigma, and humiliation related to compulsory measures (Szmukler, 2017). The strategies that I am about to present have been adopted by participants to frame and account for many of these differentiated situations along the coercion spectrum. I have attempted to select relevant examples from the field—either observed and reported in my fieldnotes or described in the interviews—allowing to account for the heterogeneity and complexities of coercion and its articulated intertwining with care in everyday practices.

6.3.1 Therapeuticization of Coercion

The first strategy by which an act of coercion can be framed as performing good care is what I will call the *therapeuticization* of that act. This operation can rest on several mechanisms: a paternalistic approach, but also a claim of the variegated beneficial consequences of the coercive intervention, and the conceptual shift which transforms restraint into an act of protection or affective support.

As the anthropologist Tanya Marie Luhrmann (2001) observes, a fundamental operation learnt by psychiatrists to come to terms with the imbalance of power in their clinical practice is the drawing of a line between the person and the illness. In this view, which resonates with a biological model of mental illness, the disorder is disconnected by the person and treated as if it had temporarily displaced him/her. This disconnection ethically sanitizes the coercive act as it allows professionals to intervene on the patient without considering the person as a sovereign decision-maker with his/her own will and agency: instead, the intervention can be framed as a therapeutic attempt to care and recuperate the person who had been temporarily subjugated by mental illness (Brodwin, 2014). The following excerpt from fieldnotes is well representative of this strategy: it concerns the program designed by psychiatrists for the post-discharge of a boy, Silvio, who does not agree with their plan and perceive it as a form of coercion.

> *Excerpt 6.20.* Silvio is laid on his bed, as usual. [As we enter the room] he sits up and says he does not want to go to the residential facility, but he knows they will force him to go: "I see it as an imposition, so I automatically fight it". Vincenzo [psychiatrist] replies it is not an imposition, "imposition is a strong word", but there are no alternatives, he already went back home after discharge one month ago, and after three weeks he had to be re-admitted again, so his solution does not work. Silvio insists that he is not free to choose, that the [community] doctor had talked about the residential facility as a proposal, and a proposal can be accepted or refused. Instead, he has no choice. Vincenzo replies that maybe "proposal" is not the right word, and suggests "offer" instead, but that can be refused too, so at the end he chooses "program", saying that a program can be discussed between

> competent people, and a patient does not have the competences to do so. Silvio says this is a life choice they are making on his behalf, depriving him of freedom. The doctor replies that freedom is a concept which is only black or white, while in psychiatry there exist grey areas, due to the fact that *illness undermines a person's capability to choose freely, so it is necessary to trust the doctors.*[14] (Pine Ward, fieldnotes)

This strategy of segregating personhood and patienthood is eloquently visible in practices and discourses concerning involuntary admission and treatment. Besides legal criteria, these measures are usually motivated—explicitly (in TSO papers) or implicitly—by the patient's lack of awareness of his/her own state of illness. Lack of insight is acknowledged as an obstacle to shared decision-making and patient-centred psychiatric practice (Seale et al., 2006). Both in the restrain and the no-restraint context, a cooperative relationship and therapeutic alliance with patients was generally preferred and pursued, by listening and taking into consideration patients' wishes and preferences, discussing treatment alternatives, and remaining open to negotiation about medication choices and the subjective relevance of their adverse effects. Also, an evolution toward more cooperative practices and fewer coercive interventions (notably involuntary treatments) than in the past was commonly perceived, referring to an increased tendency to share decisions about treatment with patients and promote the inclusion and cooperation also of their significant others: "what I observe now is that we try harder to involve family in decisions concerning the patient, especially when he is temporarily unable to decide for himself" (Fausta, nurses coordinator at the Cedar Centre). Involuntary treatment is described as a "last resort" measure, employed after gradual attempts to regain the patient's cooperation, which failed to build a therapeutic alliance. Despite this general commitment to a patient-centred

---

[14] After the visit, the doctor will explain to me that they actually have no power to force Silvio to spend some time at the residential facility if he does not want to, even if the alternative is to discharge him and probably re-admit him after some time. Nevertheless, during the visit, he attempts to obtain his collaboration by presenting the transfer to the facility as the only viable option, underlining his previous, unsuccessful attempts to decide for himself, his lack of medical competences and his reduced ability to choose for his best because of illness. This paternalistic attitude is intended here as a therapeutic intent to care and recuperate the person who had been temporarily displaced by mental illness.

approach, the need to become more directive, even coercive, when the person was judged to be too ill to participate in rational decisions, or not to have insight, was acknowledged by psychiatrists and other mental healthcare professionals as inevitable.[15]

> *Excerpt 6.21.* Davide (psychiatrist, Cedar Centre): Relationship [with patients] is asymmetrical. Then you can make it civilized or uncivilized [he laughs], like: "you have this, you do that, and shut up, because I said so!", "sorry, I'd like to ask-", "don't ask, I don't give any explanation!", this is uncivilized, ok. But the fact that *I know and you don't,* because you are unwell and I am the one who has to cure you, this is it. How can you change this? It's impossible, it makes no sense, it's a waste of energy. [...] Otherwise you go to a friend, why don't you go to a friend? That is symmetrical, you are on the same level, he knows as much as you do, maybe something more, but it's symmetrical, right? But if relationship is asymmetrical and he [the patient] comes to you ... it's inevitable that in a difficult moment YOU have to guide him. Even if this means saying: "go there", "I don't want to", "you must go there". Necessarily.

Consistent with previous literature on this topic (Seale et al., 2006), the decision to intervene coercively, by treating a patient against their will, was presented as something which can be "repaired" later, once patients are considered to have regained (partial) awareness of their condition. Even though this is not always the case, and some patients still express some resentment for the coercive episode after the crisis has passed, the coercive act can also be legitimized by asserting that the patient will eventually understand the good reasons behind a difficult medical decision, accepting that it was performed in his/her best interest. In both restraint and no-restraint contexts, the benefit and necessity of the intervention is presented as something which the person herself will retrospectively acknowledge too, allowing the therapeutic relationship to

---

[15] An alternative to this paternalistic, also involving the informal caregivers (patient's relatives), approach might include documents which have been variously called "psychiatric advance directives" or "joint crisis plans" (Henderson et al., 2008). Such instruments allow service users to state their preferences for future mental health care, especially in times of crisis, consistently with a model of shared decision making and the implementation of the United Nations Convention on the Rights of Persons with Disabilities (Szmukler, 2019).

be maintained and move forward. Evidence of this retrospective acknowledgement is sometimes found in the fact that the patient does not ask to change his/her psychiatrist after the coercive episode, even though this is not a straightforward operation (which requires discussion within the professional *équipe* to evaluate the person's motives and implications of the change) and might be hindered by dynamics intrinsic to a cohesive medical group.

Excerpt 6.22. Irene (psychiatrist, Pine Ward): I happened to do a TSO to patients and once they have regained a bit of awareness of the fact that when they had been [involuntarily] admitted nothing else could be done, our relationship was not undermined, and I keep seeing patients I have involuntarily admitted. It depends also on the relationship you have before. If you have a relationship and there is a phase of decompensation, for which you have to choose admission, then relationship can be restored, I never had particular difficulties. If the patient understands that in that moment there was nothing else you could do, in the meantime of course he will tell you whatever, but afterwards no, if there is a good relationship, I think that for our work relationship is everything, everything.

Excerpt 6.23. Chiara (psychiatrist, Tulip Centre): What usually happens is that the person understands. Maybe she doesn't know how to call what happened, she doesn't accept the name that we are suggesting, but we were there [for her].

Excerpt 6.24. Davide (psychiatrist, Cedar Centre): It is like cutting [amputating] an arm, it is the same thing. Because I can-, it is difficult to cut an arm, but if I do it at the right time you will never reproach me. It is difficult for the doctor, this is precisely the burden of medical work, unfortunately this is inevitable, the burden of medical work is to understand and bear all of the tensions you have to face when you decide, I mean, when you become aware of when you have to make a decision. And this is something that, you are alone in this, the doctor is alone. [...] Once you make the decision it is difficult that-, the other [the patient] will understand, the other understands that you did it with all the difficulty and depth which are needed, and it is difficult that he reproaches you.

Therapeuticization of the coercive act—which is also a form of ethical sanitization (Brodwin, 2014)—is also performed through the assertion of the beneficial effects it will have on the person to whom it applies. This has been observed, for example, with respect to mechanical restraint. In the Pine Ward, this measure was sometimes employed suggesting a calming effect enabling agitated patients to fall asleep. The therapeutic dimension of restraint can be both explicitly maintained and indirectly asserted by describing its beneficial effects and using terminology (e.g. prescription) which qualifies it as a medical act (see Excerpt 6.25). The following quotation is also interesting in that, similarly to discourses concerning involuntary treatment, it employs as a further element of legitimation the patient's acknowledgement—even gratitude—for the relief provided through restraint.[16]

> *Excerpt 6.25.* Gaia (nurse, Pine Ward): Sometimes [mechanical restraint] is useful to reduce excitement, because there are patients with persistent insomnia, even if you give them drugs, benzodiazepines, they won't be effective because there is a physical restlessness, so even if you take anxiolytics, hypno-inductive therapy, physical restlessness won't let you fall asleep and sleep. In those cases [mechanical] restraint can be prescribed, just for the time it takes for patient to fall asleep, and in that case he [the patient] is almost grateful because you stop him, he manages to fall asleep, then

[16] Extreme examples of patient's gratitude for the coercive act are patients' requests to be restrained. Orientations toward this issue are not homogeneous among our participants. While the request can be seen as legitimizing the coercive intervention (or even removing the coercive dimension because restraint is accepted and demanded), some interviewees have observed how such request may be the result of a habit, a mode of self-management learnt along the carrier as a psychiatric patient, which should not be fulfilled acritically by the staff without having previously tried to provide the person in distress with alternative (relational, pharmacological) forms of support. Such attempt can both result in a successful negotiation, which manages to avoid or procrastinate restraint, or it can fail if the patient adopts a behaviour which s/he knows will lead to restraint ("they know how to get restrained [...] they're more expert than us!", said Gino, nurse at the Pine Ward). A similar orientation has been observed in the no-restraint context, where requests for chemical means of control of negative feelings (e.g. anxiety) or behaviour (e.g. agitation) are generally not immediately satisfied, but alternative support—such as clinical interview with a psychiatrist—is provided ("sometimes we refuse to administer therapy because the patient abuses it, he's not able to solve the problem and medicalizes every kind of emotion", said Nadia, nurses coordinator at the Iris Ward).

doctor prescribes his unrestraining, and the patient sleeps for the whole night, you know?[17]

Also, for patients to whom pharmacological therapy can be deleterious (e.g. elderly people, or patients suffering from organic diseases), mechanical restraint is attached with a therapeutic value "by difference": it is presented as the best available intervention when other medical options are ruled out. This position is clearly expressed by psychiatrist Vincenzo (Excerpt 6.26), who nevertheless acknowledges the ambivalence of resorting to mechanical restraint since it is associated with unintended consequences too (he mentions bedsores). This qualifies it as the least bad option, which should theoretically be avoided if human resources were sufficient to assist elderly people with dementia and prevent them from falling without resorting to mechanical restraint.

Excerpt 6.26. Vincenzo (psychiatrist, Pine Ward): There can be a therapeutic use in elderly people affected by pathologies to whom too many drugs, sedative drugs, can do harm, can have side-effects on their state of consciousness, cardiac or respiratory alterations, so in these cases [mechanical] restraint allows to avoid using drugs that could compromise their situation [...]. In this sense it [mechanical restraint] also has a therapeutic value.

The therapeutic dimension of a coercive act can also be maintained by suggesting that to restrain a person may contain his/her distress, intervening on a psychological level. This is consistent with Yannis Gansel and Samuel Lézé's (2015) genealogic study of the term *contenir* and its application in mental health treatment of violent adolescents in France: moving from physical constraint to psychological holding, the measure was attached with a therapeutic role and transformed from an action of concrete control to an immaterial act of care. This change of state is most

[17] On the three night shifts I have spent on the field in the Pine Ward, I never happened to observe the interruption of mechanical restraint right after the patient has fallen asleep. Instead, restraints were normally confirmed in the evening for the following twelve hours and removed in the morning (when I have not spent the night on the ward, I observed or have been informed about this when I arrived there), even though a "state of necessity" was no longer detectable during the night. For patients "requiring" restraints to fall asleep, they were generally tied loose, suggesting a different aim than immobilization pursued for very agitated or violent patients.

notably visible in the case of manual or physical restraint, a practice that is associated more with care than coercion through a terminological shift: containment (*contenimento*) instead of restraint (*contenzione*). The following quotation I translated from Lorenzo Toresini (2007), creator and honorary president of the Club SPDC No Restraint, explains the background and rationale for this practice.

> When, in a very rare percentage of cases, a physical containment is necessary, we allow ourselves to perform holding. As it is well known, holding is a term coined by Winnicott [psychoanalyst] to indicate the physical containment of autistic children performed by their parents. A containment which, we can understand, is more emotional than physical, it is "affective". A containment that is an embrace. Usually our patients, when restraint ('*contenzione*') is needed, actually need physical containment ('*contenimento*') to be performed with our bodies. [...] [If] it is necessary to physically stop an individual in crisis [...], to "risk" your own body in a physical relation with the patient—in an interaction modality which equates professional and patient, so that "contamination" becomes theoretically possible—will be *a therapeutic measure in itself.* [...] Like with children, it is important to make them [patients] understand and feel that *(physical) and affective containment is a form of care for them.*

According to this account, the therapeutic nature of this measure is due to the physical presence and intervention of the healthcare professionals *with their own body*, contrary to mechanical restraint where (except for its initiation) containment is performed by belts (see also Chap. 6). Such opinion has been encountered on the field, both in psychiatric wards (the Iris Ward and the second no-restraint unit I visited with my research team in January 2019) and Mental Health Centres. As Nadia underlines in the last part of the quotation (Excerpt 6.27), the physical engagement of the healthcare workers requires a careful evaluation of the situation not to expose themselves to potential danger: nurses are described as finely tuned instruments (Björkdahl et al., 2010), able to read patients' signals and intervene accordingly.

> *Excerpt 6.27.* Nadia (nurses coordinator, Iris Ward): Our former head physician use to call it [holding] the "therapeutic embrace", right? [She smiles]

> That's what we do with the girl [Giulia]. Like, *I really hug you*. I mean, if you want to leave, if you are in a moment of crisis, and if I feel that I don't put myself in danger, I hug you, and sometimes people loosen up in that embrace. It is the physical contact. Sometimes physical contact is the last thing you have to use, right? The thing is to be able to understand at the right time-, which is very difficult.

> *Excerpt 6.28*. Dalila [nurse] tells me about the crisis of Santiago from yesterday. He kicked her, so Gianluca [nurse] intervened by grabbing the boy *like he embraced him* and took him to the ground, where colleagues administered intramuscular therapy, in the presence of his doctor. (Violet Centre, fieldnotes)

> *Excerpt 6.29*. To admit [Viktor], it was necessary to invoke a state of necessity and adopt a "*therapeutic embrace*", sedating the boy through an injection. (No-restraint ward, fieldnotes)

This form of physical restraint is performed to prevent the person from leaving the ward or the MHC, to deal with a moment of agitation, or to administer sedative medication with the help of the whole staff. Even when the practice is not explicitly defined as "therapeutic embrace" (*abbraccio terapeutico*), references to the act of embracing are present when narrating episodes concerning its application (see Excerpt 6.28), framing them as acts of care even when their therapeutic nature is not made explicit. The focus, here, is shifted from medicalization to an affective registry which recalls the mother–children relationship, explicitly referred to when framing restraint as protection (see Excerpt 6.31). This is related to the intimate physical interaction in which staff members and patients engage when holding is performed, which allows to represent the intervention as "caring through restraint" (Hejtmanek, 2010).

A beneficial effect on the patient's psychological state achieved through a coercive intervention has been maintained with respect to mechanical restraint too. This is explicitly claimed by nurse Sara in the following excerpt. A more nuanced and tenuous version of this belief can be found in ordinary discourses about mechanical restraint, asserting that it manages to calm patients down: here, the target can be both physical and mental agitation (anxiety), both the body and the mind.

Excerpt 6.30. Sara (nurse, Pine Ward): There are also patients who ask to be stopped, to be restrained, because probably that kind of stop also manages to stop their mind.

Mechanical restraint was also framed and performed as a beneficial act providing protection and safeguarding the patient, comparable to those of a mother with her baby. The analogy, suggested by a nurse during his interview (see Excerpt 6.31), explicitly qualifies the coercive act as an act of care, again through a terminological shift from the notion of *contenzione* (restraint) to that of *protezione* (protection). This "restraint as protection" frame can be easily applied to cases of self-harm (the person has to be "protected from herself") or night wandering and consequent risks of falling (the person has to be protected from the effects of illness), while it is less compatible with hetero-aggressiveness.

Excerpt 6.31. Cristian (nurse, Pine Ward): I think that "*contenzione*" is not a correct word. I would distinguish between "*protezione*" and "*contezione*". Often what we call "*contenzione*"—bed rails, for example, are considered a form of "*contenzione*"—is rather a form of protection ("*protezione*"), like a baby in his cot, is he restrained? The cot has bed rails! Is he detained? Is his mother a child kidnapper? No, she's caring about his safety.

With respect to pharmacological restraint, the qualification of its therapeutic dimension is not straightforward because—as we have seen at the beginning of this chapter (see Excerpt 6.1)—both curative and sedative purposes can be pursued at the same time through a single therapy administration. Even when therapy is meant to affect a patient's behaviour, though, it can be discursively held in a therapeutic registry by focusing on the beneficial consequences of medication, both for the patient (in terms of distress reduction) and for the opportunities for dialogue and communication it fosters.

Excerpt 6.32. Nadia (nurses coordinator, Iris Ward): I think that in some situations therapy can be a form of restraint. It is a form of restraint called chemical, or pharmacological, if you wish […] I think chemical restraint does exist, but I would use it, I mean, I define [therapy] as chemical restraint when it becomes a tool of control. [On the other hand] if we know that after that you [patient] will feel better and we will be able to discuss about what happened, I don't experience it as restraint.

Interviewer: Because there is a purpose?

Nadia: Not only because it has a purpose, but because it is about going through something, it is not something that ends [with administration], *I am not a vending machine* for snacks, right? The same is with drugs. I offer you some therapy because afterwards we can understand what happened, there is a path. Crisis does not begin and end there, with therapy administration, so that you feel better and I can move on with my job. I experience it as restraint and define it restraint when somehow I want to control a symptom. I don't want to control a symptom, I want to "control" a difficult moment for the patient to make him feel better. I mean, not to control, that's not the right word, I want to … help him feeling better, and if I can't do this without drugs, I offer him drugs. Not because I don't want chaos, or I don't want to work, but because somehow I want to help him.

The therapeutic dimension of sedative medication is maintained by Nadia on the basis of the relationship underlying therapy administration: when she says she is not a vending machine, namely a mere supplier of drugs, she suggests that medication is only one among many interventions performed to address crisis. To (pharmacologically) control a symptom is not described as an end in itself, but instead as a necessary step to get through crisis, restore relationship and allow its preferred therapeutic dimension to unfold.

To conclude, a softer version of therapeuticization of coercion can be performed by framing mechanical or physical restraint as necessary in assisting the administration of pharmacological therapy. In this case, the coercive act acquires a therapeutic dimension because of its role in facilitating or even allowing a therapeutic intervention (medication) to be performed. Once again, the "state of necessity" should apply to the therapy administration only, and interruption of mechanical restraint should occur right after, but this has been hardly ever observed. Psychiatrist Michela (Excerpt 6.34) provides a possible explanation, namely avoidance of several acts of restraint during the day (medication is generally administered three times a day), even though regular attempts to negotiate medication and achieve patient's cooperation to remove restraints were not always observed, weakening Michela's argumentation.

Excerpt 6.33. Irene (psychiatrist, Pine Ward): [Mechanical restraint can be] therapeutic as far as, I never happened to use it without a pharmacological administration, they usually go together, so in this sense it has a, a therapeutic value.

Excerpt 6.34. Michela (chief psychiatrist, Pine Ward): I think that the best [mechanical restraint] from an ethical point of view are those performed to administer therapy and they [patients] wouldn't accept it, because yes, you can jump on them [for forced medication], but if you, maybe you have to administer therapy three times [a day] for four days, and if every time you have to tie him, untie him, tie him again, untie him again, it definitely becomes something very distressing.

Excerpt 6.35. Livia (nurse, Pine Ward): Well, therapeutic, I don't know, it can be a coadjuvant, I mean, it's a whole, not always, but there are cases when it is part of the … therapy? I don't know if it can be called therapy, but in a case like him [Aldo] if you didn't stop him, if you only sedated him, it would have not been enough, if you didn't stop him it would have become risky, he would have fallen. I think it is a package, which sometimes requires this piece [mechanical restraint] too. Let's call it therapy, I don't know, maybe it is more of a treatment, yes, I like "treatment" better.

As a conclusive observation, we notice how restraint can be inscribed in a therapeutic, medical registry also through terminology: nurse Livia (Excerpt 6.35) chooses terms such as "coadjuvant" and "treatment", but mechanical restraint has also been described as the result of a "prescription" (see Excerpt 6.25) similarly to a drug, and its qualification as a medical act was recurrent in nurses' interviews in the Pine Ward.[18] Whether a medical act or a measure pertaining to nursing assistance, though, mechanical restraint is also linguistically retained in a registry of

[18] This definition also responds to the issue of moral and legal responsibility, which formally rests on psychiatrists: they are those who sign initiation, termination, and renovation (every twelve hours) of restraint, while nurses are asked to monitor vital parameters and care for the restrained person. In practice, decision-making concerning mechanical restraint is more blurred: nurses participate in it, for they can suggest both initiation and termination of restraint (their patients' knowledge is generally acknowledged by psychiatrists, who can benefit from it to inform their decisions); they can decide to temporarily interrupt restraint, and in situations of emergency, or night shifts, they can initiate it and inform the doctor at a later time, by phone call or in the morning (see also Excerpt 6.8).

healthcare provision, therapeutic per se or in association with other measures.

The therapeutic dimension of mechanical restraint in the Pine Ward has been explicitly denied, in the interviews I conducted, by two psychiatrists only: Michela ("I wouldn't say that [that mechanical restraint is therapeutic] because it's risky, because if you start thinking that it's therapeutic you would tie them all [she laughs], there are days when you are tempted to say: /"I tie them all"/ [laughing]", Excerpt 6.36), and Sandra ("I don't think it is a therapeutic issue. I think it is more therapeutic that a healthcare worker stays with a patient in difficulty, who's afraid to do something bad", Excerpt 6.37). Though rejecting the therapeutic dimension of mechanical restraint, they nevertheless explained and supported the reasons for its application (e.g. aggressiveness and self-harm, posing risks for themselves and others, both patients and the staff), in line with other strategies and with a context which normalizes this measure as a routine practice.

6.3.2 Proceduralization of Coercion

A second strategy by which coercion can be performed as an act of good care is that of *proceduralization* of the coercive intervention. This operation operates by sanitizing coercion not as much on an ethical than on a technical ground, providing a scientific and procedural basis for the performance of a good (i.e. procedurally correct and safe) coercive intervention.

With respect to pharmacological interventions aimed at controlling disruptive behaviour—both in terms of chemical restraint through ordinary/daily therapy and extemporaneous rapid tranquillization (see Sect. 2.3.3)—the goodness and appropriateness of the administration is generally legitimized on the basis of scientific evidence supporting the use of a given medication to treat or control a specific symptom. The following example refers to the case of a seventeen-year-old girl, Giulia, admitted to the Iris Ward after a number of serious self-harming attempts, which she tried to perform in the ward as well while expressing suicidal ideation. Such behaviour required constant shadowing and observation, and a considerable effort by the nursing staff, who suggested that activities and opportunities to temporary leave the ward would have been more beneficial to Giulia than receiving sedative medication and spending her day within the hospital. The critique was partially directed to the non-hospital actors involved in her care—community psychiatrists—but nevertheless invested SPDC psychiatrists as well, who tried to respond to the girl's challenging behaviour by pharmacological means.

> *Excerpt 6.38.* Paolo [psychiatrist] suggests introducing lithium or valproate (both are mood stabilizers). Luana [psychiatrist] said she would rather avoid valproate. Elettra and Marzia [nurses] seem sceptic, they ask the doctors if this therapy modification makes sense or if it is done because they do not know what else to do. Luana, annoyed by nurses' argumentative attitude, replies that *there is evidence in scientific literature that lithium positively affects suicidal thoughts*. Paolo adds that "here [in SPDC] there is nothing else we can do" anyway. (Iris Ward, fieldnotes)

Pharmacological choices aimed at chemically restraining the young girl's behaviour are supported by explicitly referring to pertinent scientific literature. Administration of lithium is here discussed as a response to the disruptive behaviour of a young patient which needs to be managed, but the psychiatrist Luana indirectly approaches the behavioural issue by invoking medication's scientifically proven efficacy on suicidal thoughts, which in turn induce self-injurious behaviour. Medication is supposed to affect and contain negative thoughts, but the ultimate target which induces doctors to discuss this therapy modification is behaviour. We can also observe how, while nurses prioritize their contextual understanding of the individual patient and suggest that other, non-pharmacological solutions could be more beneficial to Giulia, the psychiatrist invokes current best evidence to inform her clinical decision. This points to the old tension between phronesis (privileging clinical acumen and experience) and techne (privileging a scientific outlook), which has been defined as a inescapable dilemma in psychiatric practice (Falkum, 2008).

Even when therapy administration is not formally "correct"—it is the case of off-label medication, prescribed for unapproved purpose, population, or dosage—legitimation is claimed on a procedural basis, which allegedly guarantees patient's safety. This is accomplished through the careful and regular monitoring of specific parameters (e.g. body temperature, blood pressure, oxygenation, blood levels), aimed at checking for drug accumulation[19] and alterations which could indicate potentially dangerous side-effects. Commenting on the attention paid to such aspects, doctor Luana told me: "QTc is psychiatrists' real obsession".[20] Though it might be observed a defensive dimension in such zeal for control, a genuine interest in causing no harm or distress to the patient was detected as well: this was evident in doctors' effort to administer the minimum quantity of drug (even when this corresponded to an objectively quite elevated dosage) necessary to reach a perceivable change in patient's behaviour. An effective administration which, however, would leave the patient "too bended" (also in terms of posture) by sedative drugs, was qualified by healthcare workers as "bad care", and therefore attempted to be avoided. Good care, on the contrary, was performed as monitored, medically controlled administration, even when this was coercive (e.g. forced medication), targeted at controlling patient's behaviour (chemical restraint), or off-label.

With respect to mechanical restraint, proceduralization of the coercive act is realized by representing the practice of restraining a patient as requiring a specialized knowledge, a know-how which is typical of mental health workers, notably nurses. Such competence, or techne, is acknowledged both by some members of the SPDC's personnel and by other hospital wards' staff, sometimes asking the psychiatric ward for help to intervene on particularly difficult patients.

> *Excerpt 6.39.* Michela (chief psychiatrist, Pine Ward): Their (nurses') colleagues [of other hospital wards] are not able to restrain, for example. If a restraint happens, once it happened in the Infectious Diseases ward with a

---

[19] This happens when a drug is administered at a fixed dose at regular intervals for a prolonged period, but the previous dose has not been completely eliminated yet, resulting in a progressively higher amount of drug in the body (Swartz, 1997). In the context of this study, this represented a problem, especially in case of off-label (i.e. higher than the approved) dosage of a drug, which seemed to have no immediate effect on the patient, but—according to mental healthcare providers—might have been "accumulating" and have serious consequences over the days.

[20] QTc (QT interval corrected for heart rate) prolongation is an electrocardiogram abnormality which individuals taking psychopharmacological drugs are exposed to.

girl with TB to whom they were not able to administer therapy [...] they have those disposable strips which patients can tear, and they absolutely do not have any *manual skill.*

Interviewer: You mean, materially?

Michela: Yes, so they call them [SPDC's nurses], because we have specific belts with screws,[21] it is not easy [to use them], you know? It is not that easy.

Interviewer: I guess it's not.

Michela: And also, you have to know a modality to, I mean a praxis, because you first have to restrain one arm and then, because otherwise you hurt yourself or the patient, because there are some, some *competences* which are typical of theirs [SPDC's nurses]. [...] Because in many other [non-psychiatric] wards, it is not that they do not use restraint! [She laughs] They restrain rough-and-ready, as it is. [...] They restrain, and they restrain *badly.*

In the quotation above, psychiatrist Michela acknowledges SPDC nurses' expertise about mechanical restraint, while at the same time underlining that such practice is not performed in the psychiatric context alone but also in other hospital wards: the difference—she suggests—is that in her unit, mechanical restraint is practiced *goodly*, while elsewhere it is performed badly (i.e. without paying attention to the correct procedure to mechanically restrain the patient safely).

Interestingly, a couple of Pine Ward nurses in their interviews downplayed the specificity of this competence that psychiatrists and colleagues

[21] Restraining belts used in psychiatric wards we have observed are made of a robust fabric. They can be closed and opened through a magnetic mechanism (called "magnets", "screws", or—colloquially—"coins") that needs a particular key, possessed by nurses and usually kept with the ordinary (ward doors) keys. Because of the different contexts and situations they have to manage, non-psychiatric wards have simpler strips, described in detail by Cesare, a young nurse at the Cedar Centre previously working in an Internal Medicine Department: "A [non-psychiatric] ward has strips which are very easy to remove, they are used to avoid that a person rips everything [e.g. needles] off. [...] They are different [than those employed in the psychiatric ward], in SPDC belts have a magnet, while other wards have strips that basically are tied to the bed rails, on the wrist they have a, like a watch band, they have a softer side on the inside, like a wristband. [...] They are closed with a Velcro. If you do not have both hands restrained, it is easy to remove them. In [non-psychiatric] wards you usually restrain a single arm, the elderly man is not able to [remove the strips], because your goal is not to tie him, to immobilize him, but to avoid that he rips off the needle or the catheter or the feeding tube [...]. Our psychiatric patients are absolutely able to tear those strips" (*Excerpt 6.40*).

from other units attribute to them, maintaining that no restraint-specific knowledge is required, or that restraint is something that every nurse is trained to perform.[22] Given the moral connotation of coercive interventions, markedly mechanical restraint, these nurses' posture may be interpreted as a face-saving practice (Goffman, 1955, 1959), an operation of impression management which is typical in front of the interviewer (Cardano, 2011).

Excerpt 6.41. Livia (nurse, Pine Ward): To know how to restrain, I don't think it's such a big deal, I don't think it takes a specific competence to understand that there are wrists and ankles, you cannot restrain a shoulder, or the neck.

Interviewer: Have you seen this happen [in other wards]?

Livia: [She nods] So, when you see something like this you say: "no, wait a minute ... sorry, but you cannot restrain a patient's knee", I mean ... You seriously risk causing them harm!

Excerpt 6.42. Gaia (nurse, Pine Ward): We've been called often by other wards to restrain, or for an agitated patient, to care for him, to send one of our nurses to another ward.

Interviewer: You mean keeping that patient in that ward, but asking you to go there and restrain him?

Gaia: We had to do it even if we did not agree, because we said: "we have all been trained as nurses", even if once we did not get a [university] degree but only a nursing school diploma, we all did [studied] Psychiatry, it is not that we [SPDC nurses] come, we lay our hands on the patient and he calms down, or to restrain! It is not that [it takes some special skill] to take a belt, close it, hold a patient ... then if we talk about dialogue, about a specific approach, [that's another story] ... but sometimes they [other wards] take

[22] This is peculiar to the Italian context, where nurses working in mental health contexts get the same training in mental health as every other nurse operating in other branches: there is no specialization in mental health for graduate students. This also allows nurses to work in other medical departments and then ask to be transferred to the psychiatric ward (sometimes for reasons that have little to do with a genuine interest in psychiatry, e.g. related to the shared understanding that the SPDC is a ward where one can easily minimize their efforts and avoid relationships with patients beyond basic interaction and therapy administration). In the Pine Ward, the staff was equally divided between nurses who have been spending their entire professional career in mental health and nurses coming from different hospital wards (some of whom committed to their job and were genuinely motivated to learn to work with the psychiatric patient).

advantage of this thing, "because they work there, they are experts", it is not true, if I have to place an Angioset [venous catether] do I call an Emergency Room's nurse? No, it's not … But this is what happens.

Livia minimizes the knowledge required to correctly and safely restrain a person, somehow denying the know-how inherent to mechanical restraint; at the same time, though, she admits that nurses in other wards are not able to perform it properly. Her colleague, Gaia, acknowledges such competence but stresses that every nurse—regardless of the context where s/he works—has been taught with basic procedures (mechanical restraint but also the application of a venous catheter) and psychiatric notions (e.g. de-escalation techniques), and that therefore mental health nurses have no peculiar expertise in such practice. Her further specification when she states that: "then if talk about dialogue, about a specific approach …" appears as a further attempt to save her face, to convey an impression which is consistent with her self-image as an *ordinary nurse* (with specific relational skills, at best) rather than a *nurse specialized in mechanical restraint*.

Despite these face-saving strategies, in other moments of their interviews, the same nurses describe or refer to appropriate procedures to mechanically restrain a patient, denoting the knowledge that is involved (although tacitly) in the performance of such measure.

Excerpt 6.43. Livia (nurse, Pine Ward): *The restrained person has to be restrained correctly and safely*, because if she hurts herself while restrained, she can seriously harm herself. Because if they [restraints] are too tight, one might say: "hey, they restrained her tight", no, wait, this is not a game, we don't do this because we enjoy seeing-, but the restrained person can really hurt herself, if [restraints] are too loose she can get up, she can turn the bed, she can do whatever.

Excerpt 6.44. Gaia (nurse, Pine Ward): We were restraining this patient *in the correct position*, namely four of us, one for every limb, I was holding my limb-, no, there were three of us holding [the patient] and I had to restrain, I was the one who had to close [the belts] (*fascettare*).

Attention paid to the tightness of restraints, to the number of staff members involved in the performance of the practice, and to the monitoring of the patient while s/he is restrained, conveys the image of mechanical restraint as a safe intervention, guided by procedural rules and performed carefully, even scientifically. Furthermore, the existence of protocols regulating the monitoring of patient's vital parameters (notably blood pressure and oxygenation) while restrained, which should be performed and registered on a dedicated form in the clinical record every two hours,[23] is discursively used to relieve the distress and control bad feelings which could be associated with the adoption of a coercive measure, as the nurse Simona clearly explains in the following excerpt.

> *Excerpt 6.45.* Simona (nurse, Pine Ward): [Mechanical] *restraint has to be done well,* has to be, I mean, not too loose because the patient could try to throw himself off the bed, sprain a shoulder, twist a leg ... [...] I think it [mechanical restraint] has to be done *in a scientific way*, to be shorter [keeping patient's limbs as close as possible to the bed], attention has to be paid that it is not too loose or too tight, because if it is too loose he might free himself, if it is too tight on the following day he will have swollen hands and feet, and this is not good, so we are very careful about it. [...] I remember that some years ago I went to a training course, there were some colleagues saying: "when I restrain someone I feel bad, mmh, I suffer". Personally, I do not suffer, because it is not a forgetful restraint, it is a controlled restraint, we have a protocol.

The training course that Simona refers to is one of those which are periodically offered to the personnel of the wards considered to be at a higher risk of aggression from patients: Psychiatry and the Emergency Department. Besides theoretical courses aimed at providing general notions about de-escalation techniques, open to healthcare workers from every discipline, meetings dedicated to psychiatric and ER staff are designed to constitute practical occasions to observe and learn self-defence and immobilization manoeuvres from martial arts experts.

[23] This was not always the case, especially at night, when continuity of patient's sleep was prioritized over frequent monitoring of parameters, which would have woken the person up. On this occasions, patient's conditions were monitored during the regular checks nurses perform at night in every bedroom, usually assisted by an electric torch.

During my fieldwork, I had the opportunity to participate in one such training, organized in two separate meetings. The first one provided participants with basic defensive techniques to be adopted in case of physical assault, teaching them how to fall to the ground minimizing harm (e.g. protecting the vertebral column) and how to avoid further attacks while being on the floor. The second meeting illustrated what trainers called "immobilization techniques", aimed at actively intervening the aggressive patient to stop and eventually restrain him/her. These techniques required the cooperation of the whole group, within which practical tasks must be distributed. If the aggressive patient is standing and threatening to assault a nurse, for example, one colleague is supposed to stop him by using a sheet to lasso him,[24] while another one should grab the patient's legs to knock him off balance, and then collectively hold him on the ground. The following excerpt from fieldnotes describes how, with the collaboration of a volunteer playing the part of the patient laid on a stretcher, the trainers—Nicola and Cinzia—showed the participants how to practically immobilize a person, both manually and with the aid of common objects (e.g. bed sheets).

> *Excerpt 6.46.* Cinzia explains that to immobilise someone, the body has to be imagined as divided in three parts to be singularly blocked: the head, the chest with the arms, and the legs. Ideally, there should be one healthcare worker for each part, "even four if one of them is [as thin as] me", Cinzia specifies.
>
> Nicola shows us the first technique: the worker is standing beside the stretcher on which the patient is laying; he puts his arms on the patient, forcing him to turn his head in the opposite direction; he leans his upper body on the patient's chest and grabs the stretcher's structure, in order to use his own weight to prevent the patient from moving arms or head, or sitting up. One by one, participants try to reproduce the manoeuvre, but female workers have some difficulty. Cinzia goes behind the patient's head and shows us how, while she holds his head with both hands, she uses fingers to stretch his ears and the skin besides his eyes, to scratch him: "this is

[24] The expression refers to the procedure entailing the use of a looped rope, usually to catch animals. Comparison to animals—markedly wild animals—to underline acute patients' behaviour's unpredictability and sometimes irrationality, emerged as well in other fields within the Piedmontese context.

not nice, but while I'm here and my [male] colleagues immobilise his legs and body, I do whatever I can to disturb him". Nicola even suggests to put a mattress cover ('traversa') on the patient's face to block his view and disorient him; Cinzia comments this is risky as it could smother the patient, but Nicola says it is not possible to smother someone with a mattress cover and insists with his advice.

[...] Cristian [SPDC nurse] says that on a previous course from last year he found very useful the technique of immobilising a patient's ankles using bed sheets, and asks the trainers to show it to us. There are two procedures to do so. The first one employs the sheet of the bed on which the patient is lying: with a skilful manoeuvre, the trainer grabs the sheet's corners and uses them to wrap the patient's ankles to block them and prevent him from moving his legs. The second procedure makes use of a mattress cover, passed between the patient's ankles in a particular way (forming an "8"): not only the patient can't bend his legs (preventing him from kicking), but pain is inflicted every time the patient tries to move by tightening the grip ("stringendo la presa"). Cristian observed that this technique proved very effective and has been employed in the SPDC on several occasions, to the point that he always put some mattress covers on a bed nearby and suggests his colleagues to do the same.

Cristian asks if there are some tools to prevent a patient from raising his shoulders on the bed. He specifies that the problem is that if you tie his shoulders with a mattress cover, this might move as the patient is moving, reaching his neck and risking smothering him. He adds that it would be possible to block each shoulder independently, passing the sheet under the patient's armpit and therefore letting the neck free, but "mattress covers are too short, and even if you apply them, then you cannot knot the extremities together" (this makes me think they have been doing some experiments!). Cinzia replies that a new harness, padded but robust, has been requested by the Intensive Care Unit, and that the new tool might be extended to other wards in the future. (Pine Ward, fieldnotes)

This extensive citation reveals several interesting aspects of the restraining practice. In the first place, its performance seems related to a way of seeing the agitated person as an objectified body, an assemblage of (three) body parts, around which the resources available to the group have to be allocated. Distribution is made according to each healthcare worker's physical characteristics, such as build and strength, which are usually related to a gendered dimension. The thinnest bodies are not presented as useless but can be employed to disturb or distract the patient, making the immobilization work of the strongest colleagues easier. To frame a(n emergency) situation in such terms, and quickly act as a group accordingly, requires a vision that is specific to this community of practitioners, a professional vision which is a socially organized way of seeing and understanding (Goodwin, 1994). What this training course aims to provide is an ethnography of seeing (ibidem), which directs participants' attention to locally relevant entities (e.g. the patient's body parts, or the available objects which might be useful to the purpose of restraining, such as bed sheets), framing them through a specific coding scheme as objects of knowledge.

Besides the techniques conveyed to perform a skilful and effective restraint, a dimension of *improvisation* emerges. Cristian's observation, reported in the last paragraph of the citation, denotes how, when faced with concrete situations of emergency, he and his colleagues have been trying—or experimenting with—non-conventional (and sometimes non-safe) ways to hold a patient. At the end of the meeting, he approaches me and observes that in the SPDC, in situations when they have to restrain a patient, they usually improvise: "I call them rodeos". Reference to rodeos conveys a perception of unpredictability, because nurses never know exactly what to expect from the patient: as I have been told multiple times through informal conversations on the field, every admission, every performance of restraint is a case in its own right, and even the behaviour of patients known for thirty years is never fully predictable. Nevertheless, improvisation has not to be intended as a completely unprepared course of action performed in absolute freedom: while improvising, actors never start from scratch, but always rely on tradition, pre-assumptions and experience (Sparti, 2005). Improvisation is a practice in itself, entailing an operative, embodied knowledge associated with actions done without reflecting on how, or why, one does it: it has been called "background knowledge" (Sparti, 2013). What sociologist Davide Sparti observes about improvisation in jazz music and other fields of human activity (ibidem) can be fruitfully employed to reflect on the practice of restraint and what healthcare workers do when they have to perform it.

When nurses utilize mattress covers of bed sheets to hold a violent patient, making a deviant, exceptional use of those objects, they are improvising: muddling through an emergent situation as it unfolds, they rely on competences they have absorbed along their experience in their community of practices, and at the same time they try and experiment alternative, creative solutions (e.g. a different knot under the patient's armpit) with contingent available resources. Techniques shown by the trainers—derived from a different field, that of martial arts—are useful to ward's nurses to the extent they can be situated in their working context, be adapted to their needs, and provide their action with new possibilities by turning ordinary things into affordances (Gibson, 1977).

This mixture of competence and (skilful) improvisation emerged also in discourses of nurses from the no-restraint context. During a rich conversation we had over the night shift, Franco described how, before the abolition of mechanical restraint, in the Iris Ward they used to perform it with common but unspecific objects—again, bed sheets—which nevertheless entailed some skills (developed by using them) to prove effective.

> *Excerpt 6.47.* Mechanical restraint was usually practiced without procedures or specific and safe tools, but through improvisation. Franco [nurse] recounts how, to tie someone to the bed, they used a bed sheet. Miriam [OSS] asks him if with a simple sheet patients were not able to free themselves. Franco laughs, then replies that *if you know how to do it*, they absolutely cannot untie themselves. (Iris Ward, fieldnotes)

Also recent, currently in use practices, such as manual restraint, are guided by specific techniques, which prioritize patient's safety, and therefore allow us to inscribe them in the registry of proceduralization. These techniques are objects of training for mental healthcare workers as well, which frame good restraint as that which contains but does not hurt the restrained person. Gianluca, a nurse at the Violet Centre, explains how to accomplish this to Santiago, involuntarily treated during an important psychotic crisis, which led him to believe to have superpowers (specifically, the power to heal people) and that they could be stolen from him by people standing behind him.

Excerpt 6.48. Santiago says: "you must not stand behind me, or you steal my power". He told me the same thing some days ago, while we were having a walk in the park. Now, he is addressing Gianluca, who holds him from behind when he has to stop [physically restrain] him. Gianluca replies: "I stand behind you because when I began working in Psychiatry they taught to do so: I have to stop you without hurting you, and if I grab you from front you risk falling backwards and hitting your head". (Violet Centre, fieldnotes)

To conclude on the *proceduralization of coercion* strategy, we have seen how the performance of coercive practices—chemical, mechanical, or manual restraint—is accompanied with discourses upon techniques, skills, competences, and standard protocols, which convey an image of these interventions as scientific, correct, and safe procedures. Knowledge required to perform good restraint is both acquired and produced through formal training courses, exposure, and participation to the community's practices and experimentation (with alternative restraining tools or off-label drugs, for example). To define the coercive acts as technically good and appropriate—also by counterposing badly performed practices from other contexts—allows practitioners to relieve bad feelings associated with the use of coercion, and to present themselves as caring, attentive, and skilled healthcare providers who (even while restraining them) care for their patients.

6.3.3 Relationalization of Coercion

The third strategy allowing to perform coercion as good care is the inscription of the coercive intervention in a registry of relation, and its contamination with elements of negotiation, trust, compassion, and empathy. Here, personhood and patienthood, which we have seen to be disconnected in the first strategy of therapeuticization of coercion, are attempted to be cared for simultaneously. Of central concern to this strategy is not whether coercion is exercised and to what extent but *how* it is performed, namely how it is initiated, maintained, and subsequently processed.

With respect to the initiation of a coercive measure, it is useful to cite the words of Ernesto, nurse at the Pine Ward for nineteen years, to introduce the issue of relationalization of mechanical restraint.

> *Excerpt 6.49.* Ernesto [nurse] tells us that according to him it is not important if and how frequently mechanical restraint is used, but *how you restrain a patient.* He says that "women [female nurses] are smart" and that they can perform restraint using some tricks, such as telling the patient he has to do an ECG and then, while he is lying on the bed, applying the belts. "The patient remembers [how you restrained him]", he says. He defines this mode of restraining a "sweet" one—I recall he used the term "loving" too—which according to him is preferable than a mode based on the use of force. (Pine Ward, fieldnotes)

The operation Ernesto described as a "sweet" mode of restraining could be read otherwise as a form of deceit: the patient is asked to lie on the bed with an excuse—to do an electrocardiogram—and then restrained by taking advantage of his/her cooperation and unawareness of the nurse's real purpose.[25] Despite what may be seen as an ethically problematic conduct involving a form of deceit, it is crucial to understand what actors are privileging here: this mode of restraining is considered preferable than a violent one involving the use of physical force because what is prioritized is the *subjective experience of being restrained*, that the patient will remember for a long time. By considering violent, "hard" intervention as a potentially more traumatizing experience, this nurse is framing this "soft" initiation of restraint as an act of care, described as "sweet" or even "loving". Restraint and care are discursively and practically held together.

Attention to the modes of performing coercion, which inevitably prioritize one "good" over another (in the abovementioned example, the subjective experience of being restrained was made relevant over, for

[25] Patient's cooperation denotes that no immediate danger or "state of necessity" was present, but restraint might have been performed on a preventive basis (observed in other occasions) for an already known patient having a reputation of being at risk of falling, wandering, or tending to become agitated or aggressive.

example, transparency between patient and the nurse[26]), represents an element of what I have chosen to call *compassion*. Compassion—which is an acknowledged key element of care and healthcare relationships—is not intended here as a mental disposition or an individual feeling, but, with Lauren Berlant, as an emotion in operation: "compassion is a term denoting privilege: the sufferer is *over there*. You, the compassionate one, have a resource that would alleviate someone else's suffering" (Berlant, 2004, p. 4). Berlant's definition points to the opportunity a privileged actor (e.g. the healthcare professional) has to relieve the distress of another (the patient), acting as an ameliorative actor (ibidem). Intended as such, compassion becomes a profoundly practical matter by which the (at least) unpleasant experience of the patient—whether restrained, involuntarily hospitalized, struggling with symptoms or side-effects of medication—is acknowledged and concretely ameliorated by means that are specific to the institutional context. Acts of *practical compassion* (Brown et al., 2014)—such as a soft initiation of mechanical restraint—can then take shape also, and maybe most notably, in contexts of coercion and power unbalance, such as acute mental healthcare ones.

To care about how a coercive intervention is performed concerns involuntary treatment as well. In his interview, the community psychiatrist Giorgio described how the intervention is generally pre-arranged (except for rare emergency situations) and organized in order to avoid exposing the person to the judgement of neighbours and fellow citizens and to the resulting stigma: again, the subjective experience of the patient is prioritized and attempts to minimize the potentially traumatizing consequences of the coercive measure are made. This is achieved, for example, by executing the intervention in the Mental Health Centre or in

[26] Alternative choices might have been performed, for example by opting for a transparent discussion and explanation for the coercive act. This has been observed by the research team elsewhere on the field in the Piedmontese context, accompanied also by justification and almost apology, and is well exemplified by the strategy of *explanation* of the coercive act that I discuss further in this section.

other protected, non-public environments (such as the police barracks, in the case mentioned below[27]) where the person is willing to go.

> *Excerpt 6.50.* Giorgio (psychiatrist, Cedar Centre): What we can do in the community, contrary to the SPDC, is to choose the way that is *as painless as possible*, not to expose the person, usually we try to do it in a controlled environment, if possible here [in the MHC] [...] [With Ada] we avoided doing, intercepting the person in a public place, to avoid exposing her we organized it, asking her to come to the police barracks.

It is important to underline that the arrangement for an involuntary treatment—consisting of preparing the papers for the procedure, alerting the police and the SPDC, and mobilizing community staff, after a period of patient's non-cooperation and worsening of clinical conditions—does not necessarily result in its execution. Attempts to negotiate with the person and obtain her collaboration for voluntary admission are always pursued, both in the restraint and the no-restraint context, mobilizing resources such as the different personalities composing the *équipe* and the relationships developed over time with specific doctors or nurses, which might convince the person to accept treatment on the basis of personal trust. When persuasion does not work, or relationships are not present or weak because, for example, the person has recently become a service user, other strategies—such as show of force and implicit threat—may be performed, resulting in the admission of what have been called "coerced voluntaries" (O'Donoghue et al., 2014; see Chap. 2), which nevertheless manages to avoid violent interventions and formally involuntary admissions. The case of Ada represents an example of this mode of performing non-violent (though implicitly coercive) intervention, which is considered successful by the psychiatrist precisely because of the pre-arranged, unforced, and environmentally protected *mode* in which it has been practiced.

[27] This is an example of attunement of MHC practices to the specificity of the woman, Ada, unwilling to go to the services and living in a building and neighbourhood which were already problematic (see Chap. 5). The police barracks appeared as a neutral and protected space, where she eventually accepted to go.

Excerpt 6.51. Giorgio (psychiatrist, Cedar Centre): At the end we did not need to do anything, usually this combined show of force [of mental health services and the police] is sufficient, and also in this case [of Ada] it was diriment, there was a formal opposition which disappeared when the marshal intervened with me, so the person could not, she understood that there were motivations, or that there was an overwhelming force, so she probably decided defensively for a collaborative admission. This requires great organization, but these are the results.

Similarly to the "soft" initiation of restraint, this mode of approaching (and avoiding, if possible) involuntary treatment acknowledges personhood and the patient's subjective experience, attempting to prevent unnecessary elements of public humiliation, stigma, and use of force, which would be traumatizing and remembered for a long time.[28]

Several other examples of practical compassion in case of coerced patients have been observed on the field or described by our interviewees. The following excerpt concerns the case of a boy, admitted during a violent onset, whose aggressiveness was not adequately manageable in the psychiatric ward (not even through mechanical restraint), and required relevant dosage of sedative medication which led to his transfer to the Intensive Care Unit (ICU) for proper monitoring. As it usually happens, the boy was mechanically (other than pharmacologically) restrained there too. Maria, an OSS with a personal background on alternative (e.g. music, dance, art) therapies, narrates how she managed to start building a relationship with this patient while he was restrained, by visiting him at the ICU, massaging him, and playing some music for him, showing a compassionate attitude.

Excerpt 6.52. Maria (OSS, Pine Ward): We had admitted a boy … it was his first admission … he was very much uncompensated, he was out [of his

[28] Memories of a violent intervention can re-emerge in the doctor–patient relationship, as the description of the following episode shows. In a medical encounter at the Tulip Centre, while the psychiatrist Chiara was trying to negotiate with a patient of hers—Filippo—the administration of a therapy, she asked the man if he remembered being given depot medication in the past. Filippo recalled the occasion on which he received the depot injection, during an involuntary treatment, when—he says—he had been "taken away like a dog" by the police. Chiara seemed embarrassed by his assertion and replied saying she felt sorry for that experience.

mind], aggressive and everything, he had been [mechanically] restrained for ... a long time, every time we tried to unrestrain him- [...] Then he has been moved to the Intensive Care [Unit], because they have tried to sedate him ... and I went there every day to treat him. I used to [temporary] unrestrain one leg, massaged it, and play some music with sounds of nature, relaxing music, I did it for a pretty long time, then little by little he has been unrestrained and went back here [in the SPDC] [...] [Later, his mother] thanked me, this approach has succeeded, and it was the only thing I could-, *it was also a way to relate to him.* Because he was always, it was difficult for him to access to-, he was always on the alert, he reacted by being aggressive, than little by little he managed to, physical contact helped him a lot, to massage his head, feet, hands, legs, because *poor son, he was tied to that bed*, and it was also a particular situation because, you know, to do it here [in the SPDC] is one thing, but I had to go up there [to the ICU].

Acts of practical compassion performed by Maria qualify her as the ameliorative actor (Berlant, 2004) of the boy's condition, but also show us how a coercive intervention can represent the opportunity (or even the only possibility) to work on building a relationship with the acute patient. This argument was used in the studied contexts for both mechanical and pharmacological restraint, sometimes described as means through which communication (and therefore relation) with patients could be established in moments of crisis. As an extreme position on this opinion, a psychiatrist at the Cedar Centre, Davide, suggested that mechanical restraint is a tool among others, a communicative tool for "[unwell] people who do not understand other languages but that of the body", and for this reason its complete and indiscriminate abolition was not something he considered desirable.

The following excerpts from fieldnotes show how relation was not built but rather maintained, with Aldo—a service user known for thirty years—through acts of practical compassion while he was mechanically restrained, and how past episodes of fun, play, and shared moments during restraint were recalled as part of the history of the nurse–patient relationship.

Excerpt 6.53. After a few, Aldo comes in and asks me if I want to play cards with him. I accept and follow him to the living room. After some minutes,

Ernesto [nurse] arrives (he was probably having his lunch break in the kitchen) and starts playing with us. We chat, then Ernesto smiles and asks Aldo: "do you remember in the old ward when you were restrained by one arm and we played cards with the other [arm]?", and then: "I used to smoke my Cuban [cigar], we both smoked while we were playing, there was fog in that room!". Aldo nods. (Pine Ward, fieldnotes)

Excerpt 6.54. [It is around 23]. Giorgio hears Aldo screaming, goes to his room and asks me to follow him. Aldo is sat on his bed; the mattress is lifted, and [restraining] belts are rather loose. Giorgio brings two cups of hot chamomile tea, one for himself and one for Aldo, recommending him to wait until it cools down and not to drink it all at once. Aldo does not listen to him, takes a sip right away and starts coughing [because it is too hot]. Then, he repeatedly tries to drink again while Giorgio, who stands beside him, moves the cup away from his mouth every time, laughing and telling him how stubborn he is. They chat for a while about last football matches, then Giorgio sits on a chair near Aldo's bed and asks him what was wrong with the residential facility he was sent to. Aldo says there were cocaine and pot there. Giorgio asks if he has been using them, Aldo denies, Giorgio looks at him raising his eyebrows like he did not believe him,[29] Aldo laughs. Giorgio then proposes to unrestrain him, but Aldo shakes his head and says that it is better if he stays there [restrained]. (Pine Ward, fieldnotes)

Excerpt 6.53 tells us something about the time nurses can spend with restrained patients, ameliorating a condition which is acknowledged as delicate: "Precisely because he is restrained, he is in a moment of defence-lessness" (Simona, nurse, Pine Ward). Excerpt 6.54, on the other hand, describes how medical encounters with psychiatrists (in this case a community psychiatrist during a night shift in the ward) can take place in a relaxed, even playful atmosphere despite the situation of (normalized) coercion, and represent an occasion to discuss other aspects of the person's therapeutic path (in this case his returning to the ward after a short period spent in a residential facility). Also, it is interesting to observe patient's compliance with mechanical restraint. The psychiatrist will try

[29] Aldo has been smoking pot for years.

again later to propose Aldo to unrestrain him, but the man will keep refusing, saying: "if you untie me, I'll do something stupid". This shows that patients socialized to this kind of practice rely on restraint to avoid misbehaviour (e.g. hitting some other patient again) and somehow acknowledge its function having internalized contextual logics of control.

The last phrase of Excerpt 6.54, concerning termination of restraint, introduces another element of relationalization of coercion: that of *negotiation*. Negotiation is not only crucial to termination of restraint (which in this case is refused by Aldo) but also to temporary moments of interruption or attenuation of the restraining measure. This has been observed about pharmacological restraint (e.g. the request of a patient to have his/her sedative medication reduced because s/he felt too confused) but also about mechanical restraint, in the form of a partial or temporary removal of the restraining belts. The latter case is exemplified in the following episode: interruption of mechanical restraint is described by the nurse who performed it, Gino, as the result of an arrangement between the professional and the patient, based on reciprocal knowledge and trust, sometimes even sealed with a handshake. Emphasis in the text ("yes, he is tied, but he is considered, I mean, like a person and everything") indicates the acknowledgement and attention paid to the dimension of personhood and personal needs, which are typical of the discursive strategy of relationalization of coercion.

Excerpt 6.55. Gino (nurse, Pine Ward): [Before temporary unrestraining a patient] I try to make an arrangement.

Interviewer: How?

Gino: I mean, I go there and say: "look, it's lunchtime now", I say: "I was thinking of untying a hand of yours, sit you up, put on a bib, bring you the table with the tray, so you can manage to eat. But you know that afterwards ... I have to put the belt back, because this is not the time to take it off [permanently] yet." And I shake his hand, like: "we shake hands, because a contract is a contract". And then, normally it works, unless the patient is hallucinated and you see he throws and beats-, but then you don't even take it [the belt] off, right? You feed him. But to make him more autonomous, to let him getting up, it is better, also to make him understand that *yes, he is tied, but he is considered, I mean, like a person and everything*, he is not abandoned there, and this is true for everything, personal hygiene ...

> **Interviewer: Yes, I see someone using a urinal, someone else …**
>
> Gino: Sure. It was Saturday night, Saturday or Sunday, one of these last nights, Giuseppe was restrained, and he could not urinate, he said: "look, I can't …", I visited him, he had a slightly enlarged bladder, not so much but staying in bed in that position is annoying, so I gave him the urinal and an ice bag but it didn't work, he said: "I can't urinate if I don't put my feet on the ground", so I unrestrained him, I took off the belts from his ankles and from one arm, and left him alone, but always staying there, you know.
>
> **Interviewer: Sure.**
>
> Gino: And he says: "look, I can't because you are here and everything", so I said: "look, Giuseppe, but then we put them [the belts] back", I said: "I take all four of them off, let you go to the bathroom, we wait outside", it was me and the colleagues, I said: "we wait outside, you pee, when you're done you come back, and then I have to put them [the belts] back". We shook hands, it took no more than five minutes, he got up, went to pee, then went back to bed, put the belts back …
>
> **Interviewer: He kept his word.**
>
> Gino: Yes, and he fell asleep. Otherwise I could have said: "I don't want to do this, I put a catheter" […] It depends on the patient, on the nurse, on the relationship you have with the patient, on how the patient is in that moment, on whether you know him or not, I mean, if it was someone else, if it was not Giuseppe but a patient in the same condition of him but on his first admission, I would have not unrestrained him. […] It is based on trust, purely on trust.

Gino's account of the agreement, or contract, illustrates how trust, previous knowledge, and the specific nurse–patient relationship are the essential elements which make temporary interruption of restraint possible. Moreover, these episodes have been usually described as a sort of "test" to evaluate both clinical conditions (whether the person is calm or agitated, hallucinated or confused, hostile or agreeable with both the staff and the other inpatients) and patient's trustworthiness (to verify if, like in the case of Giuseppe, the person keeps his/her word and behaves properly, i.e. accepting the temporariness of belts removal). This narration adds to the relational dimension intersecting coercion as an element of *temporality*: definitive interruption of restraint is presented as something which is approached gradually, over a period of time during which an evolution in patient's behaviour is expected to unfold, both for clinical reasons ("[crisis] must take its course [...] time has to pass, and it is subjective", explained nurse Livia in her interview) and for the degree of collaboration showed by the person. Through attentive observation, dialogue, and tentative episodes of partial or provisional removal of the belts, the staff places the patient on this *trajectory of restraint*, evaluating whether it is "too soon" to try to remove the belts, or conversely if "the patient is converging towards unrestraining" (Simona, nurse, Pine Ward). By considering a wider time frame, the necessity of mechanical restraint is again disassociated from the immediate state of necessity, and tied to a diachronic dimension instead. From this point of view, the permanent removal of restraints appears as something the patient can also earn by proving to be trustworthy when s/he is temporarily unrestrained.

> *Excerpt 6.56.* [On Tuesday afternoon] Ernesto [nurse] tells Carlo they will unrestrain him for a snack break, but he will go back [to be restrained] by 6 p.m. "If everything runs smoothly, we unrestrain you again for dinner, ok?". Carlo nods and takes his medication, then says he needs to stretch his legs because they hurt. Ernesto adds that if he will be good, tomorrow he might be unrestrained for a longer period. [...] [On the next Thursday] we go visiting Carlo, which is on four-points restraint, sat on the bed, he wears a t-shirt and his underwear. When doctor Vincenzo asks him how he is doing, he replies he has been tied to the bed for five days. Gaia [nurse] points out: "you've been unrestrained on Tuesday afternoon". Vincenzo leans against bedrails and says to him: "*let's make a deal, you and me*". He offers to unrestrain him, then he informs him that later he will do a CAT scan, and, if he will be good, he will be left unrestrained. (Pine Ward, fieldnotes)

> *Excerpt 6.57.* Maia has been temporarily unrestrained during the morning to go to the bathroom twice. At lunchtime she asks to eat in the dining room with the other [inpatients], she's tranquil. Doctor Irene agrees to permanently unrestrain her. Alessio [nurse]: "so I go unrestrain her with a *compromise*". Edoardo [nurse]: "yes: at the first kick she's back there [restrained] again".[30] (Pine Ward, fieldnotes)

[30] The girl had been restrained in the first place because she repeatedly kicked the door or the walls, hurting herself, despite staff's presence and attempts to dissuade her.

Excerpt 6.56 shows how temporary removal of restraint, first experimented on Tuesday afternoon and then offered again two days after, is the precondition for permanent unrestraining, especially for unknown patients.[31] Improper behaviour (e.g. aggressiveness or, in the case of Maia, self-harm) while temporarily unrestrained is here defined as a violation of the agreement and faith showed by the staff, and therefore it is inscribed again in a relational registry, which justifies coercion as a consequence of disloyalty.[32]

To conclude on the agreement interpretation, it is interesting to observe that it is considered equally crucial for the staff to prove reliable and keep their word too. If, for example, a nurse promises a patient s/he will be temporarily unrestrained again, for a longer period of time, if s/he behaves properly the first time, it is relevant for the relationship and mutual trust that the nurse keeps the promise s/he made. Excerpt 6.59 exemplifies the bidirectionality of the negotiation process between patient and nurse, in which "it's all about convincing each other".

> *Excerpt 6.59.* Livia (nurse, Pine Ward): There are cases when the person is there, and I negotiate, [I mobilize our] relationship, the times gone by, I put everything [on the plate], there I trust him, [I say:] "don't mess up or I will pay for you [for having unrestrained you]", [the patient says] "I know, you don't have to worry", ok, you play your cards. Then I said: "you know that if you collaborate, I will report [to the doctors] that you behaved in a certain- [way]", *it's all about convincing each other*, so if he goes back to bed, the following day I keep my word, because the thing is that when you say something to a patient than you have to honour it.

[31] Despite nothing bad happening when Carlo was first unrestrained on Tuesday, no further attempts were made on Wednesday. Temporary unrestraining depends not only on the clinical condition of the patient, the number and conditions of the other inpatients, and the available resources in terms of nurses, but also on the initiative of the staff, who might decide to start negotiation and try to make a deal with a patient or not. This in turn depends on each professional's experience and self-confidence, and on the relationship s/he has with the specific patient: Carlo was in his first admission and was unknown to the ward; this may explain the cautious, sometimes reluctant approach of most nurses towards his temporary unrestraining.

[32] This narration somehow confers restraint a punitive dimension, despite that it has been repeatedly denied and labelled as a bad practice by the staff when explicitly thematized. Excerpt 6.58: Mario says that in other [psychiatric] wards, restraint is used as a threat ("if you do this again, we will tie you"). Doctor Sandra says that they absolutely do not intend this practice as such. Tania [nurse] comments: "that is a bad phrase" (Pine Ward, fieldnotes).

Interestingly, in the discourses of our interviewees, negotiation does not necessarily result in temporary removal of restraints. To consider and try to fulfil patients' requests—when they are compliant with mechanical restraint—can mean to maintain them restrained even if the staff does not detect a state of necessity (anymore). This was the case of Aldo described in Excerpt 6.54, but also of Maia: nurse Livia describes how, while being provisionally unrestrained to go to the bathroom, she seemed calmer than before, so she asked her if she would like to remain unrestrained, but the girl refused and was restrained again as she wished.

> *Excerpt 6.60.* Livia (nurse, Pine Ward): Half an hour [after restraint] she had to go to the bathroom, let's say after an hour. Then I told her: "listen ... if we unrestrain you to go to the bathroom, do you feel like remaining untied?", I mean, "no, no, now I want to stay in bed". [...] I asked her: "are you sure?", "yes, yes, yes, I want to remain in bed, with my, I drink some more-", alright, I told her: "because you seem calmer", "yes but I, I want to remain in bed [restrained]".

The coercive measure, presented here as something which is demanded by the patient herself, is represented as a response to the girl's needs or preferences, and therefore qualified as a good act, as an act of care and consideration for the person's desires. Shortly after this episode, around lunchtime, the girl felt like being unrestrained to go to eat in the communal dining room, and restraints were definitively removed (see Excerpt 6.57).

An alternative way in which coercive interventions can be practically incorporated in the relationship between the patient and the healthcare worker, and discursively inscribed in a relational registry, is through the *explanation* of the intervention itself, during or after its performance. By explaining the reasons behind the coercive act, the person subjected to it is once again acknowledged as such, in his/her personhood. Moreover, dialogue and exchange of respective motives become possible, fostering mutual understanding. The following example, concerning manual restraint in the context of the Violet Mental Health Centre, illustrates this reciprocal explanation of the reasons behind each actor's behaviour: the restraining intervention and the patient's aggressiveness. This was possible in a rare moment of communication with Santiago—the already mentioned Bolivian young man, involuntarily treated at the MHC for a profound psychotic crisis—during a car trip with two nurses, a rehabilitation specialist, and me. The car trip was organized to reduce the tension and "relationally contain him" (the boy seemed to enjoy escorted walks in the surrounding park and moments outside of the Centre, which were planned as frequently as possible to make his TSO more bearable). Driving around without a destination in mind, Santiago gradually relaxed, opened up, and verbalized some of his distress: the distance from his home country, the recent death of a beloved grandmother, the dependence on cannabis as a self-medication tool. As he was talking, explaining himself, and shortly after crying with his head on a nurse's shoulder, we were holding our breath, surprised by such unexpected breach into his feelings. Openness breeds openness, and a few minutes later, Santiago expressed his annoyance with being always surrounded by staff members, while they explained their reasons for—and most notably, their discomfort with—intense surveillance and coercive interventions (e.g. physical restraint) they sometimes had to perform to respond to his behaviour. Excerpt 6.61 from fieldnotes concerns the conversation about respective explanations which took place in that car.

> *Excerpt 6.61.* Dalila [nurse]: "Do you remember kicking me yesterday? It is not nice to kick a woman, don't you think?". Her tone is not of scolding, but more of an invitation to reflect, to be self-critical, discussing about Santiago's aggressive behaviour in this moment of contact and communication. Santiago replies: "you were fifty, I had to defend myself!".[33] Gianluca [nurse] intervenes, saying that if he runs away, they are forced to intervene for his own good, to stop him, even if they don't like having to do so. Santiago says: "you must not stand behind me, or you steal my power". He told me the same thing some days ago, while we were having a walk in the park. Now, he is addressing Gianluca, who "hugs" him from behind when he has to stop [physically restrain] him. Gianluca replies: "I stand behind

[33] This refers to the fact that Santiago was always escorted around the Violet Centre and its surroundings by one or more mental healthcare workers (*affiancamento*), who used to gather around him in moments of particular tension. Though not explicitly indicated as such, these moments can be seen as an example of show of force (Bowers et al., 2012) similar to the one employed (and acknowledged as such) in the Cedar Centre (see Excerpt 6.51).

you because when I began working in Psychiatry they taught to do so: I have to stop you without hurting you, and if I grab you from front you risk falling backwards and hitting your head". This discussion addressing the respective reasons seems surreal, especially considering the extremely difficult communication of these days. (Violet Centre, fieldnotes)

The need for explanation emerged also with respect to other coercive measures, such as pharmacological restraint. Sometimes explanation itself allowed to avoid violent interventions—in this case forced administration of medication—as the following episode observed at the Tulip Centre illustrates. Similarly to the non-violent admission achieved with Ada (see Excerpt 6.51), here the patient unwillingly accepts medication, persuaded by her father's and nurses' arguments (but maybe also by the implicit possibility they have to forcefully administer therapy if she refused). Explanation for the pharmacological restraint that was about to be (voluntarily or involuntarily) administered was also employed to seek for Alina's cooperation and avoid tougher interventions on her.

Excerpt 6.62. Mimmo [nurse] tells Elia [psychiatrist]: "we need to talk to Alina, she kicked Jessica out there on the footpath before. She has on-demand therapy prescribed, but *first we have to justify it to her*, we need to talk to her while her father is here, and even if she is delirious, we have to make her understand that she might hurt someone and be reported". [...] Alina is a bit hostile, but with the help of her father she listens to healthcare workers' recommendations and accepts to take medication after some insistence. (Tulip Centre, fieldnotes)

Explanation is needed also with respect to a psychiatrist's decision to involuntarily hospitalize one of his/her patient. This was perceived, both in the restraint and the no-restraint context, as a crucial element to process a certainly delicate moment for the person treated against her will. Both psychiatrists and nurses, more intensively in contact with patients during their stay, take part in this process of discussion and explanation, especially after the first, most difficult phase of the crisis had passed.

Excerpt 6.63. Nadia (nurses' coordinator, Iris Ward): In involuntary treatments, we try with involuntary treatments not to say: "ok, you're unwell,

> you have to be cured, that's it and there's nothing to discuss". "You are unwell, you have to be cured, *but we do discuss*". Even if this is a contradiction in terms, we try during involuntary treatment, both after and during the stay, to make patients understand—because [pharmacological] therapy helps, it's undeniable—and when people start to see the light at the end of the tunnel [they understand] that maybe we were not completely wrong [in thinking they had to be treated].

Exceptions to the—both practical and discursive, simultaneous or subsequent—incorporation of coercive treatment in the relationship have been observed as residual and usually criticized occurrences. In the no-restraint context, this was observed with respect to a community psychiatrist who arrived to the Iris Ward together with a community nurse to discuss with SPDC's colleagues about a patient of him, Pietro, involuntarily admitted the day before. After having talked to their colleagues, the nurse goes to Pietro's room to see him and possibly talk a bit about his situation, but the psychiatrist remains in the medical office deciding not to make himself visible to his patient. He justifies his choice by saying that it was better "not to instigate him [Pietro]" (the man had been aggressive with his general practitioner two days before and might be resentful with his psychiatrist too). After he left, the ward's nursing staff maintained this was just an excuse (the psychiatrist was afraid to meet his aggressive patient) and judged his decision as an act of bad care: a way to avoid the encounter with his patient in the tense moment due to the coercive measure adopted (i.e. involuntary treatment), and therefore a missed opportunity to explain the reasons behind it and frame it in the therapeutic relationship.[34]

In the restraint context, the most representative exception to the relationalization of coercion was that of a psychiatrist, Carmela, who decided

[34] We do not know if this was done in a second phase, maybe after Pietro's discharge, and I do not have the competence to say if the psychiatrist's decision had a clinical or personal (being scared is an admissible condition) rationale. What I wish to underline here is the shared understanding that relationship—even in tense moments related to coercion—should always come first, and it is a professional's duty to "stay in the relationship" (*stare nella relazione* was a sort of mantra in this context, something that is considered essential for a mental healthcare worker to be able to do, see also Chap. 7) and clarify the reasons behind a coercive intervention, despite the inherent difficulties. Significantly, this is consistent with the opinions expressed by two psychiatrists of the Cedar Centre (see Excerpts 6.65 and 6.66), in the restraint context.

to involuntary admit a patient of hers—Giuseppe—without signing the papers herself (so that the measure could seem decided by another doctor) and without escorting him or being present in the SPDC at his arrival. Later, during her interview, she explains this was done to preserve the patient's faith in his doctor.

> *Excerpt 6.64.* Carmela (psychiatrist, Pine Ward): The patient and his doctor, the risk is that, the problem, the concern is that he might lose faith in his doctor, while if it [TSO] is done by other members of the medical équipe, I mean, it is a narrow squeak ('ci si salva in calcio d'angolo'). In fact, I did not wanted to be present when he was admitted, even if it was me who decided, I had talked to the police marshal, to execute it [TSO] on that morning.

I considered this episode so relevant I decided to include it, though removing any reference to both the psychiatrist's and the patient's identity, in the interviews with community psychiatrists of the restraint context I met two months after, in order to understand if this tactic—not to appear as the decision-maker behind an involuntary treatment and not to meet the patient when coercively admitted—was a shared local practice or rather an individual strategy to deal with the performance of a coercive intervention. Before narrating the episode, I asked my interviewees about how, if at all, the execution of a TSO affected the therapeutic relationship with their patients. The following excerpts synthetize their answers, which indicate that their colleague's strategy is not shared at all: instead, relationship and openness are once again acknowledged as crucial elements, despite the inherent difficulties, not only to remain credible in their patients' eyes but also to help them make sense of the dramatic phase of crisis and coercive treatment.

> *Excerpt 6.65.* Davide (psychiatrist, Cedar Centre): I think that a psychiatrist has to work very hard to admit people when they need to be admitted, and it's not easy to get to that, so when the person is unwell, when she is unwell and you get her admitted she understand it was inevitable. [...] "Now I have to admit you"; [imitating an hypothetical patient:] "but I-, you are-", swearwords; "no, I'm sorry, you are unwell, I have to admit you"; "I am not unwell, you are an asshole, you are on their side"—because that's

what they say to you—"you are on their side, who sent you?"; "you are unwell". They understand it, right? So the problem with TSO, of course it is a delicate aspect, the, the imposition over the person, but it is something that if carefully considered and well safeguarded it's not, in my experience it is not something which spoils the relationship of trust. [...] I think you lose authority by doing like this [like Carmela]. [...] It's ridiculous to make someone else doing it [TSO]. He [the patient] comes to you precisely for that, so that you can help him recovering, right?

Excerpt 6.66. Giorgio (psychiatrist, Cedar Centre): Personally, if I have to do a TSO to a patient, I prefer to tell him and do it myself. Because they are people like us and, I mean, [otherwise] we are burying our head in the sand. We should declare the state of illness we observe, the difficult situation, which is also useful to process a compulsory admission, because otherwise it has little justification in the perspective of the person subjected to it. And [we should] be available to, to everything, to his requests for explanation, as far as possible, and yes, we have to be decisive and firm, [and try to pursue] solutions different than TSO, that's what has to be done, but *precisely because you are his doctor and you have a certain kind of relationship with him*, you have to try, *you have the power to explain it to him*. [...] Then you also accept criticisms, right? Which will come, but later they will be a point of departure, you know? This is it. "I had you admitted because in that moment you were unwell. I know you, you are not like that, you were unwell, I can tell you because I know you, you were like this, you did this and that", right? Somehow, to represent a history of the crisis is useful to understand, to help getting through a tough moment such as compulsory hospitalization, I mean, even when formally it is not a TSO and admission is accepted ... it is always, it is always a coercive moment, because ... it is a moment of suffering.

Giorgio's quotation helps us conclude on the relationalization of coercion strategy by highlighting some of its fundamental elements: the need to remain open and honest with the person on whom the coercive intervention has to be performed, "staying in the relationship" even when this exposes the psychiatrist to criticism and resentment; to explain the reasons behind the measure, while or after it has been applied; to acknowledge personhood and the person's need to understand, so that they can attach a meaning to the coercion experienced; to retrospectively reconstruct the history of the crisis with the patient, so that coercion can possibly make sense in his/her trajectory.[35] Relevant to our approach to coercive practices is Giorgio's observation that admission can be difficult to process and understand also when formally it is voluntarily accepted: the focus is once again placed on the subjective experience; in this case on perceived coercion (Szmukler, 2017) of coerced voluntaries (O'Donoghue et al., 2014). Besides explanation, we have seen other strategies to relationalize coercion, such as that of negotiation (of initiation, continuation, termination, or temporary interruption or attenuation of coercive measures) and acts of practical compassion (Brown et al., 2014). These strategies allow to incorporate coercion and make it compatible with the provision of good (health)care.

6.3.4 Multiplication of the Objects of Care

The fourth and last strategy employed to frame coercion as good care is the *multiplication of the objects of care*. If the first three strategies focus on the individual patient and his/her relationship with the staff, this one invests other (individual and collective, human and nonhuman) actors and considers them as legitimate recipients of care. Crucial to this vision is the acknowledgement that the aspects or objects of care are always multiple, and that they are overlapping, and simultaneously being cared for, resulting in tensions which are experimentally and locally handled as they unfold (Law, 2010).

First of all, mental health workers care for each individual patient. We have seen how this happens and is made compatible with the application of coercive measures in the previous three paragraphs concerning therapeutization, proceduralization, and relationalization of coercion. But mental healthcare workers simultaneously care for each other (for the staff) and for the other inpatients admitted to the SPDC or assisted in the Mental Health Centre. This does not only mean, as one could more easily imagine, that

[35] What Giorgio describes seems to recall the "narrative reconstruction" theorized by Gareth Williams (1984) with respect to chronic illness, which constituted a disruption in the patient's biography. To make sense of the coercive event is presented as crucial to incorporate it in one's self-narration and overcome that experience.

they have to be protected from possible aggression or annoying behaviour (e.g. screaming or wandering at night). This also means that—in our participants' notion of good care—*every* patient should be provided with the assistance s/he needs. In an organizational context characterized by lack of human resources, lack of time, and, in the case of the Pine Ward and many other Piedmontese ones, shortage of beds (resulting in the overcrowding of the units), equitable provision of care is not always achieved. Overcrowded spaces and the heterogeneous population inhabiting them are represented by our participants as inherently deleterious for vulnerable categories of patients, those who tend to withdraw from communal areas and protect themselves through isolation, such as people going through a depressive episode. Patients who are particularly unwell, or who are diagnosed with disorders usually associated with having a demanding attitude (e.g. borderline and antisocial personality disorders, or manic phases of bipolar disorder), are conversely described as annoying and difficult to tolerate by those who share the same ward with them. Nurse Gaia addresses these issues in her interview, illustrating how she (but also other colleagues of hers) tries to lighten the atmosphere in the ward by temporarily "removing" difficult patients (e.g. by escorting them out to the hospital café for a while or inviting them to spend some time in the nursing room when there are no activities to be performed there).

> *Excerpt 6.67.* Gaia (nurse, Pine Ward): Sometimes you do [invite a patient to stay in the nursing room for a while] because if he's a bad patient the others can take a breath. If you keep him there with you the other patients can take a breath, because sometimes some patients are very annoying and the others can't stand them anymore, here we have also depressed [people], we have other pathologies, and to have an antisocial, or a borderline who starts dancing the can-can [making a mess], or a manic, it's difficult, and you see that the depressed are increasingly closed in their rooms, they cannot-
>
> **Interviewer: Is it a way to protect themselves?**
>
> Gaia: Yes, exactly, exactly.

A situation of uneven provision of care among inpatients can also occur when a particularly difficult patient requires attention and time from the staff, which are inevitably subtracted from other patients. This was the case of Santiago, the man involuntarily treated at the Violet

Centre whom I frequently mentioned in this chapter. The need to have one or more nurses to stay with him all day long, and his repeated attempts to leave the Centre or to hit the staff, forced professionals to focus most of their attention on him, postponing non-urgent home visits and inevitably having less time and energy to dedicate to the other service users. In fact, in the case of a twenty-four-hour Mental Health Centre, the staff has to care for both hosted patients and ordinary users, either at home, on a day hospital program, or visiting the service for therapy administration, medical interviews, lunch, and other activities. When, in particularly critical situations such as the one I had the opportunity to observe, priorities and routines of the MHC have to be modified and adapted to the needs of one or few acute patients and issues concerning good care arise and explicitly discussed. The following excerpt refers to a staff meeting held in the Violet Centre on those intense days.

> *Excerpt 6.68.* Matilde [OSS] maintains that to do like they had to do on Sunday—when all of the four nurses had to go after Santiago as he was leaving, and therefore abandoned the Centre—is a sign of *poor quality of the service*. Doctor Claudio intervenes, saying that the fact that they managed to stop Santiago from leaving (which was the priority) is synonym with *effective and high-quality intervention*, and that it has not to be taken for granted (other times they did not manage to stop a patient who was leaving, and had to let him go [alerting the police if he was under TSO]). [...] Greta [nurse] is sceptical about how long they will be able to deal with such a difficult situation (which has already lasted for more than one week without any substantial improvement). Other patients' dissatisfaction is discussed too: Igor explicitly complained about Santiago, Corrado spoke badly of the "little man" [Santiago, who's not very tall], Camillo seems particularly sullen, and, more generally, service users seem to feel neglected because attentions are all centred on Santiago. Azzurra [psychiatrist]: "to take him [Santiago] out is one of the few things that seem to work". (Violet Centre, fieldnotes)

In the first part of the excerpt, Matilde and Claudio are discussing precisely about what kind of care the Centre was able to provide in that situation, and whether it had to be considered good or bad care. While the woman underlines the fact that, in order to care for Santiago, the staff had to leave the Centre and its users alone (even though for few minutes), Claudio affirms that the priority of the situation justified their choice, and he highlights the efficacy of the intervention in preventing an involuntarily treated patient to leave. In a context of multiple objects of care (Law, 2010), the inherent tensions and incompatibilities are attempted to be handled by ordering and prioritizing these objects, adopting a version of good care that consists in (successfully) caring for those who need it the most. This solution is not free from ambivalence and did not satisfy care providers. In the second part of the excerpt, nurses raise the issue of other users' dissatisfaction with the unequal distribution of care within the service. According to doctors, there seemed to be few alternatives: the boy was in an acute phase of illness, and besides relationally supporting him and continuously trying to adjust his pharmacological therapy, which had not achieved the expected results yet, they could not do anything else than wait while trying to do their best. Ambivalence is inherent to the provision of good care in such complex situations, where different goods have to be dealt with together, and good and bad are intertwined (Mol, 2010). Rather than discussing about a general notion of good care, namely an overall good, psychiatrist Azzurra suggests keeping experimenting and trying to handle the emerging tensions practically. A tentative solution, similar to the practice described by Gaia in the Pine Ward (see Excerpt 5.67), was that to accompany Santiago for walks in the park, or car trips, both to care for his needs (as he suffered from having to stay inside all day long) and to provide some relief to the users in the Centre while he was not there.

The issue of resources allocation for a provision of care adequate to each person's needs seemed to be relevant also in the relationship between ward and community services. In the no-restraint context, community mental healthcare workers are more frequently involved in the care of people admitted to the SPDC, especially when the ward hosts particularly critical situations and is near (or has reached) its legal capacity. As observed in Chap. 5, not all Mental Health Centres seem to equally contribute to alleviate the ward's workload. In the case described below, the MHC (not the Tulip nor the Violet one) had been asked to send a nurse to escort Marcello (a user of that service) to undergo a bronchoscopy in another hospital unit because at 8.30 in the morning the SPDC could not allocate two out of its four nurses for an activity outside of the ward. The Centre did not cooperate nor justified its refusal to help, and Marcello was eventually escorted by an SPDC nurse and the nurses' coordinator because he was feeling sick and the medical examination could not be postponed. The following excerpt from fieldnotes describes a meeting between ward and MHC staff that took place right after this episode.

> *Excerpt 6.69.* [MHC worker:] If I deprive the MHC of a nurse to send him here for Marcello, I subtract resources to territorial activities, and other patients risk ending up here [in the SPDC]". It is the too-short-blanket problem. Marzia reacts saying: "but Marcello is a difficult patient, he's part of the MHC family, and the blanket for him has to be stretched. Here in the SPDC we cannot subtract resources from the equivalent of your home visits, we have admissions, urgency, consultation in the ER, and so on". (Iris Ward, fieldnotes)

We can see how the difficulties in establishing what is "better" in this specific situation result in a friction between the ward and the community care teams. Two different modalities of ordering the objects of care, two different hierarchies, seem to emerge: while the Mental Health Centre professionals prioritize ordinary care of non-acute patients and frame their practice as a mode of indirectly caring for the ward too ("if I subtract resources to territorial activities, other patients risk ending up here", namely to be hospitalized and increase ward's workload), SPDC workers observe that their service has very little chance to defer its activities (most of which—emergencies, ER consultations—cannot be postponed). Moreover, by mentioning Marcello's belonging to the "MHC family", nurse Marzia refers to an historical conflict concerning this patient and the community service. Affected by psychosis and described as one of the most serious and aggressive cases of the whole area, Marcello is hardly ever hosted in the twenty-four-hour Mental Health Centre, but instead admitted to the ward, usually for prolonged periods of time, every time he goes through a crisis.[36] His situation raises questions concerning

[36] Over a period of nine years, Marcello has been admitted to the Iris Ward twenty-one times, six of which were involuntarily (TSO), for a maximum of three months of stay. Source of information: ward's registry of past admissions and patient's personal record, consulted on the field.

general notions of good care, which the ward's staff maintains to provide,[37] while the Mental Health Centre is accused of being rejecting and providing no therapeutic continuity to its patient.

Multiplication of the objects of care is particularly relevant for our purposes when it is related with coercive practices, which are framed as compatible with good healthcare precisely because of the multiplicity of the recipients of care. This has been observed, like the strategies illustrated in the previous paragraphs, for several restraining practices and in both contexts under scrutiny.

The first coercive practice I consider is environmental restraint, namely the locking of SPDC's or MHC's doors to prevent patients from leaving. This is a possibility that both the Iris Ward and the Mental Health Centres have, at night (when doors are regularly closed) or during the day, for limited periods of time, when particularly tense situations occur. The open-door policy applied in these contexts rests on the idea, supported by some empirical evidence (see Sect. 2.3.4 on advantages and disadvantages of these policies), that locking doors results in a restrictive therapeutic atmosphere and increased patient aggression. This implies that when the measure has to be applied, for reasons related to a temporary difficulty or to a situation peculiar of a singular patient, it is considered deleterious for the other users. The two episodes I present in the following quotations exemplify the case of adopting a restraining measure to respond to an individual moment of crisis, which nevertheless affects the whole population of the service (the ward in the first excerpt, the MHC in the second one).

[37] Marcello has been aggressive toward the SPDC staff several times, causing also some serious injuries: he almost strangled a nurse who does not work in the ward anymore, and tried to do the same with Marzia, who nevertheless tells me: "here we've been all beaten up too [like in the MHC], but along time you build a relationship again. After he grabbed my neck, I left the ward with a face that was blue, but *nevertheless* when he is here I do my job and don't back out" (*Excerpt 6.70*). Supported by her colleagues, she highlights that ward's staff keeps providing "affective" and "professional" care despite the assaults and consequent fear, while the MHC is equally scared but reacts by refusing to care for him. Consequently, Marcello seemed to rely primarily on the ward's staff, as these excerpt from fieldnotes related to the moment of his discharge show: "Marcello says goodbye to Marzia and Franco [nurses], hugs them, and asks if he can call the ward on the phone if he needs to. They reassure him: he can. He says goodbye to a couple of patients and leaves. Despite he is considered a difficult and violent patient, this moment of greeting after two months of stay is emotionally charged, both for me and the workers involved" (*Excerpt 6.71*).

Excerpt 6.72. To escort and follow him [Pietro] continuously around and outside of the ward is very demanding for the staff, who cannot carry on with ordinary activities, such as therapy administration to the other inpatients, some of whom are waiting in the hall, outside the door of the nursing room. Elettra [nurse] asks her colleagues to temporarily lock the [ward's] door to allow her to administer therapies. They agree without consulting the doctors—this is considered a nursing decision—and the door is locked. [...] After therapy administration the doors are opened again. (Iris Ward, fieldnotes)

Excerpt 6.73. Taking into consideration Santiago's attempt to leave and his persistent hostility, the three doors of the MHC are locked. This decision implies some problems for other service users, who usually enter and exit the Centre freely. The staff invites them to be patient and reassures them that this is only a temporary thing. (Violet Centre, fieldnotes)

Excerpt 6.72 is about Pietro, an involuntarily admitted patient who had already managed to leave the ward the day before, and then had been escorted back to the ward by the police after few hours.[38] Despite his previous escape, in the morning the staff successfully managed to leave the ward's doors open by carefully observing Pietro's movements around the ward, following him at a distance when he approached the stairs and elevators right outside the unit, and gathering in the hall to discourage him from leaving. After the staff meeting in the early afternoon, therapy administration is scheduled. This activity requires a dedicated nurse, who needs not to be distracted from a delicate task, and a colleague (nurse or OSS) who asks patients in the hall or their rooms to come to the nursing room one at a time. Attention and number of resources necessary to look after Pietro did not allow therapy administration to be performed, also because the risk of absconding was high: I had seen him push the button to call the elevator the second he thought he was not being observed. Nurses agreed to temporarily close the doors to administer therapies to the patients already waiting in the hall (who received an apology for the delay), and re-opened them after about an hour and a half. Excerpt 6.73 describes a similar episode:

[38] During the staff meeting, when most of the staff was gathered in the dining room, Pietro managed to distract a nurse in the hall asking her for a painkiller (he arrived at the ER with a hand almost broken) and run through the door. An OSS who was standing in the hall at some distance and the rest of the staff immediately run after him, but the man was an athlete and easily managed to leave them behind and disappear.

after Santiago's several more or less serious attempts to leave the Centre, the staff decided to temporarily lock the doors of the MHC for the staff meeting (which is held in a room near the entrance). The measure affected the other service users, both hosted on the twenty-four hours and passing through the Centre for other activities, who could not enter or leave the building without the staff's cooperation. The "unfair" restriction of their usual freedom of movement was acknowledged and repaired by the nurses, who explained to them the reasons for the temporary measure and asked for their understanding and patience. In both of these episodes, the patient's, the staff's and the other users' needs are attempted to be cared for simultaneously, by applying the environmentally restraining measure of doors locking for the shortest period of time possible, explaining motives to people subjected to it, and apologizing for unintended consequences of the tense situation (i.e. delays on the usual routine).

The second coercive practice I consider is mechanical restraint. The following excerpts from fieldnotes, inevitably related to the Pine Ward only, describe two different episodes where the multiplicity of the "objects of care" proved to be relevant for the application (or its discussion) of the restraining measure.

> *Excerpt 6.74.* Livia (nurse, Pine Ward): On Saturday the doctor came and he wanted to unrestrain Aldo and I took the liberty to say: "it's not that I don't want to [unrestrain him], but on Saturday there are [only] three of us", I mean, it's the less advisable day to try, because we had tried few days before and it went really bad.[39] [...] And we had 21 patients [the ward was overcrowded], ok? [...] I said: "I think Saturday is the less advisable day", I mean, then if we want to try now there we are all [psychiatrist included] here together we can do it, but I can't say if the ward will be [calm] like this all day long, we are in a limited number, and with a patient like her [Iris] who required a lot of time, a dedicated nurse, we went out [of the ward with her], I stayed out [with her], I mean, it is a lot of work, so if one of us is with her ... another one is with him [Aldo, if we unrestrain him] ... the third [nurse] alone with the rest of the ward can't do it.

> *Excerpt 6.75.* Gaia [nurse] says that according to her Carlo is too delirious to be unrestrained, especially because there is Diego in the ward. Livia

[39] The patient had hit a nurse few times after termination of restraint, and therefore had been restrained again.

> [nurse]: "what about stopping [restraining] Diego?". Diego is agitated, yesterday he was cross with a patient, today he picked on another, and he had been hostile with Gaia. [...] Maria [OSS] adds: "Diego is very bad ['brutto'], you know that I don't like restraints but with all due respect, he's very bad. Maybe he should be tied and be given appropriate therapy"; "Diego is a time bomb"; "Yesterday he asked me if I wanted to eat dead fish [death threat], I locked myself in here, the other patients are terrified". Doctor Vincenzo comments that if Diego broke something, they would have a justification to take him and tie him. (Pine Ward, fieldnotes)

In the first excerpt, nurse Livia describes the multiplicity of factors implied in the decision of interrupting restraint: the number of nurses and OSS on duty; the result of preceding unrestraining attempts; the number and profile of people admitted to the ward; and the overall situation on the unit. In the specific case, all of these factors seemed to discourage the staff from trying: on a Saturday, there were fewer workers than usual, many inpatients (five more than the ward's legal capacity), a demanding one (Iris) who required the almost-constant presence of a nurse with her (in or outside the ward), and a previous unrestraining attempt resulting in an assault of a colleague. To protect the staff from possible aggression, as well as other patients who would have been left with a single nurse to care for their requests and needs, the doctor's proposition is refused and termination of restraint postponed after the weekend.[40] The second excerpt from fieldnotes is about two critical patients deemed not compatible: the first one, Carlo, is restrained and the termination of the measure is not supported by nurse Gaia, both because of his persistent hallucinations and the hostile presence of Diego. The latter has been contentious with both inpatients and the staff: Maria describes them as terrified and reports about an episode when he threatened and scared her. Nevertheless, the doctor decides not to intervene with restraint because no aggressive behaviour had been actualized to justify a coercive intervention yet. To avoid increasing conflicts and chances of accidents in the ward, though, Carlo is left restrained.

[40] Because of fewer nurses on duty and a singular doctor on-call, the weekends have been described by participants as a moment when attempts to reducing coercive measures are rarely performed. Exceptions may be due to the particularly low number of inpatients, experienced and motivated workers, and/or well-known and trusted patients.

The last coercive measure, pharmacological restraint, is once again discussed by our participants in the Iris Ward with respect to Pietro, the involuntarily admitted patient who absconded from the ward the day before the exchange quoted in Excerpt 5.76.

> *Excerpt 6.76.* At the staff meeting, pharmacological therapy of Pietro is discussed. Yesterday Acuphase[41] was administered, and they thought about repeating it tomorrow, but after his escape they are considering repeating administration today. Paolo [psychiatrist] and the staff are critical toward Pietro's community psychiatrist, who never wants to use depot medication, or uses "light" drugs on tough patients [like Pietro] (Abilify[42]). SPDC's chief psychiatrist has decided to initiate Clopixol depot medication [a "heavier" drug] despite the opinion of Pietro's community psychiatrist, and Paolo expresses his support for this decision. Marzia [nurse] agrees too, then she adds: "*besides curing the patient we have not to get beaten up, we have to protect ourselves and the other patients*". The latter, she explains, have spent the whole morning holed up in their bedrooms, scared by Pietro who kept walking up and down the ward "like an animal in a cage", glaring at everyone. (Iris Ward, fieldnotes)

Administration of supplementary dosage of sedative medication is here discussed not only in relation to Pietro's clinical condition and elevated risk of absconding but also considering staff's exposure to possible assaults (the patient had been aggressive with his GP right before involuntary hospitalization) and other inpatients' fear of Pietro, which discouraged them from leaving their rooms. Contrary to environmental restraint through doors locking, which indifferently penalizes every inhabitant of the ward (whether patient or professional), the restraining measure of pharmacological therapy allows to minimize conflicts between the different goods at stake, and to simultaneously care for inpatients and the staff while (coercively) treating the person in crisis.

To conclude on the strategy of multiplication of the objects of care, I wish to underline how, besides justifying the application of coercive

[41] Acuphase is the commercial name for zuclopenthixol acetate (first-generation antipsychotic), while Clopixol depot is a long-acting medication with the same active ingredient (zuclopenthixol).

[42] Aripiprazole, a second-generation (or atypical) antipsychotic.

measures, it can also be mobilized to choose between different forms of restraint, motivating a preference. In what follows, the psychiatrist Giorgio (Cedar Centre) explains how the choice between mechanical and pharmacological restraint of a patient in the Pine Ward depends on several factors.

> *Excerpt 6.77.* Giorgio (psychiatrist, Cedar Centre): In the SPDC there are pressures, there are circumstances that require to *look at the ward as a whole*, there is a mixture of different kind of acuteness ... [There are] situations in which you have to deal with the nursing staff's expectations, expectations related to the difficulty in managing the ward, there is also this aspect, so you also pay the consequences of overcrowding, of the difficulty in looking after all of the patients, so [he sighs] there are circumstances when you cannot administer some drugs because there is a prolonged QTc, an ECG which does not allow-, so with an agitated patient you have to use mechanical instead of pharmacological restraint.

Objects of care are, once again, multiple (Law, 2010). The psychiatrist, while dealing with an agitated patient, is expected to care for: the other inpatients' needs and the heterogeneity between their conditions; the difficulties of the nursing staff in managing the ward, especially when it is overcrowded and resources do not suffice; the health status of the agitated patient, who might show altered parameters or organic diseases which make pharmacological administration risky. To look at the ward as a whole ultimately means to tinker with a multiplicity of expectations, conflicting needs, and tensions, which may motivate the use of restraining measures (or of a specific kind of restraining measure) and frame them as legitimate ways to provide, if not good, at least "good enough" or the better possible care.

6.4 Conclusion

Acute mental healthcare is characterized by the aim to provide therapeutic environment and support to people going through a crisis, which can require coercive interventions (e.g. involuntary treatment, forced medication, mechanical and other forms of restraint) overcoming a patient's will. The chapter has shown how the inherent ambivalence in pursuing such aim is dealt with, framing everyday psychiatric practice as good care. Two repertoires have been identified: that of outsourcing coercion (attributing its exercise to non-healthcare actors) and that of embedding it in the healthcare context (performing it as good care). The latter repertoire has been further articulated into four discursive and practical strategies: (1) therapeuticization of coercion; (2) proceduralization of coercion; (3) relationsalization of coercion; (4) multiplication of the objects of care.

Table 6.1 synthesizes repertoires, strategies, as well as residual elements which emerged from the analysis of the empirical data, denoting the complexities and ambivalence to hold together a coercive dimension and the provision of good mental healthcare.

Table 6.1 Combining care and coercion: Repertoires and strategies

Repertoires	Practical and discursive strategies	Key points	Residuals
Outsourcing coercion	Segregation of care and coercive functions; Attribution to different actors	Social control excluded from healthcare providers' tasks	Disagreement with other agencies (e.g. police force)
Embedding coercion	Therapeuticization of coercion	Beneficial effects of coercive intervention	Detrimental effects ("least bad" intervention)
	Proceduralization of coercion	Scientific, technically competent, safe coercion	Improvisation
	Relationalization of coercion	Acknowledging personhood and the subjective experience of the coerced person through negotiation, explanation, and acts of practical compassion	Withdrawing from relationship in case of coercion
	Multiplication of the objects of care	Others' best interest	Unequal provision of care

References

Austin, W., Goble, E., & Kelecevic, J. (2009). The ethics of forensic psychiatry: Moving beyond principles to a relational ethics approach. *The Journal of Forensic Psychiatry & Psychology, 20*(6), 835–850.

Berlant, L. (Ed.). (2004). *Compassion: The culture and politics of an emotion.* Routledge.

Björkdahl, A., Palmstierna, T., & Hansebo, G. (2010). The bulldozer and the ballet dancer: Aspects of nurses' caring approaches in acute psychiatric intensive care. *Journal of Psychiatric and Mental Health Nursing, 17*(6), 510–518.

Bowers, L., Van Der Merwe, M., Paterson, B., & Stewart, D. (2012). Manual restraint and shows of force: The City-128 study. *International Journal of Mental Health Nursing, 21*(1), 30–40.

Brodwin, P. (2014). The ethics of ambivalence and the practice of constraint in us psychiatry. *Culture, Medicine, and Psychiatry, 38*(4), 527–549.

Brown, B., Crawford, P., Gilbert, P., Gilbert, J., & Gale, C. (2014). Practical compassions: Repertoires of practice and compassion talk in acute mental healthcare. *Sociology of Health & Illness, 36*(3), 383–399.

Calabrese, J. D. (2011). "The culture of medicine" as revealed in patients' perspectives on psychiatric treatment. In M. J. D. Good, S. S. Willen, S. D. Hannah, K. Vickery, & L. T. Park (Eds.), *Shattering culture: American medicine responds to cultural diversity* (pp. 184–199). Russell Sage Foundation Publications.

Cardano, M. (2011). *La ricerca qualitativa.* il Mulino.

Falkum, E. (2008). Phronesis and techne: The debate on evidence-based medicine in psychiatry and psychotherapy. *Philosophy, Psychiatry, & Psychology, 15*(2), 141–149.

Foot, J. (2015). *The man who closed the asylums: Franco Basaglia and the revolution in mental health care.* Verso Books.

Foucault, M. (2006). *Psychiatric power: Lectures at the Collège de France 1973–1975.* Palgrave Macmillan.

Gansel, Y., & Lézé, S. (2015). Physical constraint as psychological holding: Mental-health treatment for difficult and violent adolescents in France. *Social Science & Medicine, 143*, 329–335.

Gibson, J. J. (1977). The theory of affordances. In R. Shaw & J. Bransford (Eds.), *Perceiving, acting, and knowing: Toward an ecological psychology* (pp. 67–82). Erlbaum.

Goffman, E. (1955). On face-work: An analysis of ritual elements in social interaction. *Psychiatry, 18*(3), 213–231.
Goffman, E. (1959). *The presentation of self in everyday life*. Doubleday.
Goodwin, C. (1994). *Professional vision. American anthropologist, 96*(3), 606–633.
Hamilton, B. E., & Manias, E. (2007). Rethinking nurses' observations: Psychiatric nursing skills and invisibility in an acute inpatient setting. *Social Science & Medicine, 65*(2), 331–343.
Hejtmanek, K. (2010). Caring through restraint: Violence, intimacy and identity in mental health practice. *Culture, Medicine, and Psychiatry, 34*(4), 668–674.
Henderson, C., Swanson, J. W., Szmukler, G., Thornicroft, G., & Zinkler, M. (2008). A typology of advance statements in mental health care. *Psychiatric Services, 59*(1), 63–71.
Law, J. (2010). Care and killing: Tensions in veterinary practice. In A. Mol, I. Moser, & J. Pols (Eds.), *Care in practice: On tinkering in clinics, homes and farms* (Vol. 8, pp. 57–72). transcript Verlag.
Lawn, S. J., Pols, R. G., & Barber, J. G. (2002). Smoking and quitting: A qualitative study with community-living psychiatric clients. *Social Science & Medicine, 54*(1), 93–104.
Luhrmann, T. M. (2001). *Of two minds: The growing disorder in American psychiatry*. Vintage.
Mol, A. (2002). *The body multiple: Ontology in medical practice*. Duke University Press.
Mol, A. (2010). Care and its values. Good food in the nursing home. In A. Mol, I. Moser, & J. Pols (Eds.), *Care in practice: On tinkering in clinics, homes and farms* (Vol. 8, pp. 215–234). transcript Verlag.
O'Donoghue, B., Roche, E., Shannon, S., Lyne, J., Madigan, K., & Feeney, L. (2014). Perceived coercion in voluntary hospital admission. *Psychiatry Research, 215*(1), 120–126.
Olick, K. J. (2008). From collective memory to the sociology of mnemonic practices and products. In A. Erll & A. Nünning (Eds.), *Cultural memory studies: An international and interdisciplinary handbook* (pp. 151–162). Walter de Gruyter.
Pols, J. (2003). Enforcing patient rights or improving care? The interference of two modes of doing good in mental health care. *Sociology of Health & Illness, 25*(4), 320–347.
Raboch, J., Kališová, L., Nawka, A., Kitzlerová, E., Onchev, G., Karastergiou, A., Magliano, L., Dembinskas, A., Kiejna, A., Torres-Gonzales, F., & Kjellin,

L. (2010). Use of coercive measures during involuntary hospitalization: Findings from ten European countries. *Psychiatric Services, 61*(10), 1012–1017.

Seale, C., Chaplin, R., Lelliott, P., & Quirk, A. (2006). Sharing decisions in consultations involving anti-psychotic medication: A qualitative study of psychiatrists' experiences. *Social Science & Medicine, 62*(11), 2861–2873.

Sparti, D. (2005). *Suoni inauditi. L'improvvisazione nel jazz e nella vita quotidiana*. il Mulino.

Sparti, D. (2013). On the edge. A frame analysis for improvisation. In G. Lewis & B. Piekut (Eds.), *The Oxford handbook of critical improvisation studies* (Vol. 1, pp. 182–201). Oxford University Press.

Steinert, T., Noorthoorn, E. O., & Mulder, C. L. (2014). The use of coercive interventions in mental health care in Germany and The Netherlands. A comparison of the developments in two neighboring countries. *Frontiers in Public Health, 2*, 141.

Strauss, A., Schatzman, L., Bucher, R., Ehrlich, D., & Sabshin, M. (1981). *Psychiatric ideologies and institutions*. Transaction.

Swartz, C. M. (1997). A simplified account of drug accumulation and steady-state dose equivalences. *The Journal of Clinical Pharmacology, 37*(10), 962–970.

Szmukler, G. (2017). *Men in white coats: Treatment under coercion*. Oxford University Press.

Szmukler, G. (2019). "Capacity", "best interests", "will and preferences" and the UN convention on the rights of persons with disabilities. *World Psychiatry, 18*(1), 34–41.

Toresini, L. (2007). SPDC No Restraint. La sfida della cura, in AA.VV., *I Servizi Psichiatrici di Diagnosi e Cura. L'utopia della cura in ospedale*. Edizioni Co. Pro.S, Caltagirone.

Williams, G. (1984). The genesis of chronic illness: Narrative re-construction. *Sociology of Health & Illness, 6*(2), 175–200.

Willmott, Y. (1997). Prison nursing: The tension between custody and care. *British Journal of Nursing, 6*(6), 333–336.

Wood, V. J., Curtis, S. E., Gesler, W., Spencer, I. H., Close, H. J., Mason, J. M., & Reilly, J. G. (2013). Spaces for smoking in a psychiatric hospital: Social capital, resistance to control, and significance for 'therapeutic landscapes'. *Social Science & Medicine, 97*, 104–111.

Zerubavel, E. (1979). *Patterns of time in hospital life. A sociological perspective*. University of Chicago Press.

7

Care in the Time of Crisis

Abstract The chapter addresses preferability between different coercive practices, notably mechanical restraint and the open-door policy, which mark the difference between the restraint and the no-restraint contexts empirically explored in this research.

Previous chapters have considered a number of interventions involving a coercive dimension: mechanical, pharmacological, and manual restraint, but also enforced medication, and involuntary admission and treatment. Chapter 6 has observed how such coercive measures can be performed within mental healthcare contexts by adopting repertoires which exclude or embed coercion in the provision of care, independently of the specific intervention and the (restraint or no-restraint) context considered. This last chapter wishes to address how preferability between such interventions was shaped and argued for by participants, moving from the questions suggested by Paul Brodwin to inform ethnographic research concerning ethical topics in healthcare: "Why do people ferret out one particular issue, but not another one, as raising ethical stakes? Why do they puzzle over the rightness or wrongness of this particular clinical manoeuvre, but regard that manoeuvre as unproblematic?" (Brodwin,

E. Rossero, *Care in a Time of Crisis*, https://doi.org/10.1007/978-3-031-34418-3_7

2014, p. 546). Moving from these questions, the issues of mechanical restraint and open-door policy—which most notably mark the difference between the restraint and the no-restraint contexts considered in this study—will be the focus of the following considerations. At the end of the chapter, limitations of the present study, suggestions for future research and for further discussion of today's acute mental healthcare provision will be advanced.

7.1 Preferability Between Restraining Practices

A transversal element from which I would like to begin is that of limit or, once again, boundary: in both the restraint and the no-restraint contexts, acute mental healthcare practice has been presented as having a *limit-setting function*, especially when dealing with acute phases of illness. This is evident in everyday clinical practice, when specific episodes (e.g. aggressive or self-harming behaviour) or temporal extension of a given behaviour (e.g. prolonged non-compliance with depot administration schedules or medical appointments with community services) are deemed to have "crossed a line" and may lead practitioners to decide to intervene coercively. We have seen how specific actions performed by patients can be tolerated to some point (which is not fixed but depends on a number of factors: overall situation of the ward/MHC, individual approaches of nurses or doctors on duty, availability of human and material resources), beyond which intervention is considered legitimate. In other words, what constitutes disruptive behaviour requiring coercive intervention is not pre-given nor is it necessarily shared among practitioners of the same community, but it is the result of a social process of construction (Cardano & Gariglio, 2021). Mechanical restraint in the Pine Ward, for example, could result from a specific episode or action which justified the coercive intervention in a state a necessity, such as an imminent danger to be prevented. The situatedness of the decision-making process was very evident though: psychiatrists or nurses working in the same ward may decide not to wait for disruptive behaviour to be actualized, but to intervene preventively by mechanically restraining a quiet and cooperative patient, either unknown (and therefore unpredictable) or deemed potentially aggressive on the basis of his/her reputation in previous admissions.

Excerpt 7.1. Gino (nurse, Pine Ward): If they call us from the ER and say: 'there is Rossi Mario [casual name] agitated', and we know Rossi Mario, we are less preoccupied than if they say: 'there is Bianchi Tommaso [another casual name] agitated' and we never saw him, right? You have seen it the other day when Giuseppe arrived: we know him, so we took some precautions [mechanical restraint], because we know the patient.

The constructed nature of disruptive behaviour is visible also in the fact that the need to enact a limit-setting intervention may be evaluated differently from the different actors involved in the performance of coercive measures: healthcare providers can consider the status of an involuntarily admitted patient sufficient condition to ask for police intervention, but police officers deem their presence appropriate only "if the patient smashes something or hurts somebody" (Iris Ward, fieldnotes; see also Sect. 6.2 in Chap. 6 on outsourcing coercion).

The following excerpts from fieldnotes show how the coercive intervention—in this case mechanical restraint—can be explicitly performed (or mobilized in the form of threat) to set the limit and sanction its overstepping after a specific behaviour has been enacted.

Excerpt 7.2. Maria [OSS]: "Diego is very bad ['brutto'], you know that I don't like restraints, but with all due respect, he's very bad. Maybe he should be tied and be given appropriate therapy"; "Diego is a time bomb"; "Yesterday he asked me if I wanted to eat dead fish [death threat], I locked myself in here, the other patients are terrified". Doctor Vincenzo comments that *if Diego broke something, they would have a justification to take him and tie him.* (Pine Ward, fieldnotes)

Excerpt 7.3. Hassan expresses the wish to hurt Aldo should he come near him. Cosimo [nurse] threatens him: "*If you hurt someone you force me to restrain you*, do you understand? If you hurt him, I must put the [restraining] belts". He opens his arms mimicking the position of a restrained person. (Pine Ward, fieldnotes)

Limit-demarcation can also be performed by marking the difference between the pre-intervention and the post-intervention setting: in the following example (Excerpt 7.4), we can see how—even if the restrained person is assisted and her condition relieved from suffering whereby acts of practical compassion (see Sect. 6.3.3 in Chap. 6)—such status of restraint must not become too "enjoyable" or too similar to the state of being non-restrained, not to blur the line between the two situations which would also undermine the limit-setting efficacy of performing (or threatening to perform) mechanical restraint.

Excerpt 7.4. Aldo [who is mechanically restrained] asks to play cards there, on the bed. Ernesto [nurse] says no: "it is not therapeutic, because *then you enjoy being here restrained*. You have to be stimulated to go out [leave the room] instead". (Pine Ward, fieldnotes)

The limit-setting function of the measure can also be maintained on a symbolic level. Either by calling the police, coercively admitting a patient or forcibly administering medication, effectiveness of the intervention is maintained on the basis of its ability to give the person a sense of the limit—*to mark a 'before' and an 'after'*—rather than on the actual (pharmacological or physical) restraining function (which sometimes can be avoided because the symbolic efficacy suffices).

Excerpt 7.5. Chiara (psychiatrist, Tulip Centre): In that case it was necessary to stop her and [coercively] administer sedative therapy. *The point is not its immediate effect but the fact that it marks a 'before' and an 'after'*. There, the person stops because, it's like a sensation of having crossed a line, because it is the most violent part of the question. [...] I cannot believe that the effect [of medication] is so immediate, it's that the person in that moment [of forced medication] feels that the other prevailed, so there is a moment of-, then clearly therapies are done, and they are strong in those cases, but for the purpose of switching off that kind of agitation.

Excerpt 7.6. Cesare (nurse, Cedar Centre): If we see that the situation keeps escalating, we call the police and usually the uniform, most of the times to see the police, to see the uniform is effective.

Excerpt 7.7. Chiara (psychiatrist, Red Centre): I am thinking about this girl from Burundi. She knows that there is a 'before' and there is an 'after' with respect to her crisis and her involuntary admission in the MHC, but back then she did not have insight of what happened. Now, after two years, she is starting to see it differently, but *[TSO was performed] to explain our role, to give her a sense of the limit*, you know?

Such limit-setting function has been theorized as a form of sovereign power (Foucault, 2006) aimed at modifying disruptive behaviours: it is the case of seclusion (or other coercive interventions) used as a disciplinary and punitive technology (Jacob et al., 2009). Punitive purposes aimed at "teaching a lesson" to the patient have occasionally emerged during fieldwork, in terms of threat or blackmail: "if you keep doing this, we'll end up restraining you", or "be careful, if you do this again, you'll end up restrained" (excerpted from the interview with Cristian, nurse at the Pine Ward, on punitive uses of mechanical restraint). In both restraint and no-restraint contexts, though, interventions—even when coercive—were rather used and portrayed as having other functions (e.g. therapeutic, or protecting the patient or the other patients, or allowing pharmacological therapy to be administered; see Chap. 6). This is also due to the fact that punishment was deemed ineffective and meaningless to teach something or to 'correct' behaviours attributed to the acute phase of illness and not to the person's will, as Livia, nurse at the Pine Ward, explains in the following.

Excerpt 7.8. Livia (nurse, Pine Ward): The patient is unwell, he has that kind of behaviour, even if he's a border [having borderline personality disorder] who manipulates and provokes, it is not something he does on purpose. To some extent he does, maybe someone can be a bit of a jerk, but he has that behaviour when he is not well. When he is well the patient, even border[line], does not behave like that. When they come here, they are totally uncompensated, so they are extreme, and it is not that I educate them, or that by doing that [restraining him] he understands. Until crisis is over, he does not understand anything, it is not that through restraint he understands. It is that in that moment you are not able anymore, the truth is that you are not able anymore to manage, to manage him, there is no way in, there is nothing.

Besides the practical employment of coercive intervention as a limit-setting tool, restraining measures are tied to the restoration of boundaries also on a conceptual level: the notion of boundary is embedded in that of containment, defined as "the act of controlling or limiting something or someone harmful".[1] We have seen how, in acute psychiatric practice, this concept can translate into acts of physical restraint to restore body limits in those who lack containment (e.g. a violent patient), but also to contain distress at a psychological level, allowing to frame them as legitimate clinical practices: ultimately, as acts of care (Gansel & Lézé, 2015).

Professionals describe the process of decision-making preceding interventions which imply a degree of coercion as complex, ethically charged, and sometimes hurtful for the healthcare providers themselves. They are expected to evaluate the situation and understand when a decision for a coercive intervention has to be made (see Excerpt 7.9 about involuntary admission), but also to help the coerced person understand the necessity of the intervention, by explaining the modalities and the reasons behind it in an open, frank discussion (see also Sect. 6.3.3 in Chap. 6 on relationalisation of coercion).

Excerpt 7.9. Davide (psychiatrist, Cedar Centre): It is like cutting [amputating] an arm, it is the same thing. Because I can-, it is difficult to cut an arm, but if I do it at the right time you will never reproach me. It is difficult for the doctor, this is precisely the burden of medical work, unfortunately this is inevitable, the burden of medical work is to understand and bear the tensions you have to face when you decide, I mean, *when you become aware of when you have to make a decision.* And this is something that, you are alone in this, the doctor is alone.

Excerpt 7.10. Nadia (nurses coordinator, Iris Ward): *You have to set a limit*, absolutely. In case of aggressiveness, we do not always react through pharmacological means. Not always. There can be a pharmacological response, there can be nothing, or a simple medical consult, there can be a call to the police without therapy administration, there are many things. Also we have had situations when we had to administer therapy against a person's will,

[1] Cambridge Dictionary definition (accessed on 4th December 2022): https://dictionary.cambridge.org/it/dizionario/inglese/containment.

> to... in that moment, to force them to treat themselves, because it was strictly necessary and... *this thing hurt many of us [healthcare providers]* but also led the person to understand that yes, we were enacting a form of power, but actually she would have felt worse if she did not accept therapies.

As observed by Nadia (Excerpt 7.10), interventions which may be implemented to set the limit are heterogeneous: enforced medication, call for police intervention, but also physical restraint, mechanical restraint, or involuntary treatment. Despite the transversally acknowledged need to restore a limit in situations of crisis—also through coercive interventions, and especially when the person lacks insight (Seale et al., 2006)—divergences emerge when it comes to decide whether a practice is legitimate or not. On the field, preferability of a form or restraint over another has been maintained on the basis of clinical assessments (e.g. clinical conditions which make, for example, mechanical restraint safer than sedation), personal preferences (e.g. by treating others as you would wish to be treated: "If I were him, I would rather be restrained/sedated..."),[2] or considerations pertaining to the perceived degree of force or violence involved in a given measure, which may not align with healthcare providers' preferred self-image and identity ("we do not do these things", see also next excerpt). In the Iris Ward, for example, the practice of forcing a patient to the floor to prevent him/her from leaving ("*atterramento*"), which was employed in the Violet Centre, was not accepted. In an interview with an SPDC experienced nurse, Franco, the practice was equated with mechanical restraint and deemed inconsistent with a no-restraint orientation, while community colleagues who performed it were charged with being contradictory and having an ideological attitude.

[2] This observation has been reported to me in opposite versions. In the restraint context, I have been told the following: "If I were him, I would rather be [mechanically] restrained than sedated, because it ends with the removal of the belts" (suggesting that sedative medication, on the contrary, may have undesired long-term effects). In the no-restraint context, the opposite was true: "If I were him, I would rather be sedated, so I would not remember being unwell": the focus here is on the subjective experience of the person, who is unwell and who might be further traumatized by being conscious and mechanically restrained. Different values are brought into being: preservation of (or minimization of damage to) physical integrity in the former case, attenuation of psychological harm in the latter.

Excerpt 7.11. I ask Franco [nurse] about the Santiago case, which revealed disagreement about patients' management between SPDC and the Violet MHC. Franco tells me that Santiago repeatedly left the ward, and that it is not true that they did nothing to stop him: they went after him (Franco remembers leaving the hospital with Paolo, wearing his nurse uniform, worried that something could happen to Santiago on the road, and uncomfortable about what passers-by could think and see), they obstructed his way, they tried to convinced him to go back, they alerted the police and the MHC. Claudio [community psychiatrist] wanted them to force him to the ground, and he called the ward instating to tell the doctors what to do, 'scolding' Paolo [SPDC psychiatrist] for having let the boy go. Franco: '*this is the contradiction of these ideologized luminaries, who refuse mechanical restraint but practice these things*', and: 'this is the psychiatry of great ideologists'. (Iris Ward, fieldnotes)

What makes "these things"—the practice of forcing a patient to the floor, but also mechanical restraint—inadmissible to the staff of the Iris Ward is the visibly violent dimension of such practice, sometimes referred to as "exercising a power" (see also Excerpt 7.10 above, about enforced medication). The notion of power intended by the Iris Ward staff is that of a violent power, frequently compared to the imaginaries inherited from former psychiatric hospitals ("a remnant of the asylum"), which resonates with the punishment-oriented, sovereign power theorized by Foucault (2006). More generally, the staff frames exercising a power as the imposition of a decision or intervention on a patient without acknowledging his/her personhood—wishes, preferences, subjectivity—and therefore undermining the development of a (therapeutic) relationship fostering understanding and cooperation.

Excerpt 7.12. Nadia (nurses coordinator, Iris Ward): We understood that *a power relationship is wrong*. It is counter-productive and... dangerous. We always underline that power relationship is not ok, I also say this at meetings: 'the program has not to be decided *on* the patient but *with* the patient', otherwise it is a power relationship. [...] Clearly, the patient can find himself in a condition where, in that moment, he is not able to understand what is best for him, so you guide him. But you have to consider [his] desires, wishes, right? You have to involve him, otherwise it would not work. *It is a relationship of care, it's therapeutic.* It's like with other pathologies, they used to say: 'you have cancer but I won't tell you'. He has to do chemo, how can you not tell him, for God's sake? It is the same![3] [...] Clearly our pathologies are a bit different, they invest the emotional sphere, the sphere of thought, organization, I mean, it's complicated, but you have to address, on the basis of [patient's] hidden abilities he has, or you have to develop them because he never had them, it depends. But...

Interviewer: You mean with patient's cooperation.

Nadia: Yes, absolutely, absolutely, otherwise you won't go anywhere.

As we can read from Nadia's words, the opposite of a power relationship is maintained to be a therapeutic relationship, or a relationship of care. With this expression, the nurse refers to those elements of cooperation, empathy and transparency—enacted in the strategies of relationalization of coercion, such as explanation of the coercive interventions and acts of practical compassion (see Sect. 6.3 in Chap. 6)—which are the goods, or values, prioritized by the no-restraint approach. These values are brought into being in everyday care practices, which embed specific notions of what is good to do, and become particularly visible in those situations when normative considerations are made explicit because decisions have to be made and argued for. The case of Liliana, a woman in her fifties admitted to the Iris Ward with a diagnosis of psychosis, alcohol, and drug abuse, provides an example of the "goods" that the no-restraint

[3] It is interesting to notice how medical discourse—which in this case equates mental illness and cancer or 'other pathologies'—is very present in the no-restraint context as well (especially in the hospital setting), and it is usually mobilized to shape good care as a realm separated from past custodialistic roles ("we are healthcare workers, not prison guards") and de-stigmatize mental illness itself ("SPDC was once represented as a punitive place, now we want people to understand that they come here when they are unwell, to be cured"). To frame psychiatry as a medical specialty (even if *sui generis*: see Sect. 4.3 in Chap. 4 on the construction of 'otherness-from-hospital') opens to the positive effects of medicalization (see also Cardano & Cioffi, 2016): to relieve the patient from moral responsibility and to remove blame and stigma which were (are?) posed on the person admitted to the psychiatric ward (and consequently on the professionals working there). Moreover, it allows to incorporate in mental healthcare valuable elements which have come to characterize other branches of medicine (e.g. oncology) in terms of patient's involvement and awareness, departing from the strong paternalistic approach associated—again—with old psychiatric practice. An example of prioritizing and putting into practice the value of 'patient's awareness' can be found in Excerpt 7.13 on hidden medication and its discussion.

context strives for. One evening, as I arrived to the ward for my first night shift, Liliana was feeling bad because of a difficulty in breathing and low blood saturation. She was wearing an oxygen mask, and few minutes later a doctor and a nurse from the Emergency Department, called for a specialistic consultation arrived. They visited her and decided, in agreement with the psychiatrist, that it would have been better for Liliana to spend the night in the Medicine unit where she could be properly monitored and receive prompt intervention in case of emergency. The woman, though, was very hostile towards the staff and unwilling to move to another ward despite the prolonged negotiation, reassurance, and persuasion attempts. The doctor from the Emergency Department ruled out the possibility to intervene with a short-term sedation (i.e. enforced injection of Midazolam) because of her breathing difficulties, and suggested to resort to hidden administration of oral medication instead. The following excerpt from fieldnotes describes the discussion around this topic between the doctor (whom I will call Ivan) and the Iris Ward staff.

> *Excerpt 7.13*. Ivan [Emergency Department doctor] asks whether there is something they can administer her orally to avoid [enforced] injection. Franco [nurse] is doubtful: Liliana is usually very hostile and will hardly accept new, unusual medication. Both Ivan and the nurse with him suggest, with great naturalness, to bypass the problem by hiding medication in water or fruit juice, so that she doesn't notice or protest. Franco grimaces, looks at me and gives me a hint of a smile (like: "here we go again"), then tells Ivan that those are practices from old psychiatry. Ivan and the nurse seem not to see the problem. The doctor says that just like in a state of necessity you can force an injection against the patient's will, so you can administer medication orally without her consent. Franco disagrees with his argument, saying that *this is not simply lack of consent but lack of awareness* (which, by contrast, is very present if the patient undergoes enforced medication).

Given the patient's initial refusal of oral therapy,[4] and the clinical risk associated with enforced parenteral medication, the ED doctor suggests resorting to hidden medication and ethically equates it to non-consensual

[4] The woman will eventually accept medication (her usual evening therapy slightly increased in its sedative component, Talofen) and also the transfer to the ED unit for the night, after a very prolonged negotiation with the nurse Franco way beyond the formal end of his afternoon shift.

administration through injection. In response, Franco underlines the fundamental difference between the two (both non-consensual) practices: the patient is (painfully) informed of the administration in the case of enforced medication, while s/he is completely unaware of it in the case of hidden medication. By arguing for the preferability of forced medication over hidden administration of drugs, the nurse is prioritizing the value of the patient's awareness and framing it as something they are not willing to sacrifice. While in specific situations, patient's consent can be overlooked and coercion exercised (though related to a discourse of care whereby the repertoires discussed in Chap. 6), transparency in the relationship with the patient is portrayed as something that cannot be waived. The "bad" that is attempted to be avoided here is a mode of intervention associated with "old" psychiatric practice—which did not acknowledge patients' personhood and subjectivity—and which by contrast is unproblematized (and more importantly *expected* from mental healthcare workers) by the doctor operating in a different medical specialty. The same aversion for hidden medication has been observed with respect to placebo (perceived as well as a form of deceit), both in the hospital and in the community services of the no-restraint context, maintaining that "hiding is not relationship".[5]

The goods that the no-restraint context pursues through their care practices can be ultimately synthetized by the expression, which we may call an imperative, that is "to stay in the relationship" ("*stare nella relazione*"). Such a goal is embedded, for example, in the logic of 24-hours

[5]To be clear, a singular episode of hidden medication has been observed also in the Violet Centre, with the grinding of a pill in a glass of water later administered to Santiago (involuntarily admitted patient), presented to me as an exception due to the extreme difficulty in dealing with this patient, and acknowledged as something in contrast with a therapeutic relationship. Hidden medication (sometimes referred to as "encrypted therapy") is also a practice employed, to some extent, by patients' caregivers at home, particularly with tasteless drugs (e.g. Serenase). In the Pine Ward (restraint context), hidden medication seemed more frequent, poorly problematized within the *équipe*, and performed in my presence from the very first day on the field (e.g. syrup in the soup, drops in a glass of water, drugs administered while hiding their actual name and purpose and pretended to have other purposes, e.g. En presented as a "preparation for a CT scan"). This procedure allowed healthcare workers not to engage in discussion with patients about medication they might not accept, sometimes representing a solution preferable to confrontation, or simply a convenient option. Its appropriateness was formally questioned in conversations with me by saying that "it is not ok", but nevertheless employed and even handed over to the colleagues of the following shift during meetings with other legitimate procedures.

Mental Health Centre and in the opportunity they have to host patients alternatively to hospitalization. In our interviewees' perspective, the advantage that such opportunity offers is that of "going through crisis together". To host a patient in her/his most difficult time with acute phase of illness within the MHC, avoiding transfer to a third place (the hospital ward) associated with a sense of exclusion from the community, is understood as a way to stay present—as mental healthcare workers—in the person's everyday life through difficulty, getting a first-hand perspective on the way s/he experiences crisis. Also, it is implicitly related to the knowledge MHC has of the specific person and to the competence the Centre has in dealing with (the specific) crisis, which is prioritized over the competence and specificity SPDC might have in treating acute patients. This contributes to the drawing of the institutional map (Strauss et al., 1981) that denies the uniqueness of the ward in treating crisis, which by contrast is acknowledged in the restraint context (see Chap. 5).

> *Excerpt 7.14.* Chiara (psychiatrist, Tulip Centre): [Involuntary admission in the MHC] represents the dealing with the issue of, the authenticity of the relationship, I mean: "*we will be next to you also when things will be real bad*". There is no: "after that point, you go somewhere else", or: "someone else will take care of you", mmh… Actually, you enhance the therapeutic relationship.

To stay in the relationship also means that, when coercive interventions have to be performed, *measures involving the body of mental healthcare providers themselves (e.g. manual restraint) are preferred to measures which delegate this containment function to non-human actors (e.g. restraining belts or locked doors)*. This is maintained by framing the act of manual restraint—or holding—as a moment of intimate physical interaction between staff members and patients, which shapes the event as a shared experience, recalling the expression of "going through crisis together". Intimacy, closeness, and presence entailed in manual restraint are deemed as vehicles to provide care through restraint (Hejtmanek, 2010), as well as indicators of the degree of involvement and concern expressed by healthcare workers for the restrained person. This has become evident in another episode observed in the Iris Ward, when the intervention performed by nurse Elettra to prevent a young patient from leaving was discussed in a meeting. A seventeen-year-old girl, Giulia, admitted for probable borderline personality disorder and known for repeated suicidal attempts and self-harming behaviour, had temporarily left the ward to go get some snacks from the vending machines on the ground floor, together with a nurse (Elettra) and a worker of a social cooperative involved in Giulia's therapeutic plan. Once she finished eating, she refused going back to the ward and expressed the will to leave the hospital wing. A few meters away, right in front of the entrance, a parapet separates the area from the Emergency Room and ambulance entrance located several meters below. Afraid that the girl could manage to run and exit the hospital, attempting to throw herself off that balustrade, Elettra physically restrains the girl against the wall while waiting for her colleagues to come and help in convincing her to go back to the SPDC.

> *Excerpt 7.15*. On Saturday afternoon Giulia attempted to leave: she was downstairs by the vending machines accompanied by Elettra [nurse] and a social worker, when she refused to go back to the ward and insisted to leave the hospital wing (to go toward the balustrade). Elettra asked the social worker to go upstairs to call her colleagues, but once she found herself alone and afraid that the girl could run away and throw herself off the balustrade in front of her eyes, she panicked and attempted to deal with the situation by raising her voice and pushing Giulia against the wall in a corner to prevent her from leaving. […] Elettra will then confide to Nadia [nurses coordinator] she had felt really scared, to the point of losing control and becoming aggressive. […] Nadia defends the nurse, saying that what happened [manual restraint] allows Giulia to understand that healthcare workers are people too, that they are concerned about her to the point of panicking, and that *they really care for her*. (Iris Ward, fieldnotes)

Nadia's account of how a physical reaction of manual restraint can be framed as an act of care, which conveys to the patient a sense of presence and commitment from the staff, can be read through the lenses of the repertoire of embedding coercion in the therapeutic relationship (see Sect. 6.3 in Chap. 6). Also, it is consistent with the no-restraint philosophy, maintaining that it is important to make them [patients] understand and feel that (physical) and affective containment is a form of care for them (Toresini, 2007). Here, it is presented to discuss the primary value pursued in the no-restraint context, that of "staying in the relationship", and contrast it with the (allegedly bad) mode of care they attempt to avoid by rejecting mechanical restraint, considered as an act of delegation of functions to non-human actors (even though, as we will see, this is not necessarily the case). The next paragraph will delve into this issue.

7.2 What's Wrong with Mechanical Restraint? 'Delegating' Versus 'Staying in the Relationship'

Mechanical restraint is not contemplated in the no-restraint context, even though other forms of coercive intervention (e.g. manual restraint, enforced medication) are performed. In what follows, I attempt to account for this position employing the notion of 'lieutenants' or 'non-human delegates', introduced by Bruno Latour (Johnson, 1988). The author observes that when you want to know what a nonhuman does, you have to imagine what other humans or nonhumans would have to do were this character not present (ibidem, p. 299). In the context of our research, to understand what restraining belts or permanently locked doors do we could look at the no-restraint context where they are not employed, but we can also look at the conditions for removing belts in the restraint ward: the trade-off between human/nonhuman actors emerged plastically each time the continuation or termination of restraint was discussed, by considering human resources, time and effort to be dedicated to the unrestrained person. What do humans (healthcare providers) have to do when restraining belts are not present? What do they have to do when the ward doors are open? The no-restraint identity seems to lie precisely in the relational work (we might say extra-relational work, if compared to the 'restraint' context where relation is not excluded even though mechanical restraint is employed) entailed in avoiding the use of belts and locked doors. It seems to lie in the non-delegating approach discussed in the previous paragraph, which prescribes them to "stay in the relationship", no matter what.[6] This entails that relationship has to be preserved, at least at an ideal level, also by avoiding delegating the management of crisis to other places and professional *équipes*: that is the case of 24-hour Mental Health Centres and their underlying logic of going through crisis with patients and not to entrust other services with their care.

Moreover, the no-restraint context frames this act of delegation and withdrawal from relationship as something which healthcare workers might be tempted to resort to in specific situations, should they have the opportunity to do so. This resonates with what Latour, after Madeleine Akrich (1987), has called prescription: the behaviour that nonhuman delegates impose back onto the human (Johnson, 1988). In the no-restraint participants' perspective, resorting to mechanical restraint, or keeping the ward's doors permanently locked, would open to the possibility for mental healthcare workers to withdraw from relationship, which would still be advisable but no more necessary (see Excerpts 7.16 and 7.17). Belts and locked doors would *prescribe* such withdrawal, just like the very possession of the belts (which the Iris Ward does not own anymore) would open for the possibility to use them (Excerpt 7.18), and therefore to abandon more demanding practices entailing human presence, such as manual restraint or enhanced observation ("*affiancamento*"). Prescription then becomes the moral and ethical dimension of mechanisms (Johnson, 1988, p. 301), hence a fundamental element within no-restraint normative discourse.

Excerpt 7.16. Paolo (psychiatrist, Iris Ward): I think that if you use mechanical restraint… then you don't need to stay with the person anymore, because *there is a device preventing the need to establish a relationship.*

Excerpt 7.17. Paolo (psychiatrist, Iris Ward): I am convinced that if the door was locked, they [nurses] wouldn't have this sense of responsibility for

[6] The "no matter what" specification was frequently contested when enhanced observation or coercive interventions (manual restraint, forcing the patient to the floor) entailed risks for staff safety. Indeed, to restrain or stop a patient with their own bodies could lead to injuries, minimized through the coordinated intervention of several healthcare workers. Nurses' orientations to such risks were differentiated, and decision upon the degree of physical engagement one wanted to guarantee generally left to the individual worker.

what happens [in the ward], and they would be much more retired to the [nursing] room.

Excerpt 7.18. Nadia (nurses coordinator, Iris Ward): I started from the assumption that to have them [restraining belts] means that you begin with two and then you use two hundred. So, when I arrived here, I played the extremist and said: "alright, these [the belts] are going". [...] To say: "I never use them, but I keep them here, just in case" is a teasing, because *you accept the possibility of using them.*

Juxtaposition of these two narratives—that of "staying in the relationship" and that of "delegating to non-human actors"—allows us to understand which arguments are mobilized in the no-restraint context to shape mechanical restraint and permanently locked doors as bad. Instead, no-restraint professionals advocate for practices entailing human presence and engagement with the person going through a crisis, whether coercive (holding, enforced medication) or not (dialogue, negotiation, enhanced observation or "*affiancamento*"). What I wish to underline before concluding on this issue, though, is that—on the basis of what we have observed during fieldwork—*these two narratives do not correspond nor portray the modes of dealing with crisis belonging exclusively to the restraint or the no-restraint model.* Instead, they are intertwined in everyday psychiatric practice of both contexts through a complex balancing of presence and delegation, influenced by values, routines, and organizational constraints.

Indeed, examples of delegation have been inevitably observed in the no-restraint context as well. It is the case of administering sedative medication to acute patients when dialogue and human presence do not suffice to contain their crisis; of temporarily closing the ward's doors when people other than the at-risk-of-absconding-patient need to be cared for (see Sect. 6.3.4 in Chap. 6 on the multiplicity of objects of care); of resorting to hidden medication when psychotic crisis is so deep it rules communication out. Also, it is the case of anaesthesiologic restraint, namely the transfer of a patient to the ICU for properly monitored sedation.[7] While I was on the field, such practice has been nearly implemented in the case of Santiago (which we can consider a near-miss, see Excerpt 7.22) and observed in the Iris Ward on one occasion, on my last day of fieldwork. It concerned the very particular case of a patient transferred from the jail who could not be immediately hosted in a regional REMS,[8] for lack of available beds. His temporary stay in the SPDC, decided by the judge, was arranged to involve the constant presence of two prison officers with him. Once he arrived at the Emergency Room for a first medical assessment, though, he appeared extremely disturbed, hostile, verbally and physically aggressive, to the point that prison officers escorting him had to prevent him from assaulting Paolo (Iris Ward psychiatrist) as he tried to communicate with him several times. After prolonged, unsuccessful attempts to achieve his cooperation—the man would not accept medication, medical examination (e.g. ECG), not even dialogue—the psychiatrist and the ER colleagues decided to call the intensive care specialists, and together they chose to perform rapid tranquillization on the man, while prison officers performed the most violent dimension of the intervention by forcing him to the ground and immobilizing him.[9] Once locally sedated through injections of benzodiazepines and ketamine, the man was then moved to the ICU, to be kept in an induced coma with intravenous anaesthetics (Propofol, which requires mechanical ventilation) for some days, while psychiatric medication such as haloperidol was administered to perform its curative purpose and get the patient through crisis. Such extreme form of pharmacological restraint appears not to be frequent for pure psychiatric patients, and its implementation is not regulated by protocols but requires contextual agreements with the ICU for the specific case. For our purposes, we can consider it an exceptional form of temporary delegation (to another unit,

[7] The practice concerns psychiatric patients and the management of acute phases of illness, and has to be distinguished from admission to the ICU of patients arrived to the ER after alcohol or drug abuse requiring life-saving intensive care.

[8] REMS (‘*Residenze per l'esecuzione delle Misure di Sicurezza*’) are healthcare facilities hosting people who have been found not criminally responsible for a crime or unfit to stand trial due to a mental disorder. They have replaced former OPG (‘*Ospedali Psichiatrici Giudiziari*’, namely forensic psychiatric hospitals) in 2015.

[9] This is consistent with the repertoire of outsourcing coercion discussed in Chap. 6, which can be framed as well as a form of delegation of the coercive intervention to other, non-medical figures.

to anaesthetics, sometimes to restraining belts too, applied in the ICU to the sedated patient) as well as a complete subjugation of the person's body, kept temporarily unconscious by pharmacological means. Once again, the ethical implications associated with its application have to be weighed against alternative measures—if present—which might have been performed to manage such a critical situation.[10]

On the other hand, deliberate and explicit attempts to "stay in the relationship" have been observed in the restraint context too. A clear example was provided by community psychiatrists—both Giorgio and Davide (see Excerpt 6.65 and 6.66)—when discussing about involuntary treatment and the importance of being honest with their patients, without delegating the proposal of TSO or its execution to other colleagues, 'staying in the relationship' even when this exposes the psychiatrist to criticism and resentment. Within the Pine Ward, opportunities for building a relationship with inpatients was not prevented by the sole presence of restraining belts and a closed door. Even though these devices can be seen as delegates or lieutenants—from the French 'lieu' and 'tenant': holding the place of, for, someone else (Johnson, 1988), in this case, the place of nurses—actors do not necessarily subscribe (acquiesce) to the behaviour prescribed by restraining belts or locked doors, namely withdrawal from the therapeutic relationship. Instead, they can negotiate

[10] Anaesthesiologic restraint is used in extreme, rare cases in the restraint context as well (I have been told about two recent cases). On a hypothetical level, preferability of sedation in ICU to mechanical restraint was sometimes sustained on this field for *empathic motives* (avoidance of the subjective, traumatizing experience of being mechanically restrained) or *clinical reasons* (SPDC's poor possibility to monitor vital parameters of sedated patients). This excerpt from Giorgio's interview synthetises this position: "I happened to convert mechanical restraint in anaesthesiologic restraint because it was not tolerable, this person [suffering from a cognitive impairment] did not have the instruments to understand the state of being mechanically restrained, and this condition exasperated her to the point that I, I spent the night running out of pharmacological options, so in the morning I transferred her to the ICU. [...] [Mechanical restraint] entails an important psychological trauma, and many times it is not sufficient to manage agitation, so maybe an organization entailing sedation in a proper environment where functions are monitored would be safer. I guess it would. Mechanical restraint is also... a form which has a psychic value for the person... of great relevance, so it is something very strong. The optimum would be a pharmacological restraint in an environment allowing you to perform it safely, because usually mechanical restraint supports pharmacological restraint, which can never be like that performed in the ICU. We [SPDC] are not equipped for that" (*Excerpt 7.19*). To become routine, such arrangement would require protocols between the wards or at least the availability of the ICU to cooperate, which is not always the case in either the 'restraint' or in the 'no-restraint' contexts considered.

their behaviour, adjust it to the specific situation, and they can choose deliberate de-inscription from the vision of the world that is inscribed in those objects (Akrich, 1992; Akrich & Latour, 1992). We have seen so many examples of such de-inscription. First, we encountered acts of practical compassion (see Sect. 6.3.3 in Chap. 6) through which the personhood of the coerced patient was acknowledged and relationship maintained or built, also in situations where delegation was extreme (e.g. physical contact, music-therapy, and human presence to care for a patient sedated in the ICU, see Excerpt 6.52).[11] We have described how relationship with restrained people was performed by mobilizing trust, reputation, and negotiation within situated agreements concerning temporary removal of restraints, even when delegates—catheters, diapers—would have been available (Excerpt 6.55). And we have observed multiple times that—even though a permanently locked door allows (prescribes) nurses' withdrawal from ward's communal spaces because no entrance surveillance is required—healthcare workers chose to spend time with patients, either by playing cards with them, reading magazines and horoscopes, or simply sitting in the hall chatting with them. In fact, within the hospital organization, the 'reputation' of the psychiatric ward has much to do with this degree of freedom nurses have to define the extent of their involvement with patients besides the routine clinical activities (e.g. therapy administration) entailed in their practice. This led some nurses and OSS to ask to be transferred to the SPDC to decrease their workload and reduce the technical activities they had to perform compared to other, more demanding hospital wards. It is crucial, though, not to overlook motivation, competence, and passion many participants put in their everyday work despite the delegating pressure exerted by locked doors, restraining belts and poorly involved colleagues.

To conclude, we can say that open-door policy and absence of restraining belts prescribe human presence, which nevertheless does not necessarily entail engagement and building of a relationship: healthcare

[11] Similarly, in a third 24-hour Mental Health Centre I have visited in the no-restraint context, I have been told about how, on the occasions when patients with organic or respiratory issues have to be treated in the hospital ICU, community nurses do spend time with them, for therapeutic purposes and to prevent them getting mechanically restrained, even though human presence is neither necessary nor prescribed by the intensive care setting.

workers in the Iris Ward could occasionally sit in the hall to observe the ward without actually relating with patients,[12] or enhanced observation of a patient ("*affiancamento*") may turn into mere surveillance devoid of verbal interaction and other activities.[13] Analogously, permanently locked doors and the possibility to resort to mechanical means of restraint do introduce the opportunity to reduce relational work and engagement with patients, but do not automatically translate into delegation *tout court*.

References

Akrich, M. (1987). Comment décrite les objets techniques. *Technique et Culture, 5*, 49–63.

Akrich, M. (1992). The de-scription of technical objects. In W. Bijker & J. Law (Eds.), *Shaping technology/building society: Studies in sociotechnical change* (pp. 205–224). MIT Press.

Akrich, M., & Latour, B. (1992). A summary of a convenient vocabulary for the semiotics of human and nonhuman assemblies. In W. Bijker & J. Law (Eds.), *Shaping technology/building society: Studies in sociotechnical change* (pp. 259–264). MIT Press.

Brodwin, P. (2014). The ethics of ambivalence and the practice of constraint in us psychiatry. *Culture, Medicine, and Psychiatry, 38*(4), 527–549.

Cardano, M., & Cioffi, M. (2016). Una differenza senza nome. Narrazioni autobiografiche di dislessici adulti. *Rassegna Italiana di Sociologia, 57*(2), 263–292.

Cardano, M., & Gariglio, L. (2021). The neoliberal politics of otherness in Italian psychiatric care: Notes on a team ethnography in six acute psychiatric wards. In J. Gabe, M. Cardano, & A. Genova (Eds.), *Health and illness in the neoliberal era in Europe*. Emerald Publishing.

[12] *Excerpt 7.20*. Paolo (psychiatrist, Iris Ward): How many times does it happen that workers stay there [in the hall] without doing shit? [...] There are moments when you realise that they sit there in the hall and don't do, they do nothing, there are no patients. Those could be moments dedicated to staying with people, have them tell you some things, and try to build with people a stronger alliance.

[13] *Excerpt 7.21*. Franco [nurse]: "Why don't we try to use the worker of the social cooperative who assists her [Giulia] to do something besides the guardian?" (Iris Ward, fieldnotes).

Foucault, M. (2006). *Psychiatric power: Lectures at the Collège de France, 1973–1974*. Palgrave Macmillan.
Gansel, Y., & Lézé, S. (2015). Physical constraint as psychological holding: Mental-health treatment for difficult and violent adolescents in France. *Social Science & Medicine, 143*, 329–335.
Hejtmanek, K. (2010). Caring through restraint: Violence, intimacy and identity in mental health practice. *Culture, Medicine, and Psychiatry, 34*(4), 668–674.
Jacob, J. D., Gagnon, M., Perron, A., & Holmes, D. (2009). Sovereign power, spectacle and punishment: A critical analysis of the use of the seclusion room. *International Journal of Culture and Mental Health, 2*(2), 75–85.
Johnson, J. (1988). Mixing humans and nonhumans together: The sociology of a door-closer. *Social Problems, 35*(3), 298–310.
Seale, C., Chaplin, R., Lelliott, P., & Quirk, A. (2006). Sharing decisions in consultations involving anti-psychotic medication: A qualitative study of psychiatrists' experiences. *Social Science & Medicine, 62*(11), 2861–2873.
Strauss, A., Schatzman, L., Bucher, R., Ehrlich, D., & Sabshin, M. (1981). *Psychiatric ideologies and institutions*. Transaction.
Toresini, L. (2007). SPDC No Restraint. La sfida della cura. In AA.VV., *I Servizi Psichiatrici di Diagnosi e Cura. L'utopia della cura in ospedale*. Caltagirone, Edizioni Co.Pro.S.

8

An Empirical Ethics Approach to Acute Psychiatric Care: Advancing "Situated Suggestions"

Abstract Given the different values embedded and prioritized in care and coercive practices of the two—"restraint" and "no-restraint"—contexts discussed in this book, this final chapter wishes to discuss the contribution that sociological research can give to the (debated) practices I have explored, according to what has been observed on the field and the discussion developed in the previous sections. In order to do so, I adopt the approach of empirical ethics (Pols, Towards an empirical ethics in care: Relations with technologies in health care. *Medicine, Health Care and Philosophy, 18*(1), 81–90, 2015), which does not aim to prescribe general solutions or abstract recommendations, but rather situated suggestions which take into consideration the specificity of the empirical context. In this perspective, practices, and values that I have previously described can be compared, and their intra-normativity and intra-goodness reasoned about.

In the no-restraint context, the value of "staying in the relationship" with acute patients can lead to problematic results when the physical integrity and emotional state of healthcare workers (particularly nurses) are exposed to danger deemed unnecessary or excessive. This was observed

E. Rossero, *Care in a Time of Crisis*, https://doi.org/10.1007/978-3-031-34418-3_8

with respect to the case of Santiago, involuntarily treated at the Violet Mental Health Centre after a period of hospitalization. Even though his permanence in the Mental Health Centre (MHC) was framed as an opportunity, his care providers had to go through crisis with him, his aggressiveness and frequent attempts to leave the Centre required staff's engagement through their own bodies. No serious accidents or injuries happened, but nurses complained about minor harms they suffered from (e.g. kicks, punches, back and shoulder pain reported after forcing and holding Santiago to the floor to prevent him from leaving), and most notably about the perceived elevated dangerousness of the situation, both in terms of potential aggressions (especially at night, when there are only two nurses in the Centre, and the doctor is available on-call) and possible negative outcomes of a substantial pharmacological therapy. The latter was administered at dosages and combinations that both psychiatrists and nurses considered very relevant, continuously increased and modified by inserting or excluding drugs because no effects seemed to be achieved. Eloquently, in an informal conversion, a nurse operating in the Violet Centre observed: "it's impressive to read his therapy and know that he breaths autonomously" (i.e. that he is not mechanically ventilated in an ICU). Preoccupation with adverse effects of massive medication was expressed by nurses and their coordinator during *équipe* meetings as well, but the ultimate decision clearly rested on psychiatrists, who collectively decided on Santiago's therapy and its adjustments. An example of combined therapy administered for some days consisted of quetiapine, olanzapine, promazine, biperiden, valproate, and delorazepam. As a sociologist, I do not have the knowledge necessary to evaluate pharmacological therapy, but I collected information from psychiatrists operating in other services, informing me that combined antipsychotics (polypharmacy) are risky, require strict monitoring, and that international guidelines suggest avoiding their use. I found evidence of this in available guidelines, such as the most recent *Maudsley Prescribing Guidelines in Psychiatry* (2018), stating that there is little evidence of the efficacy of combined antipsychotic medications, whereas there is evidence supporting the potential for harm suggesting that the use of combined antipsychotics should be avoided. Despite this evidence, the common prescription of combined antipsychotics seems resistant to change. Guidelines suggest, as a minimum requirement, that patients treated with combined antipsychotics should be monitored for adverse effects (including an ECG) and for any beneficial effect on symptoms (Taylor et al., 2018, p. 22). In the Mental Health Centre, as previously mentioned, possibilities for medical assessment and monitoring are limited, particularly for electrocardiograms (ECGs) which cannot be performed. This opens up for discussion about how safely these combined and high-dose treatments can be administered in poorly monitored community settings, and to which extent this option is preferable (and to whom) than hospitalization and/or utilization of restraining means different than pharmacological ones (e.g. mechanical restraint), at least in terms of patient's safety.

This question leads us to the restraint context, where—during interviews or informal conversations—the staff frequently expressed their preference for mechanical restraint over elevated doses of sedative medication, deemed clinically dangerous. In the Pine Ward, a patient going through a deep psychotic crisis, showing aggressiveness and frequently attempting to leave, such as Santiago, would have been very probably mechanically restrained.[1] This is also due to the fact that administration of three antipsychotics is considered too risky for the patient and, also, for the psychiatrist who prescribes them, should there be serious adverse effects s/he could be held accountable for. A stronger defensive attitude

[1] This hypothesis was confirmed also by Gianluca, a nurse working in the Violet Centre, but previously operating in a restraint psychiatric ward, who told me that, where he worked in the past, someone like Santiago would have been definitely mechanically restrained: "with three colleagues you take him, you tie him and you solve the problem". In the Violet Centre, he then added, efforts are put on relationship and shadowing ("*affiancamento*"), which is much more demanding for healthcare workers. Gianluca does not support mechanical restraint nor was he suggesting that Santiago should have been contained that way. What he meant is that a contextual problem, such as frequent attempts to leave or aggressive behaviour, is quickly "solved" when the person gets mechanically restrained, while using relational and manual means entails continuative and sometimes exhausting effort which does not necessarily work (e.g. the patient could manage to leave anyway). Nevertheless, Gianluca was curious about the advantages of this approach: he asked to be transferred in the no-restraint context for this reason, but has been working there for a few times and did not feel ready to take a definitive position or express a comprehensive opinion. His position as a "novice" locates him in an intermediate position between "outsider" and "insider", allowing him to critically observe and deconstruct the representations of the community he has just joined and to guide the researcher's attention to specific aspects he is in a position to see. The degree of insight potentially related to these *marginal figures*, and the opportunity and resource they constitute for the researcher to "see otherwise", has been described in Cardano (2011) and in turn inspired by Robert Park's reflections on the "marginal man" (1928).

was observed in the restraint context with respect to medication but also to patients' permission to temporarily leave the ward, also due to previous adverse events (e.g. the suicide of a patient who had been allowed to go home for the weekend while admitted to the Pine Ward), which I have been told to account for the staff's "rigidities": we know that within communities stories concerning errors and past accidents contribute to produce and circulate practical knowledge (in this case about safety), and to orient individual action as well as practice (Gherardi, 2006). The no-restraint context, on the contrary, appeared less risk-aversive—both in hospital and in the community settings—as risky therapy administration (acknowledged as such by the doctors themselves) and other episodes (e.g. walks or car trips with involuntarily admitted patients) seem to suggest. Usually, in the words of my participants, this flexibility was motivated by mental illness itself and the necessity they felt to adjust to the individual patient's needs, history, and subjective condition. A similar need for flexibility was supported also by nurses deemed "more permissive" in the restraint context, maintaining that risk was part of their job to the extent that human behaviour is never completely predictable, and that to work with human beings inevitably entails taking some risks. Not every professional operating in the services we observed, though, agreed to expose him/herself to the same degree of risk, opening for collective debate within the *équipes* and for differentiated levels of engagement of individual members of the staff, who retained some autonomy in deciding whether or not they felt like taking part in each intervention (e.g. the car trip, or accompanying a patient for a walk).[2]

An apparently more relaxed though competent use of sedative drugs and combined antipsychotics and other drugs for patients treated in the "no-restraint" rather than the "restraint" context was observed also in the hospital setting. With respect to sedative therapy administered regularly with curative medication, I had a dedicated discussion with a nurse working in the Iris Ward but previously employed in a restraint psychiatric

[2] The issue of risk, particularly with respect to interventions that reduce the restraining dimension (e.g. permissions to leave the ward, open doors, avoidance of mechanical restraint), has a long tradition in psychiatric practice, debated openly since *The Negated Institution* (Basaglia, 1968) and related also to the legal consequences psychiatrists and healthcare workers can encounter in case of incidents. A defensive approach is one possible answer to such issues.

unit in a different region, Dario. When asked to compare the two work experiences, he told me that "here [in the Iris Ward] you work better, it is completely different, there is less tension, and to have the door open does not lead to the perception of increased workload" (Iris Ward, fieldnotes). Dario also told me that: "relational containment is not enough and that patients are more sedated than in restraint wards". Such observations are consistent with the staff's general opinion concerning a more relaxed atmosphere related to the open-door policy, and about the importance of pharmacological tools besides relational ones; nevertheless, workers operating in the Iris Ward for a long time or their entire professional life appeared less aware of this dimension of sedation and could not make comparisons such as those expressed by this Dario (a "marginal man", Park, 1928). With respect to PRN medication for crisis management, in the Iris Ward, patients showing aggressiveness or agitation or willing to leave when under TSO (*Trattamento Sanitario Obbligatorio*, i.e. involuntary admission and treatment) are regularly treated with "the usual triplet" (expression used by Nadia, nurses coordinator at the Iris Ward)—namely, haloperidol, promazine, and delorazepam—and, on their arrival or after aggressive episodes, with zuclopenthixol acetate.[3] Administration is performed in a hospital setting, which can be considered safer and more medically equipped than a community one. Nevertheless, the psychiatric ward has been regularly described—both in the Pine and the Iris Ward—as a poorly controlled environment, where no continuous monitoring of vital signs is possible since no monitoring devices are available. This problem became very evident with respect to Santiago, involuntarily admitted to the SPDC for some days before being transferred to the Violet Centre, because he was administered with

[3] Guidelines indicate that zuclopenthixol acetate (Acuphase) should never be administered for rapid tranquillization and at the same time as other parenteral antipsychotics or benzodiazepines, which may lead to over-sedation difficult to reverse (Taylor et al., 2018). This was regularly done in the Iris Ward, indicating at least a risk-taking procedure. In the restraint context I included in this study, Acuphase is considered an obsolete drug (it is a typical, first-generation antipsychotic) and it is not used anymore (even though other typical antipsychotics are). This indicates also different pharmacological orientations or cultures between the two contexts compared: specific imaginaries and attributes appeared to be related with specific drugs (e.g. Leponex was considered the "last resort" indicating the seriousness of a patient's condition, Abilify was sometimes compared to "fresh water"), and the choice between different treatment options seemed imbued with ethical other than clinical considerations, which could be interesting to investigate ethnographically, together with clinicians and other experts.

increasingly high-dose and combined medications without achieving any significant effect. During my interview with Paolo, psychiatrist at the Iris Ward, I asked him about the opportunity to resort to anaesthesiologic restraint—namely treatment with anaesthetics in the Intensive Care Unit—which is not a routine option for psychiatric patients in this context. As Excerpt 6.22 shows, he has considered this solution with a colleague of his, precisely because of the clinical risks associated with uncontrolled therapy administration and the possible legal consequences for the prescribers (the patient was then moved to the community Centre and the solution not implemented).

> *Excerpt 8.1.* Paolo (psychiatrist, Iris Ward): We have thought about that in a discussion with Luana [psychiatrist]: "what the fuck are we doing here? If this continues like this, we are risking, *we are using all the drugs at inhumane doses.* If something happens to him, it's on us".

While in the restraint context (monitored) mechanical restraint is employed and deemed preferable to elevated and hence risky pharmacological administration, the no-restraint ward refuses mechanical restraint on an ethical rather than clinical ground: no interviewee or other participant ever claimed than high-dose or combined drugs administration was *clinically safer* than the application of mechanical means of restraint. Instead, the issue of "staying in the relationship" was mobilized, indicating an understanding of mechanical restraint which involves complete withdrawal from relationship/delegation to restraining belts, abandonment, brutality, and abuse. Fieldwork in the Pine Ward and other Piedmontese SPDCs, though, indicates that this measure does not necessarily have to be performed to include such features. More importantly, its application does not necessarily exclude relationship: healthcare providers can attempt to maintain and mobilize it through negotiation, explanation, human presence, and compassionate acts aimed at acknowledging and ameliorating the subjective condition of the restrained person (see Chap. 6). Potentially, the measure can be applied for a very short time, and members of the staff or other external caregivers can be allowed to remain with the coerced person, avoiding isolation and withdrawal from the relationship when crisis occurs. Such options are sometimes hindered by organizational and contextual factors—including ward's overcrowding and heterogeneity of psychiatric and non-psychiatric patients—as well as cultural features which occasionally led to the normalization of mechanical restraint and lack of reflexivity and to a general propensity for the defensively preferable option.

A crucial aspect that emerged from fieldwork and that I consider relevant to stress is the influence that actors external to the mental health services have in "creating" the psychiatric patient. Psychiatry appears increasingly exposed to heterogeneous requests concerning a number of issues (e.g. substance abuse, homelessness, poverty, domestic violence, migration) and populations (e.g. minors and adolescents, migrants), as well as requests to exert social control over behavioural issues of very different origin. The very boundaries of the discipline are drawn and defended within daily negotiations with several agencies and other medical specialties, both in the community and within the hospital. The outcomes of such negotiations rest also on power dynamics between the different services and units, as well as on routines which are never deterministic or conclusive when it comes to decide, for example, about the admission of a patient accessing the Emergency Room. Choices made in the ER by professionals who operate in it influence life in the SPDC, not only in terms of inpatient profile and composition, but also with respect to the measures adopted to manage crisis, which can be syntonic with the ward sensibility (mechanical restraint in the Pine Ward was generally "inherited" by the ER from which the patient was transferred), or not (in the no-restraint context, psychiatrists frequently had to remove restraints from patients in the ER when going there for consultation).

What seems reasonable to suggest in consideration of these factors—local sensibilities and moral imperatives, organizational routines, multiplicity of actors and places involved in dealing with crisis—is a coordinated and multi-specialist approach to acute (psychiatric or otherwise unspecified behavioural) conditions, which assures the highest possible standards in terms of clinical safety, allowing regular access to the Intensive Care Unit for going through the first moments of acute crisis in an accurately monitored environment. Such an option is consistent with the preservation of patients' safety, which seemed relevant in both the studied contexts, while at the same time compatible with the ethical imperative of limiting the most traumatizing and coercive aspects of treating crisis, such as the experience of mechanical restraint,[4] repeated enforced medication and physical engagement with the staff. Treatment in the ICU does not necessarily exclude relationship and assistance by mental health professionals, responding also to the ethical preference for human presence expressed in the no-restraint context (and, to some extent, in the restraint one: see, for example, Excerpt 6.52 concerning the therapeutic activities Maria performed with a patient admitted to the ICU). This option is proved viable by a third Mental Health Centre that I had the chance to visit in Friuli Venezia Giulia, which does not have any SPDC nearby, and treats acute patients in the twenty-four-hour MHC or, when needed, in the local ICU though having a staff member permanently present next to the admitted person (also to avoid mechanical restraint which would be used there if no caregiver was present). Since treatment in the ICU does not necessarily imply complete unconsciousness (i.e. coma induced by anaesthetics), but can involve different degrees of sedation, the opportunity for SPDC or MHC professionals to assist the person and maintain relationship seems valuable for those contexts pursuing presence and wishing to "go through crisis together". Moreover, this would have direct effects on the numerousness and most notably profile of the population hosted in the SPDC, where people could be admitted after the first most critical moments of acuteness and benefit from a less tense environment. This in turn could influence the ward's atmosphere, for both inpatients and the staff, allowing for a decrease in restrictions (e.g. permanently locked doors, usually attributed to the most critical patients but affecting all of them) and possibly a reduction of both mechanical and pharmacological restraints. This combination of clinical monitoring and opportunity to maintain relationship—together with the positive consequences it might have on the overall situation in psychiatric wards—qualifies the Intensive Care Unit as a possible solution, whose utilization could be evaluated and reasoned about by psychiatrists, anaesthesiologists, and other specialists, in consideration of each person's subjective condition.

[4] In the SPDC, the mechanically restrained person is not kept permanently unconscious by anaesthesiologic means, because of the already mentioned lack of vital signs monitoring devices and ventilators. Though, when there are no organic conditions advising against pharmacological intervention, s/he can be treated with sedative medication (both IM and IV) to reduce agitation, also as a compassionate intent to ameliorate his/her condition of being restrained: I have observed this both in the Pine Ward and, with the rest of the research team, in other contexts in Piedmont.

The last dimension which I think could (and probably should) be taken into account pertains to the person's preferences about his/her own treatment. These could be elaborated and formalized within documents which have been variously called psychiatric advance directives, anticipatory care planning, or joint crisis plans (Henderson et al., 2008). Such instruments allow service users to state their preferences for future mental healthcare, especially in times of crisis, consistent with a model of shared decision-making and the implementation of the United Nations Convention on the Rights of Persons with Disabilities (Szmukler, 2019). In fact, we have observed on the field that professionals' attempts to provide good care through everyday practices do not necessarily result in outcomes that service users consider good for themselves. This has become evident when care-receivers had the chance to speak for themselves and express their preferences on a given treatment, or judgement on the healthcare workers' behaviour. Excerpt 8.2 expresses Giuseppe's disappointment with psychiatrist Carmela's decision not to sign his TSO proposal and not to be present at the time of his involuntary admission to the ward and preventive mechanical restraint. While her choice was intended as a way to preserve the therapeutic relationship with the patient, avoiding being explicitly associated with coercive aspects of treatment, the man probably sees it as a lack of interest in his condition and re-reads her past visits as opportunistic.

> *Excerpt 8.2.* Giuseppe [involuntarily admitted] says he's very bothered by the fact that his psychiatrist [Carmela] did not even show up. He's bothered but not angry. He sarcastically adds: "when I brought her cheese [that he produces], she came to take it!" (fieldnotes by Mario Cardano, day of joint observation in the Pine Ward)

Also, with respect to measures adopted to deal with crisis, patients' preferences might emerge though they were not always given space in the context of acute mental healthcare. The following episode, observed in the Pine Ward, consists of a short conversation between an inpatient, Diego, and a nurse, Carmine. Few minutes before, Carmine saw and heard Diego hitting a glass door in the ward hall and told him to stop, which he immediately did. Having observed other patients getting mechanically restrained because of aggressiveness or other behaviours, he then comes to the nursing room to say that he would rather be pharmacologically sedated than "tied to the bed" should he break something. This informal advance directive is not only ignored but delegitimized by the nurse, according to a paternalistic and authoritative approach which sees the psychiatrist as the only decision-making figure on the scene.

> *Excerpt 8.3.* Diego arrives to the nursing room. He says: "If I broke a glass, I'd want the injection [sedative medication], not being tied to the bed [mechanically restrained]". Carmine [nurse] replies that if he broke a glass, the decision about the consequences would be up to the doctor, not him. (Pine Ward, fieldnotes)

These last considerations remind us that the "modes of doing good" (Pols, 2003) investigated in this research—which to some extent differentiate or intersect in the restraint and the no-restraint contexts—are defined, practised, and argued for by the group of professionals operating in each setting. Care practices, though, see the encounter of multiple actors, who contribute to the shaping of problems and solutions, as well as to the notion(s) of good care. The main limit of this study, I think, is the missing voice of one of these actors—service users—whose perspectives on what constitutes good and bad care are fundamental in understanding our object of analysis deeper and in articulating suggestions for future changes.[5] Their lived experiences and the way they are acknowledged or rather marginalized and delegitimized in healthcare contexts as a mere expression of pathology constitute an interesting epistemological challenge to the researcher. This issue has been recently tackled by convict

[5] Agreements with the local ethical committees did not allow us to interview patients during the time they spent in the hospital, due to the vulnerable (clinical and psychological) condition they were experiencing. The research team working on psychiatric interventions in Piedmont did conduct some interviews with service users after discharge. With respect to my study, I had many informal conversations with some people I met on the field that I still keep in contact. After discharge, I attempted to involve Giuseppe, involuntarily admitted to the Pine Ward during our period of fieldwork, in an interview about his experience, attempt which repeatedly failed despite his apparent willingness to take part in the research. We kept in contact and still talk to each other through periodic phone calls, in which he tells me about his life, and also his frequent (involuntary) admissions and experience as a service user. Frequent hospitalization and periods he spent in different healthcare facilities—together with the outbreak of the Covid-19 pandemic—have made our encounter difficult to arrange so far. Future interviews with him and other service users will hopefully be arranged, in order to collect their perspectives and lived experience of care and coercion.

criminology, which relies on first-hand experience of prisoners to produce scientific knowledge about the penitentiary (Sterchele, 2020). The fundamental question it poses—"can the 'psychiatric prisoner' speak?" (ibidem)—points to the hierarchies of credibility theorized by Howard Becker: in any system of ranked groups, members of the highest group have the right to define the way things really are, so that credibility and the right to be heard are unequally distributed through the ranks of the system (1967, p. 241). By listening to the discourses of the convict (or, in my case, of the inpatient) population, the ethnographer can challenge these hierarchies and s/he can distance him/herself from the dominant, clinical and at times disqualifying account provided by high-ranked groups (i.e. prison officers, psychiatrists, and other mental healthcare workers). Moreover, to make weak voices heard becomes particularly relevant in the field of care and empirical ethics, aimed at articulating carers and patients as relational beings (Pols, 2015; Schicktanz et al., 2012). If we consider care practices as shaped by both groups, then insights, interests, and meanings carried by the patients offer us a unique perspective on our object of study. I believe this is of peculiar importance in healthcare contexts characterized by great power imbalances, asymmetries, and dependence, such as the psychiatric one.

Also, further research should be conducted to explore the perspectives of the units and agencies involved in the construction and management of psychiatric crisis, and in caring for subjects who are frequently treated in psychiatric wards: the professionals operating in the Emergency Room, the Intensive Care Unit and other hospital wards, other community (social, addictions) services, as well as the police officers in charge for executing involuntary admissions and frequently assisting healthcare workers in the performance of coercive treatments. A comprehensive, multivocal understanding of situated routines, needs, strivings, and organizational constraints and infrastructures will hopefully be useful to formulate and translate from different contexts localized suggestions, and help researchers contribute to the improvement work (Pols, 2015)[6] that acute mental healthcare could benefit from.

[6] See also Jeannette Pols (2018) intervention on *Somatosphere: Science, Medicine and Anthropology* about empirical ethics (accessed on 4th December 2022): http://somatosphere.net/2018/a-readers-guide-to-the-anthropology-of-ethics-and-morality-part-iii.html/.

References

Basaglia, F. (Ed.). (1968). *L'istituzione negata*. Einaudi.

Becker, H. S. (1967). Whose side are we on? *Social Problems, 14*(3), 239–247.

Cardano, M. (2011). *La ricerca qualitativa*. il Mulino.

Gherardi, S. (2006). *Organizational knowledge: The texture of workplace learning*. John Wiley & Sons.

Henderson, C., Swanson, J. W., Szmukler, G., Thornicroft, G., & Zinkler, M. (2008). A typology of advance statements in mental health care. *Psychiatric Services, 59*(1), 63–71.

Park, R. E. (1928). Human migration and the marginal man. *American Journal of Sociology, 33*(6), 881–893.

Pols, J. (2003). Enforcing patient rights or improving care? The interference of two modes of doing good in mental health care. *Sociology of Health & Illness, 25*(4), 320–347.

Pols, J. (2015). Towards an empirical ethics in care: Relations with technologies in health care. *Medicine, Health Care and Philosophy, 18*(1), 81–90.

Pols, J. (2018). A Reader's Guide to the Anthropology of Ethics and Morality – Part III: Empirical ethics and the study of care. Available online on the website *Somatosphere. Science, Medicine and Anthropology*, at the following link: http://somatosphere.net/2018/a-readers-guide-to-the-anthropology-of-ethics-and-morality-part-iii.html/

Schicktanz, S., Schweda, M., & Wynne, B. (2012). The ethics of 'public understanding of ethics' – Why and how bioethics expertise should include public and patients' voices. *Medicine, Health Care and Philosophy, 15*(2), 129–139.

Sterchele, L. (2020). Can the "psychiatric prisoner" speak? Notes from convict criminology and disability studies. In J. I. Ross & F. Vianello (Eds.), *Convict criminology for the future*. Routledge.

Szmukler, G. (2019). "Capacity", "best interests", "will and preferences" and the UN convention on the rights of persons with disabilities. *World Psychiatry, 18*(1), 34–41.

Taylor, D. M., Barnes, T. R., & Young, A. H. (2018). *The Maudsley prescribing guidelines in psychiatry*. John Wiley & Sons.

Appendix A

The Ethnographic Fieldwork: Methodological Information

The overall period of participant observation consisted of about a hundred days on the field, from January 2019 to January 2020. A day of observation means a day on the field: this can consist in a different number of hours and in different—singular but more often multiple—shifts (morning, afternoon, and night). In order to have a more complete perspective on the activities in our contexts of observation, nights and holidays have been part of the fieldwork too. In these specific moments, the number of the staff units in the ward or Mental Health Centre is lower than the usual, while psychiatrists are absent and available on-call in case of need. The conduction of the participant observation developed along the following timetable (Table A.1).

Access to the field followed different trajectories according to the specific context of observation. In Piedmont, access to the Pine Ward was guaranteed by the previously accepted research protocol that has been

E. Rossero, *Care in a Time of Crisis*, https://doi.org/10.1007/978-3-031-34418-3

Table A.1 Participant observation timetable

	Period	Days of observation
Pine Ward	March–May 2019	34
Cedar Centre	July–August 2019	12
Violet Centre	September 2019	10
Tulip Centre	October 2019	10
Iris Ward	November 2019	24
Other[a]	January 2019–January 2020	12
		102

[a]By "Other" I mean days of observation conducted in other psychiatric wards in Piedmont, within the broader study "Psychiatric Interventions. About TSO and Mechanical Restraint" (see the following footnote)

designed for the research "Psychiatric Interventions: About TSO and Mechanical Restraint".[1] The Cedar Centre was not contemplated by that study; the ethical committee of the local health authority approved the research protocol separately. The Friulian context, on the other hand, was completely unexplored. During the summer of 2019, the director of the Mental Health Department and, subsequently, the head of each service considered have been contacted to present the study and officially authorized the conduct of the study.

During my fieldwork, I have conducted a total of thirty-six discursive interviews with psychiatrists (thirteen), nurses' coordinators (five), nurses (thirteen), and healthcare assistants (five). In the Pine Ward, the purposeful selection of the interviewees took into consideration gender, seniority, and experience with the practice of interest, namely, mechanical restraint. The relevance of the gender of mental healthcare workers and other

[1] "Psychiatric Interventions. About TSO and Mechanical Restraint" is a multidisciplinary study on involuntary admission and treatment of people suffering from mental illness, and the practice of mechanical restraint adopted in emergency psychiatric ward. It is a multicentric, retrospective and prospective study combining quantitative research—dedicated to the study of the clinical and socio-demographical profile of those who are subjected to the mentioned practices—and qualitative research—a team ethnography of six psychiatric wards in Piedmont designed to investigate the organizational and cultural aspects of the coercive practices under scrutiny. The group devoted to the qualitative part of the study was composed by the following members: Mario Cardano (Principal Investigator, sociologist); Alessandra Algostino (jurist); Raffaella Ferrero Camoletto (sociologist); Marta Caredda (jurist), Claudio Carezana (psychiatrist); Luigi Gariglio (sociologist); Maria Grazia Imperato (nurse working in a psychiatric ward); Cristina Pardini (jurist); Valeria Quaglia (sociologist); Vladimiro Zagrebelsky (jurist); and myself. To read about results, see Cardano et al. (2020), Maina et al. (2020), and Cardano and Gariglio (2021).

socio-demographic characteristics of the staff is well known (Bregar et al., 2018). This is true not only because women and men can differ in their physicality, which in turn can influence their attitude towards violent behaviour and its escalation, but also because different expectations are placed upon them within their working environment according to their gender (see Chapter 5, Section 5.3.2 and Excerpt 5.46 on how gender and physicality are involved in the practice of immobilization and the performance of mechanical restraint). Seniority was taken into consideration because it can be associated both with the normalization of coercive measures observed and practised along one's career, and with the experience of burnout which in turn can hinder the development of empathic therapeutic relationships (Morse et al., 2012). The third criterion—involvement in the adoption of mechanical restraint—allows interviews to focus on specific and actual rather than virtual situations. This criterion is met by every worker of the Pine Ward, because of the routine use of the measure; what I tried to do was to select those interviewees that practised restraint during my period of observation, in order to ask them more specific and "situated" questions. These three criteria—both theoretical and empirical—apply to the selection of nurses and healthcare assistants, because they represent the most numerous professional groups and it would have not been possible to interview all of them within the available time. Psychiatrists, on the contrary, constituted a smaller group and I have been able to interview all of them (five). In the Iris Ward, I selected the interviewees using nearly the same criteria already employed within the "restraint" context: gender, seniority, and experience with critical situations (which in the Pine Ward would probably have led to the use of mechanical restraint). The shorter period of time I spent on this field resulted in a smaller number of interviews, with a relatively heterogeneous sample: two nurses (a young woman recently hired and a man with a very long experience in that ward from before the abandonment of mechanical restraint), two psychiatrists (both men, but different in age and previous working experience), two healthcare assistants (a man and a woman), and the female nurses' coordinator (probably the ward's most determined defender of the "no-restraint" model).

At the Cedar Centre, I interviewed two male psychiatrists and the male director of the Mental Health Department, two male nurses and the female nurses' coordinator with a long experience as a psychiatric nurse. I was able to vary seniority as well as heterogeneity of previous experience. In the Tulip and the Violet Centres, my period of observation was very concentrated and much of the information were gathered through informal conversations during the conducting of other activities (i.e. reception and provision of support by phone, surveillance of the Mental Health Centre, or MHC, car rides). Here I interviewed three psychiatrists (two women and one man), two nurses' coordinators (both female), one nurse, and one healthcare assistant.

In the following tables, I provide a synthetic representation of the sample of my interviewees, first for those who work in the psychiatric wards and then for those employed in the Mental Health Centres (Tables A.2 and A.3).

Each interview has been conducted in the psychiatric ward or MHC while the interviewee was on shift. The temporal length of each interview varied between one hour and one hour and a half. Each interview has been recorded with the consent of the interviewee. A letter covering the issue of informed consent was provided to each participant prior to the interview. Recordings of the interviews have been transcribed *verbatim* for analysis.

Interviews transcripts, together with fieldnotes and some natural documents I considered relevant to include (e.g. a book published by the MHD in the no-restraint context, materials such as forms and protocols collected during fieldwork), constituted the textual data I analysed. The process of data analysis was informed by theory- and data-driven categories or codes. Consistent with the lean version of Template Analysis

Table A.2 Interviewees—psychiatric wards

	Gender		Seniority (in SPDC)		
	F	M	< 5 years	5–15 years	>15 years
Psychiatrists	4	3	3	–	4
Nurses	5	5	3	2	5
Healthcare assistants	2	2	2	–	2
Nurses' coordinators	2	–	–	1	1
	13	10	8	3	12
	23		23		

Table A.3 Interviewees—Mental Health Centres

	Gender		Seniority (in CSM)		
	F	M	< 5 years	5–15 years	>15 years
Psychiatrists	2	4	2	2	2
Nurses	1	2	1	–	2
Healthcare assistants	1	–	–	–	1
Nurses' coordinators	3	–	–	1	2
	7	6	3	3	7
	13		13		

(King, 2012), I began with defining a set of categories, derived from both my research questions and the relevant literature, and applying them to a subset of my empirical material, in order to preliminarily assess their suitability and fruitfulness. Consequently, categories which seemed not to fit in have been discarded or better specified, while new categories suggested by the reading of the empirical data themselves were included in the original template. This iterative process confers the analytical procedure the necessary flexibility to approach qualitative data, adapting the analytical categories to the specificities of the empirical material, and allowing unexpected elements and new themes to emerge from data. It is worth noticing that, given the heterogeneity of qualitative data, each piece of textual material can be coded using one or more categories, and that it has a fuzzy-membership relation with it (Cardano, 2020). After the coding process, I compared textual segments concerning different contexts (in the case of fieldnotes) or actors (in the case of interviews) coded with the same analytical categories, in order to identify differences and similarities. Relevant elements emerging from most eloquent cases were then compared and eventually confirmed by returning and re-reading of the extended material. The whole coding and analytical procedures were conducted with the aid of a computer-aided-qualitative-data-analysis software (CAQDAS), NVivo, intended as a helpful tool to manage and keep track of considerable extension of data.

References

Cardano, M. (2020). *Defending Qualitative Research: Design, Analysis and Textualization*. Routledge.

Cardano, M., Algostino, A., Caredda, M., Gariglio, L., & Pardini, C. (2020). *La contenzione del paziente psichiatrico. Un'analisi sociologica e giuridica*. Bologna: il Mulino.

Cardano, M. & Gariglio, L. (2021). The Neoliberal Politics of Otherness in Italian Psychiatric Care: Notes on a Team Ethnography in Six Acute Psychiatric Wards. In Gabe, J., Cardano, M., & Genova, A. (Eds.). *Health and Illness in the Neoliberal Era in Europe*, Bingley (UK): Emerald Publishing.

King, N. (2012). Doing Template Analysis. In Symon, G., & Cassell, C. (Eds.), *Qualitative Organizational Research*, London: Sage Publications, 426–450.

Maina, G., Rosso, G., Carezana, C., Mehanović, E., Risso, F., Villari, V., … & Cardano, M. (2021). Factors associated with involuntary admissions: A register-based cross-sectional multicenter study. *Annals of General Psychiatry*, 20(1), 1–11.

Appendix B

Informed Consent: Letter for the Interviewees

[Name of the city] ____________

Dear Mr./Ms. ____________________

Thank you for having accepted to participate to this interview on your professional practice in the [name of the service] where you work.

With this declaration, signed by the Principal Investigator of the research and the interviewer, the research team commits to use the information you provide for solely scientific purposes. Analysis of the data will respect the principles of protection and confidentiality, indicated in the protocol approved by the ethical committee.

According to the *principle of protection*, the analysis of the empirical material and its use for scientific publications will be conducted to exclude every possible harm to the participants in this study, both healthcare staff and patients, whose dignity will not be offended.

According to the *principle of confidentiality*, information obtained from this interview will be analysed and used for scientific publications without any reference to the services and people involved. Identification will be prevented by using pseudonyms and, if necessary, by altering details

E. Rossero, *Care in a Time of Crisis*, https://doi.org/10.1007/978-3-031-34418-3

(e.g. sex or age of the participant) in order to protect the anonymity of individuals and institutions.

The interviewer

Eleonora Rossero

Appendix C

Notation for Interviews Transcription and Quoted Excerpts[1]

Questions (interviewer's speech) and answers (interviewee's speech)	Questions and other interventions pronounced by the interviewer are written in bold, to distinguish them from the interviewees' speech. Interviewees' speech is written using a normal font. Each segment of conversation is preceded, in the excerpts included in this dissertation, by the name (pseudonym) of the interviewee. His/her role and service are specified at the beginning of the excerpt only. Gaia (nurse, Pine Ward): We've been called often by other wards to restrain, or for an agitated patient, to care for him, to send one of our nurses to another ward. **Interviewer: You mean keeping that patient in that ward, but asking you to go there and restrain him?**

(*continued*)

[1] Drawn from the Atb ("*Analisi delle transizioni biografiche*") notation in Cardano (2011, pp. 301–306).

E. Rossero, *Care in a Time of Crisis*, https://doi.org/10.1007/978-3-031-34418-3

(continued)

Direct speech / Polyphony	Direct speech (either hypothetical or quoted from someone else's discourse) reported by the interviewee is indicated between inverted commas. Doctors take us into consideration and say: "no, we do not unrestrain him".
Names (people, services, cities)	Identification of places, individuals, and institutions is prevented by omitting real names and substituting them with [xxx's name]. In [name of the city] it had ten beds.
Emphasis	Parts of the discourse emphasized by the interviewee are between slashes, while expressions pronounced with a high tone of voice are reported in capital letters. When a community doctor is on duty, he spends a lot of time here, in the ward /with us/ [emphasized], not in the external medical office. They come and see them in THAT moment, right?

Index[1]

[1] Note: Page numbers followed by 'n' refer to notes.

E. Rossero, *Care in a Time of Crisis*, https://doi.org/10.1007/978-3-031-34418-3

P

R

T

W

FSC
www.fsc.org
MIX
Papier | Fördert
gute Waldnutzung
FSC® C083411

Kolibri 360 GmbH
Ferdinand-Jühlke-Straße 7
99095 Erfurt, Deutschland
produktsicherheit@kolibri360.de